Mosby's

Review Questions & Answers

for Veterinary Boards

Small Animal Medicine and Surgery

Mosby's

Review Questions & Answers

for Veterinary Boards

Small Animal Medicine and Surgery

Edited by

Paul W. Pratt, VMD

second edition

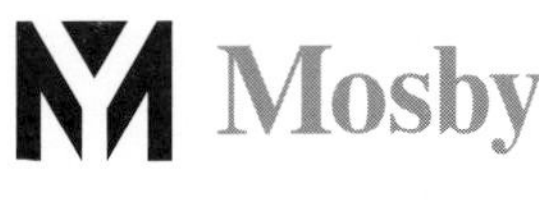

An Affiliate of Elsevier

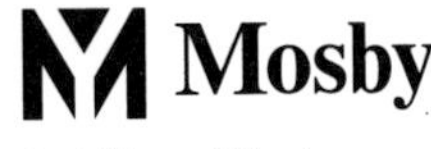

An Affiliate of Elsevier

Publisher: John A. Schrefer
Executive Editor: Linda L. Duncan
Senior Developmental Editor: Teri Merchant
Project Manager: Linda McKinley
Production Editor: Julie Zipfel
Editing and Production: Top Graphics
Design: Renée Duenow
Manufacturing Manager: Linda Ierardi
Cover design: Jennifer Marmarinos

SECOND EDITION

Printed in the United States of America

Mosby, Inc.
11830 Westline Industrial Drive
St. Louis, Missouri 63146

Library of Congress Cataloging-in-Publication Data

Small animal medicine and surgery / edited by Paul W. Pratt.—2nd ed.
p. cm.—(Mosby's review questions & answers for veterinary boards)
Includes bibliographical references.
ISBN-13: 978-0-8151-7465-3 ISBN-10: 0-8151-7465-9
1. Veterinary medicine—United States—Examinations, questions, etc. 2. Veterinary surgery—United States—Examinations, questions, etc. 3. Pet medicine—United States—Examinations, questions, etc.
I. Pratt, Paul W. II. Series.
SF759.S535 1997
636.7'089'076—dc21 97-34834

ISBN-13: 978-0-8151-7465-3
ISBN-10: 0-8151-7465-9

09 08 07 06 / 9 8

Contributors

Introduction

Paul W. Pratt, VMD
Executive Editor, Mosby–Year Book, St. Louis, Missouri

Jeffrey L. Rothstein, DVM, MBA
Hospital Director, Elm Animal Hospital, Roseville, Michigan

Anesthesiology

Sheilah A. Robertson, BVMS(Hons), PhD, Dipl ACVA
Associate Professor, Department of Small Animal Clinical Sciences, College of Veterinary Medicine, Michigan State University, East Lansing, Michigan

Cardiology

N. Sidney Moise, DVM, MS, Dipl ACVIM
Associate Professor, College of Veterinary Medicine, Cornell University, Ithaca, New York

Dentistry

Robert Bruce Wiggs, DVM, Dipl AVDC
Adjunct Assistant Professor, Baylor College of Dentistry, Texas A&M University, College Station, Texas

Dermatology

Karen A. Moriello, DVM, Dipl ACVD
Clinical Associate Professor of Dermatology, School of Veterinary Medicine, University of Wisconsin, Madison, Wisconsin

Hematology

Susan M. Cotter, DVM, Dipl ACVIM
Professor of Medicine, Section Head, Small Animal Medicine, School of Veterinary Medicine, Tufts University, North Grafton, Massachusetts

W. Jean Dodds, DVM
President, HEMOPET, Santa Monica, California

Medical Diseases

Sharon K. Fooshee, MS, DVM, Dipl ACVIM, ABVP
Animal Health Center, Franklin, Tennessee

Dennis W. Macy, DVM, MS, Dipl ACVIM
Professor, College of Veterinary Medicine, Colorado State University, Fort Collins, Colorado

Sandra R. Merchant, DVM, Dipl ACVD
Associate Professor, Dermatology, School of Veterinary Medicine, Louisiana State University, Baton Rouge, Louisiana

Fred W. Scott, DVM, PhD, Dipl ACVM
Professor of Virology, Emeritus, College of Veterinary Medicine, Cornell University, Ithaca, New York

Robert G. Sherding, DVM, Dipl ACVIM
Professor and Department Chairperson, Veterinary Clinical Sciences, Ohio State University, Columbus, Ohio

Joseph Taboada, DVM, Dipl ACVIM
Associate Professor, Small Animal Internal Medicine, Director of Professional Instruction, Department of Veterinary Clinical Sciences, School of Veterinary Medicine, Louisiana State University, Baton Rouge, Louisiana

James P. Thompson, DVM, PhD, Dipl ACVIM, ACVM
Associate Dean for Students and Instruction, College of Veterinary Medicine, University of Florida, Gainesville, Florida

Carrie B. Waters, DVM
College of Veterinary Medicine, University of Missouri, Columbia, Missouri

Michael D. Willard, DVM, MS, Dipl ACVIM
Professor, Department of Small Animal Medicine and Surgery, College of Veterinary Medicine, Texas A&M University, College Station, Texas

Nephrology and Urology

Kenneth C. Bovée, DVM, MMedSc, Dipl ACVIM
Professor of Medicine, University of Pennsylvania, Philadelphia, Pennsylvania

Neurology

Anne Elisabeth Chauvet, DVM, Dipl ACVIM
Clinical Instructor, Neurology/Neurosurgery, School of Veterinary Medicine, University of Wisconsin, Madison, Wisconsin

Oncology

Susan M. Cotter, DVM, Dipl ACVIM
Professor of Medicine, Section Head, Small Animal Medicine, Tufts University, School of Veterinary Medicine, North Grafton, Massachusetts

Evan T. Keller, DVM, PhD, Dipl ACVIM
Director, Glennan Labs, Eastern Virginia Medical School, Norfolk, Virginia

Ophthalmology

Dennis E. Brooks, DVM, PhD, Dipl ACVD
Associate Professor, Ophthalmology Service Chief, College of Veterinary Medicine, University of Florida, Gainesville, Florida

Preventive Medicine

Paul C. Bartlett, DVM, MPH, PhD
Professor, College of Veterinary Medicine, Michigan State University, East Lansing, Michigan; President, American College of Veterinary Preventive Medicine

Craig N. Carter, DVM, MS
Head, Epidemiology and Informatics, Texas Veterinary Medical Diagnostic Laboratory, Texas A&M University, College Station, Texas

Johnny D. Hoskins, DVM, PhD, Dipl ACVIM
Consultant, Internal Medicine of Dogs and Cats, Baton Rouge, Louisiana

Surgical Diseases

Ronald M. Bright, DVM, MS, Dipl ACVS
Alumni Distinguished Service Professor, Professor of Surgery, Department of Small Animal Clinical Sciences, College of Veterinary Medicine, University of Tennessee, Knoxville, Tennessee

Philip A. Bushby, DVM, MS, Dipl ACVS
Professor, Academic Program Director, College of Veterinary Medicine, Mississippi State University, Mississippi State, Mississippi

Jacqueline R. Davidson, DVM, MS, Dipl ACVS
Assistant Professor, Companion Animal Surgery, School of Veterinary Medicine, Louisiana State University, Baton Rouge, Louisiana

Joseph Harari, MS, DVM, Dipl ACVS
Director of Surgery, Rowley Memorial Animal Hospital, Springfield, Massachusetts

Darryl L. Millis, MS, DVM, Dipl ACVS
Assistant Professor, Department of Small Animal Clinical Sciences, College of Veterinary Medicine, University of Tennessee, Knoxville, Tennessee

James K. Roush, DVM, MS, Dipl ACVS
Associate Professor, Department of Clinical Sciences, College of Veterinary Medicine, Kansas State University, Manhattan, Kansas

Theriogenology

Katrin Hinrichs, DVM, PhD, Dipl ACT
Associate Professor, School of Veterinary Medicine, Tufts University, North Grafton, Massachusetts

Preface

This series of five review books was developed to help candidates prepare for scholastic, licensure, and certification examinations. Although the books are not definitive texts, they can help candidates organize their study preparations and detect areas in which more study is required.

The five-volume series contains over 8,100 questions, each with an accompanying answer. A short explanation or rationale is provided for every answer. New to this edition are additional sections on specialties, thousands of new questions, and updating of all questions according to current medical and surgical practices.

I am indebted to our group of 150 eminently qualified contributors, who have taken the time from their busy professional and personal lives to carefully craft questions on their respective subject areas. Their enthusiasm and ingenuity in developing challenging questions are evident throughout the five volumes. Although I had considered myself fairly well read in our field, I was humbled by the depth and breadth of knowledge illustrated in their questions.

We have gone to great effort to root out all errors and ambiguous statements. Despite these precautions, however, a number of flaws undoubtedly have escaped notice. We would be grateful if readers would notify us of any errors, ambiguities, or questionable statements in these books. We also encourage readers to send their comments or criticism on any aspect of these books. In this way we can improve the quality of future editions.

Paul W. Pratt, VMD
Santa Barbara, California

Contents

Introduction

P.W. Pratt and J.L. Rothstein

State and national board examinations have long been surrounded with mystery, misunderstanding, and anxiety. Preparing for licensure examinations can be an intimidating task. Faced with stacks of textbooks and lecture notes, you may find it difficult to know where to begin and how to study in an organized, productive fashion. Also, anxiety about examinations can interfere with your preparations.

To help candidates prepare for licensure examinations, Mosby has published a series of review volumes. *Mosby's Review Questions & Answers for Veterinary Boards* comprises five volumes to prepare candidates for the National Board Examination (NBE) in veterinary medicine. *Mosby's Review for the Clinical Competency Test* is a two-volume work that prepares candidates for the Clinical Competency Test (CCT) in veterinary medicine.

- *Candidates sitting for national and state board examinations* will find these review books a valuable resource because they comprehensively cover all subject areas included on veterinary licensure examinations.
- *Veterinary students* can benefit by using these books as practice tests during courses and also to review material before final examinations as each course is concluded.
- *Practicing veterinarians* will find the books useful for continuing education. Veterinarians moving to a new locale can use them to prepare for licensure examinations in their new state or province. The books also aid preparation for specialty board certification, particularly for certification by the American Board of Veterinary Practitioners (ABVP).
- *Foreign graduates* can use these review books as they prepare for the Education Commission for Foreign Veterinary Graduates (ECFVG) certification examination.

What Is Covered in These Books?

The five volumes of *Mosby's Review Questions & Answers for Veterinary Boards* contain more than 8,000 multiple-choice questions covering nearly every aspect of veterinary medicine. The series includes volumes on *Basic Sciences, Clinical Sciences, Small Animal Medicine and Surgery, Large Animal Medicine and Surgery,* and *Ancillary Topics.*

What Types of Questions Are Included in These Books?

The questions in these books were prepared by highly qualified authors, including veterinary educators, content-area specialists, and experienced clinicians. The questions have been carefully constructed to test factual knowledge, reasoning skills, and clinical judgment. They will also help pinpoint deficiencies in a candidate's studies. The questions are original, and none have been knowingly "recycled" from previous national or state licensure examinations; however, certain overlap is unavoidable and not necessarily a disadvantage.

All the questions on the National Board Examination are multiple choice. Questions in these books present five answer choices. Each question has only one correct answer. There are no "trick" questions.

How to Use These Books

Mosby's Review Questions & Answers for Veterinary Boards was meant to be used in reviewing for final examinations or licensure examinations. Before you begin a section of questions, review your texts and course notes pertaining to that subject area. Then approach each section as you would an actual examination:

- *Carefully read each question.* Look for such key words as "most," "best," "least," "always," "never," and "except." Consider only the facts presented in the question, and don't make assumptions and inferences that may not be true.
- *Carefully evaluate each answer choice.* Each question has only one correct answer, with four incorrect answers or "distractors." If more than one answer choice appears to be correct, closely examine them for clues that would eliminate any as incorrect. Most of the questions ask you to find a single correct answer among four incorrect answers. However, some questions ask you to find an exception. For these questions the answer you are seeking is the single incorrect answer among four correct answers.
- *Select an answer by circling the letter preceding your answer choice.* If you do not wish to mark the book, use the blank answer sheets in the back of the book for practice tests.
- *Compare your answers with the correct answers.* The correct answers are listed separately at the end of each section. All answers are accompanied by an explanation as to why a specific answer is correct or why the other four choices are incorrect.
- *Identify your "weak" areas.* If you cannot correctly answer most of the questions in a particular subject area, spend extra time reviewing that subject before your actual examination. If you do not understand the rationale of why certain answers are correct or incorrect, consult the references in the Recommended Reading list at the beginning of each section.

Structure of the NBE

The National Board Examination (NBE) in veterinary medicine was developed to assess a candidate's ability to evaluate and manage clinical cases, such as those encountered by an entry-level veterinarian in practice. The NBE is given in conjunction with the CCT, in April and December of each year. Each year more than 3,000 candidates take the NBE and CCT.

The NBE currently consists of 400 multiple-choice questions. The 4-hour examination is given in two parts of 200 questions each; candidates are given 2 hours to complete each part (2 hours in the morning, 2 hours in the afternoon). Only 360 of the questions are used in the final scoring; 40 questions are deleted in final scoring, based on analysis of candidates' responses. The first part of the NBE is concerned with gathering diagnostic data, such as the history and findings of diagnostic tests. The second part is concerned with identifying the problem, patient management, and follow-up care.

NBE questions cover all the organ systems and special sense. Approximately 29% of the questions are on small animals (dogs and cats), 21% on food animals (cattle, pigs, sheep, goats, and poultry), 14% on horses, 3% on companion birds, 3% on exotic animals, and 31% on non-species-specific topics. Each question lists five answer choices, of which only one is correct.

Following is a list of diseases or conditions that are reasonably likely to appear on the NBE. NOTE: *This list is for general guidance only and is certainly not all inclusive; conditions not listed could also be included on the NBE.*

- *Dogs and cats:* Renal failure, diabetic ketoacidosis, hyperadrenocorticism, hypoadrenocorticism, hyperthyroidism, hypothyroidism, gastric dilatation-volvulus, foreign bodies, pyometra, reproduction, osteochondritis dissecans, ununited anoconeal process, fractured medial coronoid process, patellar luxation, cruciate ligament rupture, hip dysplasia, malignant lymphoma, seizures, nutrition, food allergies, alopecia, atopy, scabies, demodicosis, ringworm, allergic dermatitis, autoimmune disease, glaucoma, retinal disorders, cystitis, urolithiasis, anemia, congestive heart failure, heartworm disease, cardiomyopathy, canine distemper, feline respiratory disease complex, asthma, feline leukemia virus infection, feline immunodeficiency virus infection, feline infectious peritonitis, toxoplasmosis, rabies, kennel cough, parvovirus infection, shock, and fluid therapy.
- *Cattle:* Traumatic reticuloperitonitis, vagal indigestion, abomasal ulcers, abomasal displacement, bloat, cecal torsion, Johne's disease, foot-and-mouth disease, bluetongue, rinderpest, malignant catarrhal fever, bovine virus diarrhea, listeriosis, thromboembolic meningoencephalitis, grass tetany, polioencephalomalacia, pseudorabies, reproduction, postparturient paresis, bovine respiratory syncytial virus infection, infectious bovine rhinotracheitis, parainfluenza virus-3 infection, pasteurellosis, *Micropolyspora faeni* infection, pulmonary emphysema and edema, tracheal edema, calf scours, black leg, tetanus, botulism, malignant edema, enterotoxemia, anthrax, anaplasmosis, tuberculosis, pyelonephritis, lymphosarcoma, ketosis, urolithiasis, vesicular stomatitis, mastitis, actinobacillosis, actinomycosis, leptospirosis, infectious keratoconjunctivitis, squamous cell carcinoma, anaplasmosis, necrotic pododermatitis, winter dysentery, nutrition, feed additives, white muscle disease, hypovita-

minosis A, trichomoniasis, brucellosis, lead poisoning, urea poisoning, warfarin toxicity, and lightning stroke.

- *Horses:* Fractures (miscellaneous), navicular disease, laminitis, thrush, pedal osteitis, osselets, ringbone, bucked shins, splints, curb, sole abscess, azoturia, wound repair, colic, dentistry, reproductive disorders, neonatal isoerythrolysis, equine viral arteritis, equine herpesvirus-1 infection, influenza, equine infectious anemia, encephalomyelitis (EEE, WEE), strangles, heaves, guttural pouch mycosis, choke, laryngeal hemiplegia, Potomac horse fever, babesiosis, joint and navel ill, tetanus, botulism, sarcoid, local and general anesthesia, recurrent uveitis, foal diarrhea, and nutrition.
- *Pigs:* Clostridial enteritis, colibacillosis, proliferative enteritis, salmonellosis, swine dysentery, cryptosporidiosis, coccidiosis, whipworm infection, epidemic diarrhea, rotaviral enteritis, transmissible gastroenteritis, actinobacillosis, pasteurellosis, atrophic rhinitis, mycoplasmal pneumonia, Glasser's disease, swine influenza, pseudorabies, porcine reproductive and respiratory syndrome, erysipelas, *Streptococcus suis* type-2 infection, group-E streptococcal infection, thromboembolic meningoencephalitis, salt poisoning, heat stroke, greasy pig disease, sarcoptic mange, parvovirus infection, leptospirosis, hog cholera, swine vesicular disease, African swine fever, eperythrozoonosis, iron deficiency, brucellosis, mulberry heart disease, osteochondritis dissecans, sanitation, ventilation, and farrowing management.
- *Sheep and goats:* Foot-and-mouth disease, bluetongue, dermatophilosis, lead poisoning, and orf.
- *Exotic animals and poultry:* Distemper in ferrets, insulinoma in ferrets, hypovitaminosis C in guinea pigs, wet tail in hamsters, snuffles in rabbits, psittacine beak and feather syndrome, Pacheco's disease in birds, and Newcastle disease in poultry.

How to Prepare for Licensure Examinations

Develop a Strategy

You can begin your preparations for licensure examinations by developing a study plan and a strategy for taking the tests. Studying the many subjects covered in the examinations is only one element of the strategy. Before you begin studying, determine which tests you will be required to take. State/provincial and national jurisdictions often have different licensure requirements. For example, all jurisdictions require the NBE, and all except the District of Columbia and the Virgin Islands require the CCT. Depending on the state(s) you plan to practice in, you may need to pass their state board examinations (see Table 1).

Are You Eligible to Take the Examinations?

Determine if you are now or when you will be eligible to sit for the required examinations. Many states allow junior (third-year) veterinary students to take board examinations (see Table 1). For many students this is an ideal time to take the national board examinations. As juniors, students are heavily involved in classroom study and the information is relatively fresh in their minds. They have also begun their exposure to clinical practice through rotations in the university's veterinary teaching hospital. Additionally, many students favor taking the board examinations at this time because there is relatively little pressure to pass; if they do not pass the first time, they can take the tests again during their senior year.

Know When and Where the Examinations Are Offered

Determine the dates, times, and locations of upcoming licensure examinations. Not all states administer the examinations, and they offer them on various dates. Also, the cost for taking the examinations may vary substantially from one state to the next; knowing this ahead of time might influence your decision on which state examinations to take.

Many candidates delay their initial fact finding until a few weeks before the examinations are offered. Such procrastination is unwise and unnecessarily stressful; it may take several months to obtain all pertinent information regarding state requirements, dates tests are offered, and registration requirements and costs for taking the tests. Don't waste your energy worrying about whether you will be permitted to take the test or if you will be registered on time. Gather this information well ahead of time so you can devote your full energy to studying for the examinations. Table 1 lists the licensure requirements for various jurisdictions. Table 2 lists the addresses and telephone numbers for state and provincial licensing boards.

6 Months Before the Examination

Become familiar with the examination requirements: Obtain information on the NBE and CCT from the Professional Examination Service (PES, 475 Riverside Drive, New York, NY 10115; telephone 212-870-3161). Candidates may also obtain a practice NBE and CCT from PES. This practice material provides insight into the subject areas emphasized on the examinations and shows you how the NBE and CCT are structured.

Gather specific information on licensure requirements, examination dates, and costs for each state where you would like to gain licensure (Tables 1 and 2). For more detailed information, consult the *Directory of Veterinary License Requirements,* available from the American Association of Veterinary State Boards (AAVSB, P.O. Box 1702, Jefferson City, MO 65102; telephone 573-761-9937).

Develop a master study plan: Your study plan should include:

- A list of subjects to review and emphasize
- A realistic time frame for review of specific subjects
- A general study schedule
- Resources for studying (materials, study aids, groups, review sessions, etc.)

3 Months Before the Examination

Register for the examinations: Make final decisions about which examinations to take and then register for them. This process is often more complicated and time-consuming than you might think. Many state licensure boards require registration no later than 2 months before the examinations are given, so allow yourself ample time to register. Many state boards accept only certified checks. Some have exacting requirements you must fulfill before they will let you sit for the tests. Avoid problems and reduce anxiety by taking care of these details well ahead of time.

Reevaluate your study plan: Develop a fairly rigid study schedule for the last few months of study before the examination, allotting sufficient study time for both the NBE and CCT. Begin to focus more on review sessions with other people and study groups. It is easy to become bored with studying alone during the several-month preparation period. Diversifying your study techniques helps maintain your interest level and improves retention of subject information.

Maintain a positive frame of mind: Many candidates are overwhelmed by the immense amount of material they must review. The period of preparation for licensure examinations can be stressful; however, you can redirect the stress to your benefit. Develop a positive attitude and consider the examinations a challenge.

In preparing for the examinations, you will learn many useful things and you will review information learned earlier but since forgotten. Ultimately, all the information reviewed during your preparations will serve you well, during the remainder of your veterinary education and in the practice of veterinary medicine. By taking a positive approach and beginning your preparations early, you can reduce your level of stress and do a better job preparing for the examinations.

Resources for Study

Following are some resources to help you prepare for licensure examinations:

Review Books and Other Written Materials

- General texts on specific subject areas (e.g., internal medicine, surgery, etc.)
- Board review books (e.g., five volumes of *Mosby's Review Questions & Answers for Veterinary Boards,* two volumes of *Mosby's Review for the CCT*)
- Practice NBE and CCT examinations (available from PES)
- Old licensure examinations (unofficial and in circulation among students)
- Class notes (from veterinary school courses or continuing education courses)
- Review articles in veterinary journals (e.g., from *Compendium on Continuing Education for the Practicing Veterinarian, Veterinary Medicine*)

Review With Other Candidates, Review Courses

- Study with a group of other candidates
- Study with a partner
- Review sessions hosted by faculty
- Licensure examination review courses, offered commercially (e.g., course offered by Dr. Richard Stobaeus, Animal Care Clinic and Conference Center, Brunswick, GA; telephone 912-264-2258)

Conclusion

Careful preparation is the key to passing the licensure examinations. Review the subject matter and know the licensing requirements of the states in which you want to practice. Become familiar with the structure of the NBE and CCT and how they are scored. Take the practice NBE and CCT to learn how best to select answers. These preparations will reduce your anxiety and let you concentrate on passing the examinations.

What happens if you do not pass the licensure examinations on your first attempt? Certainly, not everybody passes on the first try. Try to determine the areas in which you fared poorly, and concentrate on these areas when studying for the next examination. If you fail the licensure examinations several times, it would be wise to consider a licensure examination review course. The key is to develop a good strategy as outlined here. With a positive attitude and a well-considered study plan, you should do well.

We hope these review books will serve as a foundation for your continued success.

TABLE 1

Licensure Examination Requirements for Various Jurisdictions

Jurisdiction	NBE/CCT offered?	State exam required?	Junior test scores accepted?
Alabama	Yes	Yes	Yes
Alaska	Yes	Yes	Yes
Alberta	Yes	Yes	No
Arizona	Yes	Yes	Yes
Arkansas	Yes	Yes	Yes
British Columbia	Yes	Yes	No
California	Yes	Yes	No
Colorado	Yes	No	No
Connecticut	Yes	No	Yes
Delaware	Yes	No	No
District of Columbia	No	Yes	Yes
Florida	Yes	Yes	No
Georgia	Yes	Yes	No
Hawaii	Yes	Yes	No
Idaho	No	Yes	Yes
Illinois	Yes	No	No
Indiana	Yes	Yes	Yes
Iowa	Yes	Yes	No
Kansas	Yes	Yes	Yes
Kentucky	Yes	Yes	Yes
Louisiana	Yes	Yes	No
Maine	No	Yes	Yes
Manitoba	Yes	Yes	No
Maryland	No	Yes	Yes
Massachusetts	Yes	Yes	Yes
Michigan	Yes	No	Yes
Minnesota	Yes	Yes	Yes
Mississippi	Yes	Yes	Yes
Missouri	Yes	Yes	Yes
Montana	No	No	Yes
Nebraska	No	No	Yes
Nevada	No	No	No
New Brunswick	Yes	Yes	No
New Hampshire	No	No	Yes
New Jersey	No	No	No
New Mexico	No	No	Yes
New York	Yes	Yes	No
North Carolina	Yes	Yes	Yes
North Dakota	No	No	Yes
Nova Scotia	Yes	Yes	No
Ohio	Yes	Yes	Yes

This information was compiled in 1997. Check with the appropriate state or provincial licensing agency for the latest information.
The NBE is required by all jurisdictions except the District of Columbia and the Virgin Islands.
The NBE and CCT are offered in April and December every year.
Passing scores are the same in all jurisdictions.
Some state and provincial examinations cover only jurisprudence issues. Check with individual licensing boards.

Jurisdiction	NBE/CCT offered?	State exam required?	Junior test scores accepted?
Oklahoma	Yes	Yes	Yes
Ontario	Yes	Yes	Yes
Oregon	Yes	Yes	Yes
Pennsylvania	Yes	Yes	Yes
Puerto Rico	Yes	Yes	No
Quebec	Yes	Yes	No
Rhode Island	No	Yes	No
Saskatchewan	Yes	Yes	No
South Carolina	No	Yes	No
South Dakota	No	Yes	Yes
Tennessee	Yes	Yes	Yes
Texas	Yes	Yes	Yes
Utah	No	Yes	Yes
Vermont	No	Yes	No
Virgin Islands	Yes	Yes	No
Virginia	Yes	Yes	Yes
Washington	Yes	Yes	No
West Virginia	No	Yes	Yes
Wisconsin	Yes	Yes	Yes
Wyoming	No	Yes	Yes

TABLE 2

Addresses of State and Provincial Licensing Boards

United States

Candidates interested in practicing in the United States should contact state licensing boards at the following addresses:

Alabama
Board of Veterinary Medicine
PO Box 1968
Decatur AL 35602
(205) 353-3544

Alaska
Division of Occupational Licensing
Department of Commerce & Economic Development
PO Box 110806
Juneau AZ 99881
(907) 465-5470

Arizona
Veterinary Medical Examining Board
Room 230
1400 W. Washington
Phoenix AX 85007
(602) 542-3095

Arkansas
Veterinary Medical Examining Board
1 Natural Resources Drive
Little Rock AR 72215
(501) 224-2836

California
Board of Examiners in Veterinary Medicine
Suite 6
1420 Howe Ave.
Sacramento CA 95825
(916) 263-2610

Colorado
Veterinary Medical Examining Board
Suite 1310
1560 Broadway
Denver CO 80202
(970) 894-7755

Connecticut
Board of Veterinary Medicine
PO Box 340308
Hartford CT 06134
(860) 509-7560

Delaware
Board of Veterinary Medicine
PO Box 1401
Dover DE 19903
(302) 739-4522

District of Columbia
Board of Veterinary Examiners
Room 913
614 H St. NW
Washington DC 20001
(202) 727-7184

Florida
Board of Veterinary Medicine
1940 N. Monroe St.
Tallahassee FL 32399
(904) 487-1820

Georgia
State Examining Boards
166 Pryor St. SW
Atlanta GA 30303
(404) 656-3912

Hawaii
Board of Veterinary Examiners
Box 3469
Honolulu HI 96801
(808) 586-2694

Idaho
Board of Veterinary Medicine
PO Box 7249
Boise ID 83707
(208) 332-8588

Illinois
Veterinary Licensing and Disciplinary Board
Department of Professional Regulation
320 W. Washington
Springfield IL 62786
(217) 782-1663

Indiana
Health Professions Bureau
Room 041
402 W. Washington St.
Indianapolis IN 46204
(317) 233-4407

Iowa
Board of Veterinary Medicine
2nd Floor
Wallace Building
Des Moines IA 50319
(515) 281-5305

Kansas
Board of Veterinary Examiners
10475 Purple Sage Rd.
Wamego KS 66547
(913) 456-8781

Kentucky
Board of Veterinary Examiners
PO Box 456
Frankfort KY 40602
(502) 564-3296

Louisiana
Board of Veterinary Medical Examiners
Suite 604
200 Lafayette St.
Baton Rouge LA 70801
(504) 342-2176

Maine
Division of Licensing and Enforcement
Department of Professional and Financial Regulation
State House Station 35
Augusta ME 04333
(207) 624-8603

Maryland
State Board of Veterinary Medical Examiners
50 Truman Pkwy.
Annapolis MD 21401
(410) 841-5862

Massachusetts
Board of Registration in Veterinary Medicine
Room 1516
100 Cambridge St.
Boston MA 02202
(617) 727-3080

Michigan
Board of Veterinary Medicine
Department of Commerce
PO Box 30018
Lansing MI 48909
(517) 373-9102

Minnesota
Board of Veterinary Medicine
Room 540
2829 University Ave. SE
Minneapolis MN 55414
(612) 617-2170

Mississippi
Board of Veterinary Medicine
209 S. Lafayette St.
Starkville MS 39759
(601) 324-9380

Missouri
Veterinary Medical Board
PO Box 633
Jefferson City MO 65102
(314) 751-0031

Montana
Board of Veterinary Medicine
Department of Commerce
Lower Level, Arcade Building
111 N. Last Chance Gulch
Helena MT 59620
(406) 444-5436

Nebraska
Bureau of Examining Boards
Department of Health
PO Box 95007
Lincoln NE 68509
(402) 471-2115

Nevada
Board of Veterinary Medical Examiners
Suite 246, Bldg O
4600 Kietzke Lane
Reno NV 89502
(702) 322-9422

New Hampshire
Board of Veterinary Medicine
PO Box 2042
Concord NH 03302
(603) 271-3706

New Jersey
Board of Veterinary Medical Examiners
PO Box 45020
Newark NJ 07101
(201) 504-6500

New Mexico
Board of Veterinary Examiners
Suite 400-C
1650 University Blvd. NE
Albuquerque NM 87102
(505) 841-9112

New York
Board of Veterinary Medical Examiners
Room 3043
Cultural Education Center
Albany NY 12230
(518) 474-3867

North Carolina
Veterinary Medical Board
PO Box 12587
Raleigh NC 27605
(919) 733-7689

North Dakota
Veterinary Medical Examining Board
c/o Board of Animal Health
6th Floor
600 E. Boulevard Ave.
Bismarck ND 58505
(701) 328-4567

Ohio
Veterinary Medical Board
16th Floor
77 S. High St.
Columbus OH 43266
(614) 644-5281

Oklahoma
Board of Veterinary Medical Examiners
PO Box 54556
Oklahoma City OK 73154
(405) 843-0843

Oregon
Veterinary Medical Examining Board
Suite 407
800 NE Oregon St.
Portland OR 97232
(503) 731-4051

Pennsylvania
Board of Veterinary Medicine
PO Box 2649
Harrisburg PA 17105
(717) 783-1389

Puerto Rico
(809) 725-7904

Rhode Island
Division of Professional Regulation
Department of Health
Room 104
3 Capitol Hill
Providence RI 02908
(401) 277-2827

South Carolina
Board of Veterinary Medical Examiners
PO Box 11329
Columbia SC 29211
(803) 734-4176

South Dakota
Board of Veterinary Medical Examiners
411 S. Fort St.
Pierre SD 57501
(605) 773-3321

Tennessee
Board of Veterinary Medical Examiners
283 Plus Park Blvd.
Nashville TN 37217
(615) 367-6282

Texas
Board of Veterinary Medical Examiners
Sutie 2-330
333 Guadalupe
Austin TX 78701
(512) 305-7555

Utah
Division of Occupational and Professional Licensing
Box 146741
Salt Lake City UT 84114
(801) 530-6740

Vermont
State Veterinary Board
Office of Professional Regulations
109 State St.
Montpelier VT 05609
(802) 828-2875

Virgin Islands
Board of Examiners for Veterinary Medicine
Office of the Commissioner
Department of Health
48 Sugar Estate
St. Thomas VI 00802
(809) 774-0117

Virginia
Board of Veterinary Medicine
4th Floor
6606 W. Broad St.
Richmond VA 23230
(804) 662-9915

Washington
Veterinary Board of Governors
1300 E. Quince
Olympia WA 98504
(360) 664-8869

West Virginia
Board of Veterinary Medicine
1900 Kanawha Blvd.
South Charleston WV 25305
(304) 558-2016

Wisconsin
Veterinary Examining Board
PO Box 8935
Madison WI 53708
(608) 266-2811

Wyoming
Board of Veterinary Medicine
2nd Floor
2020 Carey Ave.
Cheyenne WY 82002
(307) 777-6529

Canada

Candidates interested in practicing in Canadian provinces should contact those licensing boards at the following addresses:

Alberta
Board of Veterinary Medical Examiners
#100
8615 149th St.
Edmonton, Alberta T5R 1B3
(403) 489-5007

British Columbia
Board of Veterinary Medical Examiners
Suite 155
1200 W. 73rd Ave.
Vancouver, British Columbia V6P 6G5
(604) 266-3441

Manitoba
Veterinary Medical Board
Agricultural Services Complex
545 University Crescent
Winnipeg, Manitoba R3T 5S6
(204) 945-7651

New Brunswick
Board of Veterinary Medical Examiners
PO Box 1065
Moncton, New Brunswick E1C 8P2
(506) 851-7654

Nova Scotia
Board of Veterinary Medical Examiners
15 Cobequid Rd.
Lower Sackville, Nova Scotia B4C 2M9
(902) 865-1876

Ontario
College of Veterinarians
2106 Gordon St.
Guelph, Ontario N1L 1G6
(519) 824-5600

Quebec
General Director and Secretary
Board of Veterinary Medical Examiners
Suite 200
795 Avenue du Palais
St. Hyacinthe, Quebec J2S 5C6
(514) 774-1427

Saskatchewan
Board of Veterinary Medical Examiners
Unit 104
112 Research Dr.
Saskatoon, Saskatchewan S7N 3R3
(306) 955-7862

Mosby's

Review Questions & Answers

for Veterinary Boards

Small Animal Medicine and Surgery

SECTION

1

Anesthesiology

S.A. Robertson

Recommended Reading

Hall LW, Clarke KW: *Veterinary anaesthesia,* ed 9, London, 1992, Bailliere Tindall.

Muir WW, Hubbell JA: *Handbook of veterinary anesthesia,* ed 2, St. Louis, 1996, Mosby.

Thurman JC et al: *Lumb and Jones' veterinary anesthesia,* ed 3, Baltimore, 1996, Williams & Wilkins.

Practice answer sheet is on page 283.

Questions

1. *Intravenous administration of atropine causes an increase in heart rate by:*
   a. stimulating the sympathetic ganglia
   b. causing release of epinephrine from the adrenal glands
   c. causing central stimulation of the vagus nerve
   d. allowing accumulation of acetylcholine at nerve terminals because of its anticholinesterase properties
   e. blocking acetylcholine at the postganglionic termination of cholinergic fibers in the autonomic nervous system

2. *The recommended dosage of a premedicant for a 25-kg dog is 4 mg/kg. The drug is formulated as a 2% solution. How many milliliters of the drug should be administered?*
   a. 0.5 ml
   b. 5 ml
   c. 3.1 ml
   d. 2 ml
   e. 50 ml

25 kg x 4 mg/kg = 100 mg
100 mg x ml/20 mg = 5 ml

3. *You are preparing to anesthetize a dog with a history of epilepsy. Which agent should **not** be included in the anesthetic protocol?*
   a. midazolam
   b. thiopental
   c. etomidate
   d. ketamine - reported to lower seizure threshold
   e. oxymorphone

4. *What is the most common change in cardiac rhythm following intravenous administration of xylazine?*
   a. bradycardia often accompanied by first- or second-degree atrioventricular block
   b. supraventricular tachycardia
   c. bradycardia, accompanied by frequent premature ventricular contractions
   d. bigeminy
   e. atrial premature contractions

5. *Which agent should **not** be used to anesthetize greyhounds?*
   a. propofol
   b. ketamine
   c. isoflurane
   d. thiopental
   e. tiletamine-zolazepam

6. *Injection of 4 ml of 2% lidocaine into the epidural space of an 18-kg dog at the lumbosacral junction is most likely to produce:*
   a. rapid onset of respiratory paralysis
   b. loss of motor and sensory innervation to both pelvic limbs
   c. loss of sensation in the pelvic limbs but preservation of motor function
   d. increased anal sphincter tone
   e. sensory blockade sufficient for thoracic surgery

7. *Medetomidine is a newer sedative-analgesic agent licensed for use in dogs. To which group of drugs does it belong?*
   a. opioids
   b. dissociative agents
   c. phenothiazines
   d. α_2-adrenergic agonists
   e. α_2-adrenergic antagonists

8. *Which agent would be **least** useful in reversing the effects of an overdose of xylazine?*
   a. yohimbine
   b. tolazoline
   c. naloxone
   d. atipamezole
   e. idazoxan

9. *Early signs of lidocaine toxicity in dogs are usually manifested by:*
   a. central nervous system signs
   b. acute anaphylaxis
   c. respiratory arrest
   d. profound cardiac depression and ventricular arrhythmias
   e. methemoglobinemia

10. *What is a common side effect of xylazine administration in cats?*
    a. excitement
    b. tachycardia
    c. vomiting and retching
    d. hypoglycemia
    e. muscle rigidity

11. *A dog undergoes prolonged orthopedic surgery for repair of a fractured femur. Which protocol could provide 12 to 18 hours of postoperative analgesia?*
    a. oxymorphone given intramuscularly at 0.1 mg/kg at the end of surgery
    b. using intravenous ketamine as part of the induction protocol
    c. 2% lidocaine given epidurally at 1 ml/5 kg at the end of surgery
    d. morphine given epidurally at 0.1 mg/kg at the end of surgery
    e. butorphanol given intramuscularly at 0.1 mg/kg before surgery

12. *A 2.5% solution contains:*
    a. 2.5 mg/ml
    b. 250 mg/ml
    c. 25 mg/ml
    d. 25 g/ml
    e. 0.25 mg/ml

13. *What is the most common arrhythmia associated with intravenous use of thiopental in dogs?*
    a. second-degree atrioventricular block
    b. atrial fibrillation
    c. bigeminy
    d. ventricular tachycardia
    e. third-degree atrioventricular block

14. *Which protocol is **not** recommended to provide anesthesia sufficient for surgical repair of a skin laceration in a reptile?*

    a. ketamine given intramuscularly
    b. mask induction and maintenance with isoflurane
    c. local anesthesia using 2% lidocaine injected around the laceration
    d. rapid cooling by whole-body immersion in ice water
    e. mask induction and maintenance with halothane

15. *The effects of systemically administered meperidine (Demerol) in a cat could be reversed with:*

    a. neostigmine
    b. yohimbine
    c. dantrolene
    d. atipamezole
    e. naloxone

16. *You rapidly infuse an intravenous bolus of propofol (10 mg/kg) in a dog, and the dog becomes unconscious. What side effect are you most likely to observe in this unconscious patient?*

    a. gross, purposeful movement
    b. vocalization
    c. apnea
    d. vomiting
    e. tachypnea

17. *Epinephrine is often added to the local anesthetic agent lidocaine. The epinephrine has the effect of:*

    a. shortening the duration of action of the lidocaine
    b. increasing the likelihood of systemic uptake and lidocaine toxicity
    c. decreasing the pain associated with injection
    d. prolonging the duration of action of lidocaine
    e. promoting wound healing at the site of injection

18. *What is a major advantage of propofol as an anesthetic induction agent?*

    a. It is effective via both the intravenous and intramuscular routes.
    b. The vial has a long shelf life, and once it is open it can be stored at 4° C for 1 week, thereby reducing waste.
    c. It can be given rapidly by the intravenous route without producing cardiopulmonary depression.
    d. It is an ideal agent for repeated daily use in cats, such as those undergoing radiation therapy every day for 1 week.
    e. Recovery is smooth and rapid.

19. *What is the primary reason for using diazepam in conjunction with ketamine in cats?*

    a. to counteract the salivation associated with ketamine
    b. to provide additional analgesia
    c. to counteract the tachycardia associated with ketamine
    d. to counteract the muscle rigidity associated with ketamine
    e. to decrease the tissue irritation associated with intramuscular or intravenous administration of ketamine

20. *Pancuronium and atracurium produce muscle relaxation by:*

    a. acting at the neuromuscular junction to prevent acetylcholine from occupying the triggering sites of acetylcholine receptors
    b. mimicking the action of acetylcholine at the neuromuscular junction
    c. acting at the internuncial neurons in the spinal cord
    d. inhibiting the action of acetylcholinesterase at the neuromuscular junction
    e. preventing rapid influx of sodium into nerve axons that produce the action potential

Correct answers are on pages 4-5.

21. *Which agent has been approved by the U.S. Food and Drug Association (FDA) for use in fish, provided they are not used for human consumption within 21 days?*
    a. tricaine methanesulfonate (MS - 222)
    b. diethyl ether
    c. urethane
    d. quinaldine
    e. benzocaine dissolved in acetone

22. *When using a Bain coaxial system for delivery of oxygen and inhalant agents to small animal patients, rebreathing of carbon dioxide is prevented by:*
    a. removal of carbon dioxide via a chemical reaction with sodalime in the absorber
    b. one-way valves that vent the exhaled gases to the atmosphere
    c. continuous high flow rates of fresh gas
    d. periodic emptying of the rebreathing bag
    e. providing a flow rate of oxygen that equals oxygen consumption by the patient

23. *Telazol is licensed for use in dogs and cats. It is a combination of:*
    a. diazepam and tiletamine
    b. zolazepam and ketamine
    c. midazolam and ketamine
    d. zolazepam and tiletamine
    e. fentanyl and droperidol

24. *In dogs, intrathecal injection of radiographic contrast media may produce seizures in the postanesthetic period. If such a seizure were to occur, the most appropriate course of action would be to:*
    a. sedate the dog with intravenous acepromazine
    b. administer intravenous diazepam
    c. collect a blood sample to check the blood glucose level
    d. administer diazepam rectally
    e. reanesthetize the dog with isoflurane by mask

25. *You are asked to anesthetize a dog for splenectomy because of hemangiosarcoma. Which combination of preanesthetic and induction agents would be most appropriate for this dog?*
    a. acepromazine and thiopental
    b. xylazine and thiopental
    c. meperidine and diazepam with ketamine
    d. meperidine and thiopental
    e. acepromazine and propofol

Answers

1. **e** The actions described in answers a, b, and d would also increase the heart rate, but this is not how atropine acts. Although atropine can produce a central effect (answer c), this results in an initial slowing of the heart before the systemic effects increase the heart rate.
2. **b** The dose (in milligrams) required is as follows: $4 \times 25 = 100$ mg. A 2% solution contains 20 mg/ml; $100 \div 20 = 5$ ml.
3. **d** Ketamine has been reported to cause seizures in some dogs and cats known to be epileptic. Ketamine used alone may also lead to seizurelike activity (muscle rigidity, twitching).
4. **a** Bradycardia is common after xylazine administration. Initially there is bradycardia with hypertension (hypertension is caused by xylazine's peripheral actions), followed by bradycardia and a decrease in cardiac output and blood pressure. Xylazine has central α_2-adrenoreceptor agonist actions and also enhances vagal tone.
5. **d** Greyhounds have prolonged and stormy recoveries from thiobarbiturate anesthesia. This is a result of altered hepatic metabolism, rather than a result of their lean body mass and lack of fat for redistribution. Recovery from propofol is smooth, but it takes longer in greyhounds than in other dogs.
6. **b** Lidocaine results in loss of both motor and sensory function. A dosage of 1 ml of 2% lidocaine per 4.5-kg body weight produces anesthesia of both pelvic limbs and abdomen caudal to the first lumbar vertebra.

7. **d** Along with xylazine, medetomidine is an α_2-adrenergic agonist.
8. **c** Naloxone is an opioid antagonist. The other agents listed all have some ability to reverse α_2-adrenergic agonist agents.
9. **a** CNS signs of toxicity (tremors, seizures) usually occur before cardiopulmonary depression. Allergic reactions are more likely with ester-type local anesthetics; lidocaine is an amide. Methemoglobinemia is most often associated with prilocaine.
10. **c** Vomiting and retching are caused by stimulation of the brain's chemoreceptor trigger zone.
11. **d** Epidural morphine may provide analgesia up to 24 hours (usually 12 to 18 hours). Epidural lidocaine provides analgesia only up to 2 hours. Analgesia from oxymorphone and butorphanol lasts less than 6 hours. Ketamine is also short acting and predominantly provides somatic analgesia.
12. **c** A 2.5% solution contains 25 mg/ml.
13. **c** Various cardiac arrhythmias may occur with thiopental, but bigeminy is the most common. On an ECG strip, bigeminy is a normal PQRS complex alternating with a ventricular premature complex. This rhythm may last up to 20 minutes and may be associated with decreased cardiac output and systemic blood pressure.
14. **d** Rapid cooling can slow the reptile's activity and has been used as a means of restraint; however, this does *not* provide analgesia. Laceration repair would be painful under such conditions.
15. **e** Meperidine (Demerol) is an opioid agonist and may be antagonized with naloxone, an opioid antagonist. Neostigmine is an anticholinesterase. Yohimbine and atipamezole are α_2-antagonists. Dantrolene is a drug specifically used to treat malignant hyperthermia.
16. **c** Apnea is commonly associated with rapid administration of propofol. The induction dose should be administered slowly, over a period of at least 1 minute.
17. **d** Epinephrine causes vasoconstriction at the site of local injection, prolonging the duration of action of the local anesthetic (decreased uptake). Decreased uptake also decreases the likelihood of systemic toxicity. The vasoconstriction and decreased blood flow, however, may impair wound healing. Addition of bicarbonate to local anesthetics may decrease the pain of injection.
18. **e** Propofol is only effective by the intravenous route and not intramuscularly. Once a vial is opened (answer b), it must be used within 6 hours because it contains no preservative and the formulation (egg lecithin emulsion) is an ideal bacterial growth medium. Rapid administration results in apnea. Cats given propofol daily become lethargic, show malaise, and develop various degrees of Heinz-body anemia.
19. **d** Diazepam is a centrally acting muscle relaxant that counteracts the muscle rigidity caused by ketamine alone.
20. **a** Nondepolarizing muscle relaxants (e.g., atracurium, pancuronium) have affinity for the acetylcholine receptor but do not trigger it. They prevent the acetylcholine molecules from occupying the trigger sites. This is competitive inhibition.
21. **a** All of these agents can be used to anesthetize fish, but only tricaine methanesulfonate has FDA approval.
22. **c** A Bain coaxial system has no soda-lime canister. Carbon dioxide removal depends on high fresh gas flow rates to vent exhaled gases to the scavenger system. Recommended flow rates are 100 to 200 ml/kg. Metabolic oxygen requirements are 4 to 6 ml/kg/min.
23. **d** Zolazepam is a benzodiazepine (along with diazepam and midazolam). Tiletamine is a dissociative agent in the same group of drugs as ketamine.
24. **b** Diazepam is the drug of choice for initial treatment of seizures. It can be given rectally, but onset of action is faster by the intravenous route. Acepromazine is contraindicated because it may lower the seizure threshold. Hypoglycemia would be an unusual cause of seizures following myelography. Isoflurane would induce anesthesia but is not a specific treatment for the seizure activity.
25. **c** Splenic hemangiosarcomas tend to be very friable and are likely to bleed if pressure is applied or if the spleen changes size rapidly. Acepromazine causes relaxation of the splenic capsule and sequestration of red blood cells within the spleen. Thiopental causes splenic engorgement. Both these agents may precipitate bleeding from the tumor. Xylazine may decrease the weight of the spleen secondary to a decrease in systemic vascular capacity. Opioids, propofol, and diazepam with ketamine have minimal effect on splenic size.

NOTES

SECTION

2

Cardiology

N.S. Moise

Recommended Reading

Edwards NJ: *Bolton's handbook of canine and feline electrocardiography,* ed 2, Philadelphia, 1987, WB Saunders.

Fox PR: *Canine and feline cardiology,* New York, 1988, Churchill Livingstone.

Keene BW, Hamlin RL: *Small animal cardiology,* Philadelphia, 1997, WB Saunders.

Tilley LP: *Essentials of canine and feline electrocardiography: interpretation and treatment,* ed 3, Baltimore, 1992, Williams & Wilkins.

Miller MS, Tilley LP: *Manual of small animal cardiology,* ed 2, Philadelphia, 1995, WB Saunders.

Smith FWK, Tilley LP: *Rapid interpretation of heart sounds, murmurs, and arrhythmias,* Baltimore, 1992, Williams & Wilkins.

Practice answer sheet is on page 285.

Questions

1. *Which drug is an angiotensin-converting enzyme inhibitor?*
   a. hydralazine
   b. prazosin
   c. enalapril
   d. nitroglycerin
   e. propranolol

2. *Which combination of drugs may elevate serum potassium levels?*
   a. furosemide and hydrochlorothiazide
   b. enalapril and spironolactone
   c. hydralazine and furosemide
   d. digoxin and furosemide
   e. enalapril and digoxin

3. *Digoxin toxicity is most likely to be induced by treatment of animals with:*
   a. hypokalemia and renal disease
   b. hyperkalemia and hyperthyroidism
   c. hyperkalemia and liver disease
   d. hyponatremia and hyperkalemia
   e. hypercalcemia and hypoadrenocorticism

4. *Which of the following is most likely to be found in dogs with chronic heart failure?*
   a. increased serum dobutamine level
   b. decreased serum insulin level
   c. decreased serum angiotensin II level
   d. decreased serum renin level
   e. increased serum aldosterone level

Correct answers are on pages 10-11.

5. *Which of the following is **not** an action of digoxin?*
   a. increases the rate of sinus node discharge
   b. decreases serum renin and aldosterone levels
   c. causes positive inotropism
   d. increases parasympathetic tone
   e. increases atrioventricular conduction time (slows conduction velocity)

6. *Which condition is associated with a diastolic murmur?*
   a. mitral insufficiency
   b. pulmonic stenosis
   c. patent ductus arteriosus
   d. aortic insufficiency
   e. ventricular septal defect

7. *Which condition is associated with bounding pulses and a wide pulse pressure?*
   a. subaortic stenosis
   b. patent ductus arteriosus
   c. valvular pulmonic stenosis
   d. tricuspid insufficiency
   e. atrial septic defect

8. *Which association between electrocardiographic findings and cardiac changes is most accurate?*
   a. deep S wave in lead I with left ventricular enlargement
   b. wide QRS complex in lead II and a deep S wave with left ventricular enlargement
   c. tall R wave in lead II with left ventricular enlargement
   d. tall P waves in lead II with left ventricular enlargement
   e. wide P waves in lead II with right ventricular enlargement

9. *Differential cyanosis (cyanosis in one part of the body but not another) is associated with:*
   a. subaortic stenosis
   b. right-to-left shunting with patent ductus arteriosus
   c. left-to-right shunting with ventricular septal defect
   d. right-to-left shunting with atrial septal defect
   e. tricuspid dysplasia

10. *A 10-year-old male Labrador retriever has a 2-month history of episodes of dyspnea that worsen with exercise. The owners observe that during these episodes the dog makes a loud, harsh sound. On physical examination the dog has obvious stridor but no signs of pulmonary edema. The most likely cause of these signs is:*
    a. congestive heart failure
    b. pneumonia
    c. infectious tracheobronchitis
    d. tracheal collapse
    e. laryngeal paralysis

11. *A 4-year-old male cat is admitted with hind limb paralysis. The owners returned home from work and found the cat crying as if in pain. The femoral pulses are absent, and the nail beds of the hind limb digits are purple. Of the following courses of action, which is **least** appropriate?*
    a. Perform emergency surgery to relieve acute caudal aortic thromboembolism.
    b. Make thoracic radiographs.
    c. Perform an echocardiographic examination.
    d. Treat the cat with aspirin.
    e. Treat the cat with heparin.

12. *A 3-year-old Pomeranian has a honking cough that worsens with excitement. A grade-II systolic murmur is heard loudest at the fifth intercostal space on the left. The most likely cause of the cough is:*
    a. pulmonary edema
    b. tracheal collapse
    c. pneumonia
    d. laryngeal paralysis
    e. pleural effusion

13. *Golden retrievers, Newfoundlands, German shepherds, and boxers are predisposed to:*
    a. tricuspid dysplasia
    b. subaortic stenosis
    c. patent ductus arteriosus
    d. valvular pulmonic stenosis
    e. mitral insufficiency

14. *In dogs with mitral insufficiency and dilative cardiomyopathy, treatment with which drug improves clinical signs and prolongs life?*
   a. furosemide
   b. enalapril
   c. hydralazine
   d. digoxin
   e. nitroglycerin

15. *A 5-month-old cat has a grade-III systolic murmur heard at the fourth intercostal space on the right hemithorax. The electrocardiogram is normal, but thoracic radiographs show generalized cardiomegaly, with enlargement of the pulmonary artery and veins and slight pulmonary edema. The most likely cause of these signs is:*
   a. heartworm disease
   b. mitral insufficiency
   c. ventricular septal defect
   d. subaortic stenosis
   e. patent ductus arteriosus

16. *An English bulldog has a grade-IV systolic murmur with a point of maximum intensity over the cranial left third intercostal space. The dog's femoral pulses are adequate. The electrocardiogram shows a deep S wave in leads I, II, III, and aV_F and a mean electrical axis of 160 degrees. The most likely cause of these findings is:*
   a. subaortic stenosis
   b. pulmonic stenosis
   c. ventricular septal defect
   d. patent ductus arteriosus
   e. atrial septal defect

17. *Which drug is usually indicated in treatment of dangerous ventricular tachycardia?*
   a. digoxin
   b. lidocaine
   c. atropine
   d. propranolol
   e. diltiazem

18. *Which drug is a calcium channel blocker used in treatment of hypertrophic cardiomyopathy in cats?*
   a. atenolol
   b. diltiazem
   c. digoxin
   d. propranolol
   e. procainamide

19. *Concerning adjustment of digoxin doses, which statement is most accurate?*
   a. The dose should be decreased with renal disease and increased in aged animals.
   b. The dose should be increased in aged animals and based on the animal's estimated lean body weight.
   c. The dose should be decreased with renal disease and based on the animal's estimated lean body weight.
   d. The dose should be increased with renal disease and decreased in aged animals.
   e. The dose should be decreased with renal disease and based on the animal's actual body weight.

20. *Which of the following most accurately describes the side effects of propranolol?*
   a. vomiting, diarrhea, seizures
   b. listlessness, anorexia, bradycardia
   c. seizures
   d. seizures, tachycardia, nervousness
   e. vomiting, diarrhea, depression

21. *An owner telephones regarding her dog with dilative cardiomyopathy. For the past 10 days the dog has been treated with digoxin, furosemide, and enalapril. The owner complains that the dog is vomiting, has diarrhea, and will not get up. The dog is drinking water and appears hydrated. What is the most likely cause of these signs?*
   a. excessive diuresis with furosemide
   b. toxicity from the digoxin
   c. progression of the disease process, with ischemia or thromboembolism
   d. unrelated gastrointestinal disease
   e. toxicity from concurrent use of enalapril with furosemide

Correct answers are on pages 10-11.

22. *Dilative cardiomyopathy in cats is most commonly associated with a dietary deficiency of:*
    a. taurine
    b. carnitine
    c. guanine
    d. selenium
    e. cobalt

23. *Which of the following is **not** associated with heartworm infection?*
    a. pulmonary hypertension
    b. no clinical signs
    c. dilatation of the pulmonary arteries
    d. right ventricular hypertrophy
    e. systemic hypertension

24. *A 12-year-old German shepherd has a sudden onset of weakness, dyspnea, and exercise intolerance. The femoral pulses are weak and the heart rate is regular at 190 beats/min. The heart sounds are muffled. You observe jugular vein distention and suspect ascites. The mucous membranes are pale pink. The most likely cause of these signs is:*
    a. auricular hemangiosarcoma
    b. splenic lymphoma
    c. dilative cardiomyopathy
    d. hypertrophic cardiography
    e. benign (idiopathic) pericardial effusion

25. *Of the following cardiac anomalies, which is **not** part of the complex known as tetralogy of Fallot?*
    a. ventricular septal defect
    b. cor triatriatum
    c. pulmonary stenosis
    d. dextroposition of the aorta
    e. right ventricular hypertrophy

Answers

1. **c** Enalapril is an angiotensin-converting enzyme inhibitor.
2. **b** Enalapril decreases levels of aldosterone and causes potassium retention. Spironolactone is a potassium-sparing diuretic.
3. **a** Hypokalemia increases binding of digoxin to myocytes and therefore increases toxicity. Because digoxin is cleared by the kidneys, renal disease increases digoxin levels and toxicity.
4. **e** Serum aldosterone concentrations are elevated because of stimulation of the renin-angiotensin-aldosterone system.
5. **a** Digoxin can decrease the sinus rate.
6. **d** Aortic insufficiency is characterized by a diastolic murmur.
7. **b** Animals with patent ductus arteriosus have a large difference between systolic and diastolic blood pressures.
8. **c** Left ventricular enlargement produces a tall R wave in lead II.
9. **b** The ductus arteriosus leaves the aorta after the brachiocephalic trunk and subclavian artery; therefore the head is oxygenated and cranial tissues are pink, whereas the caudal body is cyanotic.
10. **e** Laryngeal paralysis is common in older Labrador retrievers. Affected dogs characteristically show upper airway obstruction that causes noise known as stridor.
11. **a** Surgery to resolve thromboembolism has a high mortality.
12. **b** Collapsing trachea characteristically occurs in this breed. Affected animals have a honking cough.
13. **b** These breeds are predisposed to subaortic stenosis.
14. **b** Enalapril is indicated in treatment of mitral insufficiency.
15. **c** Ventricular septal defect is relatively common in cats. The location of this murmur is consistent with a ventricular septal defect. The radiographs confirm the volume overload state.
16. **b** The point of maximum intensity is over the pulmonic valve, and the ECG shows marked right heart enlargement. Also, English bulldogs are predisposed to pulmonic stenosis.
17. **b** Lidocaine can slow the rate of ventricular contraction.
18. **b** Diltiazem is a calcium channel blocker.

19. **c** The dose of digoxin should be decreased in animals with renal disease and based on lean weight.
20. **b** Propranolol can cause malaise, anorexia, and bradycardia.
21. **b** These signs suggest digoxin toxicosis.
22. **a** Taurine deficiency can precipitate dilative cardiomyopathy in cats.
23. **e** Hypertension is not seen in heartworm infection.
24. **a** Hemangiosarcoma of the right auricle is a common cause of pericardial effusion in German shepherds.
25. **b** Cor triatriatum is not part of the tetralogy of Fallot anomaly. In cor triatriatum the pulmonary veins enter an accessory left atrium. The true left atrium and the accessory left atrium connect through a narrow opening, obstructing pulmonary venous return.

NOTES

NOTES

SECTION

3

Dentistry

R.B. Wiggs

Recommended Reading

Crossley DD, Penman S: *Manual of small animal dentistry,* Gloucestershire, United Kingdom, 1995, British Small Animal Veterinary Association.

Emily PP, Penman S: *Handbook of small animal dentistry,* ed 2, Oxford, 1994, Pergamon Press.

Harvey CE, Emily PP: *Small animal dentistry,* St. Louis, 1993, Mosby.

Holstrom SE et al: *Veterinary dental techniques,* Philadelphia, 1992, WB Saunders.

Kertesz P: *A colour atlas of veterinary dentistry and oral surgery,* St. Louis, 1993, Mosby.

Norsworthy GD: *Feline practice,* Philadelphia, 1993, Lippincott.

Wiggs RB, Lobprise HB: *Veterinary dentistry: principles and practice,* Philadelphia, 1997, Lippincott.

Practice answer sheet is on page 287.

Questions

1. *Teeth are suspended in surrounding hard tissues by the:*
   a. cementum
   b. gingiva
   c. alveolar bone
   d. periodontal ligament
   e. pulp

2. *The fluid found in the sulcus surrounding teeth is produced by the:*
   a crevicular epithelium
   b. parotid salivary gland
   c. lingual epithelium
   d. sublingual salivary gland
   e. zygomatic salivary gland

3. *Oral parakeratinized tissue is much tougher than nonkeratinized tissue. Which of the following is* ***not*** *keratinized?*
   a. free gingiva
   b. gingival margin
   c. alveolar mucosa
   d. attached gingiva
   e. gingival papilla

For questions 4 through 8, select the correct answer from the five choices below.

a. dental elevator
b. probe
c. curette
d. explorer
e. sickle scaler

4. *Used to scale below the gum line (subgingival)*

5. *Used to scale above the gum line (supragingival)*

6. *Aids in removal of a tooth*

7. *Used to check teeth for decay, canal exposures, and cavities*

8. *Used to check the depth of the gingival sulcus*

9. *How often should curettes and hand-scaling instruments be sharpened?*
   a. with each use
   b. once daily
   c. once weekly
   d. once monthly
   e. when chipped or broken

10. *As an animal ages, several classic changes occur in the normal tooth and its supporting system. Which of the following most accurately describes these changes?*
   a. enlargement of the pulp cavity, thickening of the dentin, and loss of definition of the lamina dura
   b. narrowing of the pulp cavity, thickening of the dentin, and loss of definition of the lamina dura
   c. narrowing of the pulp cavity, thinning of the dentin, and loss of definition of the lamina dura
   d. enlargement of the pulp cavity, thickening of the dentin, and thickening of the lamina dura
   e. narrowing of the pulp cavity, thinning of the dentin, and thickening of the lamina dura

11. *Periodontal disease is a disease of the structures that support the tooth. Approximately what percentage of dogs and cats older than 3 years of age have periodontal disease of a degree that would benefit from treatment?*
   a. 5% to 10%
   b. 10% to 15%
   c. 15% to 25%
   d. 25% to 50%
   e. 70% to 85%

12. *What is the major underlying cause of periodontal disease in dogs?*
   a. endocrine disorders
   b. viral infections
   c. trauma
   d. bacterial infections
   e. fungal infections

13. *What is the primary factor contributing to periodontal disease?*
   a. tartar
   b. plaque
   c. calculus
   d. salivary polysaccharides
   e. salivary minerals

14. *All the following predispose to periodontal disease* ***except:***
   a. overcrowded and rotated teeth
   b. retained deciduous teeth
   c. hard, crunchy diet
   d. malocclusions
   e. some endocrine and systemic diseases

For Questions 15 through 17, select the correct answer from the five choices below.

a. polishing
b. sulcal lavage
c. subgingival curettage
d. scaling
e. root planing

15. *Curettage of rough and diseased cementum*

16. *Curettage of the sulcal epithelium*

17. *Flushing of the sulcus with a solution*

18. *Periodontal disease or injury resulting in communication between the oral cavity and a cavity dorsal to the upper corner incisor of a dog is most likely to lead to formation of:*
    a. an oronasal fistula
    b. an oroantral fistula
    c. a periodontal fistula
    d. an endodontic fistula
    e. a gingivobuccal fistula

19. *Periodontal disease or injury resulting in communication between the oral cavity and a cavity dorsal to the upper canine tooth of a dog is most likely to lead to formation of:*
    a. an oronasal fistula
    b. an oroantral fistula
    c. a periodontal fistula
    d. an endodontic fistula
    e. a gingivobuccal fistula

20. *Periodontal disease or injury resulting in communication between the oral cavity and a cavity dorsal to the upper fourth premolar tooth of a dog is most likely to lead to formation of:*
    a. an oronasal fistula
    b. an oroantral fistula
    c. a periodontal fistula
    d. an endodontic fistula
    e. a gingivobuccal fistula

21. *In which species are incisors an open-rooted type of tooth that continually grows throughout the animal's life?*
    a. cats
    b. dogs
    c. rabbits
    d. ferrets
    e. squirrel monkeys

22. *Which substance should **not** be used for routine brushing of the teeth of a 14-year-old dog with congestive heart failure?*
    a. enzymatic toothpaste
    b. baking soda
    c. 0.12% chlorhexidine gluconate solution
    d. 0.4% stannous fluoride gel
    e. zinc ascorbate solution

23. *Enamel hypoplasia of the permanent teeth of dogs may be associated with any of the following **except:***
    a. viral infection
    b. high fever
    c. vitamin C supplementation
    d. trauma
    e. fluorosis

24. *An adult dog is presented for treatment of a tooth with a broken crown and exposed pulp. The injury occurred several weeks before presentation. What is the most appropriate treatment?*
    a. composite filling
    b. application of a crown
    c. extraction or root canal therapy
    d. amalgam filling
    e. glass ionomer filling

25. *All the following are indications for tooth extraction **except:***
    a. advanced periodontal disease
    b. retained deciduous teeth
    c. abscessed tooth
    d. chipped tooth without pulpal exposure or pulpitis
    e. root fractured near the periodontal sulcus

Correct answers are on page 16.

Answers

1. **d** The periodontal ligament connects the root's cementum to alveolar bone.
2. **a** Epithelium lines the sulcus, producing fluid rich in immunoglobulins.
3. **c** The parakeratinized attached gingiva helps protect the nonkeratinized alveolar mucosa.
4. **c** A curette with a rounded toe is safer to use subgingivally.
5. **e** A sickle scaler with a sharp tip and edges should be used supragingivally.
6. **a** An elevator is used to loosen the periodontal ligament for tooth extraction.
7. **d** An explorer has a sharp, hooked end.
8. **b** A probe is marked in millimeters to measure pockets.
9. **a** Instruments must be sharp to remain effective.
10. **b** Increased dentin narrows the pulp cavity. Older animals have loss of definition of the lamina dura.
11. **e** Over 70% of cats and 80% of dogs have stage-I or more severe periodontal disease.
12. **d** Bacteria in plaque cause the initial infection.
13. **b** Plaque is associated with bacterial infection.
14. **c** Crowding facilitates retention of plaque and inflammation. Hard, crunchy foods help reduce plaque and calculus accumulation.
15. **e** Root planing involves use of a curette in several different directions to scale the root.
16. **c** Subgingival curettage involves use of a curette to gently remove diseased tissue from the sulcus lining.
17. **b** Sulcular lavage flushes out debris, plaque, and prophylaxis paste.
18. **a** This causes fistulation into the rostral nasal cavity.
19. **a** This causes fistulation into the rostral nasal cavity.
20. **b** This causes fistulation into the maxillary sinus.
21. **c** Lagomorph incisors are continually growing and open rooted.
22. **b** Baking soda (sodium bicarbonate) can cause sodium loading.
23. **c** Enamel hypoplasia is caused by an insult during tooth development. Vitamin C supplementation should cause no insult.
24. **c** Pulpal tissue exposed for several weeks is infected and necrotic. It should be removed and the cavity filled with inert material, or the tooth should be extracted.
25. **d** Without pulpal insult, the tooth should be preserved.

NOTES

SECTION

4

Dermatology

K.A. Moriello

Recommended Reading

Griffin CE et al: *Current veterinary dermatology,* St. Louis, 1992, Mosby.

Scott DW et al: *Muller and Kirk's small animal dermatology,* ed 5, Philadelphia, 1995, WB Saunders.

Willemse T: *Clinical dermatology of the dog and cat,* Baltimore, 1991, Williams & Wilkins.

Practice answer sheet is on page 289.

Questions

1. *Concerning dermatophyte cultures, which statement is* ***least*** *accurate?*
   a. Cultures of samples obtained by hair-coat brushing with a toothbrush are the most reliable method for cats, especially suspected asymptomatic carriers.
   b. When culturing isolated lesions from dogs, it is best to swab the area with alcohol to minimize the number of contaminant fungi.
   c. A red color change on dermatophyte test medium is diagnostic for a dermatophyte.
   d. Dermatophyte test medium contains Sabouraud's dextrose agar, a pH indicator (phenol red), and antibacterial and antifungal agents.
   e. Fungal pathogens are never heavily pigmented, either macroscopically or microscopically.

2. *Concerning intradermal testing in dogs and cats, which statement is* ***least*** *accurate?*
   a. Antihistamines and acepromazine may cause a false-negative reaction.
   b. Oral or parenteral glucocorticoids, but not topical glucocorticoids, may cause a false-negative reaction.
   c. Fear, pseudopregnancy, or estrus may cause a false-negative reaction.
   d. Inflammation associated with severe superficial pyoderma may cause a false-positive reaction.
   e. Testing with antigen mixtures, outdated allergens, or overdiluted allergen concentrations may cause a false-negative reaction.

Correct answers are on pages 21-22.

3. *Concerning the structure and function of the skin in dogs and cats, which statement is **least** accurate?*
   a. Langhans' cells are part of the skin pigmentary system.
   b. The epidermis of dogs and cats is thinner than that of people.
   c. Melanocytes are fewer in number in feline skin than in canine skin.
   d. Cats and dogs do not have eccrine sweat glands in haired skin.
   e. The tail gland (supracaudal gland, preen gland) in dogs and cats produces an oily substance believed to be important in olfactory recognition.

4. *"Hot spots" are intensely pruritic areas of self-trauma. Concerning pyotraumatic dermatitis or "hot spots," which statement is **least** accurate?*
   a. Flea infestation, ear mite infestation, atopy, and anal sac problems are possible underlying causes of pyotraumatic dermatitis.
   b. Dogs with recurrent areas of pyotraumatic dermatitis, especially on the face, may be atopic.
   c. "Hot spots" in dogs with a thick or long hair-coat (e.g., golden retrievers) are treated differently from those in short-haired dogs.
   d. *Staphylococcus intermedius* is the bacterium most commonly isolated from the lesions.
   e. Glucocorticoids and topical astringents are the treatments of choice for "hot spots."

5. *The most common underlying cause of deep pyoderma in dogs is:*
   a. demodicosis
   b. dermatophytosis
   c. inadequately treated superficial pyoderma
   d. *Proteus* infection
   e. hypothyroidism

6. *Of the following sets of diseases and causative microorganisms, which set is **incorrect?***
   a. cat bite abscess, *Pasteurella multocida*
   b. feline dermatophytosis, *Microsporum canis*
   c. bubonic plague, *Yersinia pestis*
   d. Lyme disease, *Ixodes dammini*
   e. bacterial granulomas (botryomycosis), coagulase-positive staphylococci

7. *Which of the following is not a superficial mycosis of cats or dogs?*
   a. *Microsporum canis* or *Microsporum gypseum* infection
   b. candidiasis
   c. otic *Malassezia* infection
   d. cutaneous *Malassezia* infection
   e. sporotrichosis

8. *A trauma-induced chronic subcutaneous nodule-mass with a fistulous tract that contains granules is known as:*
   a. a kerion
   b. a mycetoma
   c. a foreign body
   d. phaeohyphomycosis
   e. a histiocytoma

9. *A dog has extreme pruritus of the feet, with some foot pads crusted and some not crusted. The **least** likely cause of these signs is:*
   a. hookworm dermatitis
   b. *Pelodera* dermatitis
   c. irritant contact reaction
   d. contact allergy
   e. biotin deficiency

10. *Concerning mite infestations in cats and dogs, which statement is **least** accurate?*
    a. Cheyletiellosis is characterized by scaling, with or without pruritus.
    b. Scabies in dogs is an intensely pruritic skin disease with a predilection for thinly haired areas of the body.
    c. *Otodectes* infestations in cats and dogs require treatment of the ears and the body for eradication.
    d. Demodicosis is a contagious mite infestation.
    e. Notoedric mange in cats has a predilection for the head, and mites are easily found on skin scrapings.

11. *Which of the following has **not** been implicated in the pathogenesis of flea-allergy dermatitis?*
    a. type-1 hypersensitivity
    b. type-4 hypersensitivity
    c. late-phase immediate hypersensitivity reactions
    d. cutaneous basophil hypersensitivity
    e. type-3 reactions

12. *Concerning atopy in dogs or cats, which statement is **least** accurate?*
    a. Atopy is a familial disease with definite breed predispositions in dogs, such as terriers.
    b. Atopic animals typically show facial, pedal, axillary, and inguinal pruritus, but some dogs may show only pruritus of the ears.
    c. Clinical signs may be seasonal or nonseasonal.
    d. The primary skin lesions in atopy are hair loss, superficial pyoderma, miliary dermatitis, and seborrhea.
    e. Treatment for nonseasonal atopy includes hyposensitization, which may take as long as 9 months to produce a response.

13. *A 6-year-old Persian cat is depressed, slightly anorectic, and lame. Findings of physical examination are unremarkable except for the skin. You find marked crusting of the inner aspect of the pinnae, intact pustules, periocular and nasal crusting, and exudative paronychia. The hair coat is matted, with marked exfoliation. Results of a complete blood count, serum chemistry panel, and urinalysis are within normal limits. An antinuclear antibody test is negative. Cytologic examination of the contents of an intact pustule reveals full fields of neutrophils, no bacteria, and rafts of acantholytic cells. Histopathologic examination reveals subcorneal and intragranular pustular dermatitis with acantholysis but no evidence of bacteria. Direct immunofluorescence testing reveals deposition of immunoglobulins intercellularly. The most likely cause of these findings is:*
    a. systemic lupus erythematosus
    b. pemphigus foliaceus
    c. discoid lupus erythematosus
    d. pemphigus vulgaris
    e. drug eruption

14. *Concerning eosinophilic granuloma complex in cats, which statement is **least** accurate?*
    a. The treatment of choice is levamisole.
    b. Linear granuloma is the only form of this complex that is a true granulomatous skin disease.
    c. Recurrent eosinophilic plaques are often a manifestation of atopy and/or flea-allergy dermatitis.
    d. Squamous-cell carcinomas may develop at the margin of indolent ulcers.
    e. Peripheral eosinophilia does not always accompany lesion development.

15. *The most definitive test for thyroid disease in dogs is:*
    a. total baseline thyroid hormone concentrations
    b. free serum thyroxine (T_4) and triiodothyronine (T_3) concentrations
    c. thyroid-stimulating hormone response test
    d. thyroid biopsy
    e. thyrotropin-releasing hormone response test

16. *Which of the following is **not** a cutaneous sign of hyperadrenocorticism in cats or dogs?*
    a. calcinosis cutis
    b. thin, fragile skin
    c. symmetric alopecia
    d. hypertrichosis
    e. comedones

Correct answers are on pages 21-22.

17. *Concerning dermatoses related to sex hormones in dogs, which statement is **least** accurate?*

a. Hyperestrogenism is used to describe a syndrome of vulvar enlargement, gynecomastia, bilaterally symmetric alopecia, and abnormal estrous cycles; the treatment of choice is ovariohysterectomy.
b. Estrogen-responsive dermatosis is used to describe bilaterally symmetric alopecia in the genital and perineal regions of spayed bitches. This alopecia may become generalized. The vulva and nipples are infantile.
c. Male feminization occurs in male dogs with certain types of Sertoli-cell tumors and is characterized by bilaterally symmetric alopecia, gynecomastia, a pendulous prepuce, and attraction of other male dogs.
d. Testosterone-responsive dermatosis is usually seen in older castrated dogs. Bilaterally symmetric alopecia in the perineal and genital regions may progress to involve the trunk and legs.
e. The test of choice for sex hormone–related dermatoses is measurement of serum or plasma concentrations of androgens, estrogens, and progesterone.

18. *Cutaneous asthenia is characterized by:*

a. alopecia
b. abnormal skin elasticity and fragility
c. exfoliation
d. abnormal haircoat shedding and hair replacement
e. hyperesthesia and self-trauma

19. *Concerning color-dilution alopecia, which statement is **least** accurate?*

a. The disease is hereditary.
b. It has been documented in blue, red, and fawn Doberman pinschers; blue dachshunds; chow chows; standard poodles; blue great Danes; Italian greyhounds; and whippets.
c. The defect in melanization and critical structure of the hair results in abnormal hair color.
d. Clinical signs include papules, cystic hair follicles, alopecia, seborrhea, and recurrent pyoderma.
e. Clinical signs are evident within the first year of life.

20. *Concerning primary seborrhea and secondary seborrhea in dogs, which statement is most accurate?*

a. Primary seborrhea is pruritic, whereas secondary seborrhea is not pruritic.
b. Primary seborrhea is a disorder of keratinization inherent to the epidermal cells.
c. Primary seborrhea is generally greasy, whereas secondary seborrhea is exfoliative.
d. Secondary seborrhea is an inherited exfoliative condition that occurs primarily in Arctic breeds of dogs.
e. Secondary seborrhea is usually treated with dietary zinc supplementation and lime sulfur dips.

21. *Concerning acne on the skin of cats, which statement is **least** accurate?*

a. It is characterized by comedones on the chin and lip margins.
b. Unlike the syndrome in dogs and people, this condition tends to occur most commonly in adult cats.
c. Severely affected cats may develop suppurative folliculitis and furunculosis requiring antibiotic therapy.
d. Lesions should be scraped for *Demodex* mites, a fungal culture should be performed to rule out dermatophytosis, and cytologic examination of follicular debris should be performed to rule out bacterial or yeast infections.
e. It must be treated to prevent complications.

22. *Which of the following has **not** been associated with zinc-responsive dermatoses in dogs?*

a. oversupplementation of young growing dogs with vitamins and minerals
b. diets with high calcium levels or a high proportion of cereal grains
c. prolonged enteritis or diarrhea
d. generic dog food with a high phytate content or poor nutritional composition
e. hereditary predisposition in dachshunds and collies

23. *A 12-week-old Labrador retriever puppy is extremely depressed and anorectic. It has a rectal temperature of 104.5° F and the skin is painful to the touch. The ears, face, and muzzle are swollen, and intact vesicles and pustules are present. There is periocular swelling and ulceration. Marked generalized lymphadenopathy is present, and numerous lymph nodes have abscessed. Nodular draining lesions are present on the trunk. According to the owner, lesions developed 4 days after vaccination. A complete blood count reveals leukocytosis and neutrophilia. Lymph node aspiration reveals suppurative inflammation. Cytologic examination of material from a pustule shows degenerative neutrophils but no bacteria. A skin scraping is negative for* Demodex *mites. The most likely cause of these findings is:*
   a. occult juvenile demodicosis
   b. juvenile cellulitis
   c. septicemia
   d. systemic lupus erythematosus
   e. drug reaction

24. *A 10-year-old white cat is presented to you for examination. The cat's ear margins are red, crusty, ulcerative, and bleeding. Closer examination reveals small ulcers and proliferative masses on the cat's nose. The most likely cause of these lesions is:*
   a. basal-cell tumor
   b. squamous-cell carcinoma
   c. mast-cell tumor
   d. seborrheic dermatitis
   e. sunburn

25. *Which of the following is **not** a common skin tumor of cats?*
   a. basal-cell carcinoma
   b. squamous-cell carcinoma
   c. fibrosarcoma
   d. mast-cell tumor
   e. lipoma

Answers

1. **c** The red color indicator in dermatophyte test medium is not diagnostic for a pathogen. It only indicates that the organism is using the protein in the agar. Definitive diagnosis of a dermatophyte infection requires microscopic examination of the specimen.
2. **b** Topical (ocular, otic, cutaneous) glucocorticoid preparations can cause false-negative skin test reactions.
3. **a** Langhans' cells are important immune cells in the skin.
4. **e** "Hot spots" are areas of bacterial infection and require antibiotic therapy, especially in long-haired dogs. These lesions are best treated with at least 3 weeks of antibiotic therapy. In some instances, a short course of glucocorticoid therapy may be needed while the cause of pruritus is treated (e.g., fleas). Astringents are best avoided in treatment of these lesions because they impede wound healing and epithelialization of the lesion. The area should be kept clean with an antibacterial scrub and kept moist with an antibacterial cream.
5. **a** Demodicosis is the most common cause.
6. **d** *Ixodes dammini* is a tick that acts as the vector for the causative agent of Lyme disease, *Borrelia burgdorferi.*
7. **e** Sporotrichosis is an intermediate mycosis. Animals are infected by traumatic inoculation of the organism into the skin.
8. **b** Mycetomas are characterized by cold, subcutaneous swellings with draining fistulous tracts containing granules. They can resemble bacterial granulomas or botryomycosis.
9. **e** Zinc deficiency is the most common nutritional cause of crusted foot-pad lesions. The pruritus in zinc deficiency is caused by secondary bacterial skin infection. Biotin deficiencies have only been reported experimentally.
10. **d** Demodicosis in dogs is not considered a contagious mite infestation. Mites are transmitted during the first few days of life.
11. **e** Type-3 reactions are antigen-antibody reactions and are not involved in the pathogenesis of flea-bite hypersensitivity.

12. **d** Primary skin lesions in atopy are rare. Alopecia, superficial pyoderma, and seborrhea are all secondary to the self-trauma associated with the pruritus that accompanies this disease.
13. **b** The clinical signs, histopathologic findings, and results of direct immunofluorescence testing are most consistent with pemphigus foliaceus.
14. **a** This disease complex may be caused by any number of allergic diseases. It is best to determine and treat the underlying cause of the pruritus (e.g., food allergy, atopy, flea allergy). If antiinflammatory drugs are required, glucocorticoids should be given.
15. **d** Although it is invasive, thyroid biopsy is the best method of evaluating the function and structure of a dog's thyroid gland.
16. **d** Hypertrichosis is the most common clinical sign of hyperadrenocorticism in horses but not in dogs or cats.
17. **e** Serum sex hormone concentrations do not correlate with clinical signs and/or the responsiveness of these animals to neutering or hormone replacement. The dysfunction is believed to be at the cell receptor level or caused by an abnormal metabolite of the hormone.
18. **b** Cutaneous asthenia is an inherited collagen defect that results in abnormally loose and extendable skin. Affected animals are unsuitable as pets because of impaired wound healing.
19. **e** Clinical signs do not develop until the animal is at least 3 years of age.
20. **b** Primary seborrhea is a disorder of keratinization.
21. **e** Not all affected animals should be treated. If the lesions are not severe, no treatment is necessary. There is no evidence that early or aggressive treatment alters the course of the disease. Cats with severe folliculitis/furunculosis should be treated with topical hot packs and a course of systemic antibiotic therapy.
22. **e** Zinc-responsive dermatosis is hereditary in Siberian huskies and Alaskan malamutes and requires lifelong therapy in these dogs. With the other four causes, therapy may be temporary, depending on whether the underlying cause can be eliminated.
23. **b** Juvenile cellulitis is an idiopathic skin disease of young dogs. The lesions are almost always sterile and affected dogs do not respond to antibiotic therapy. Corticosteroids are used in treatment.
24. **b** Squamous-cell carcinoma is the most likely cause. The lesions have become ulcerative and destructive, suggesting an active neoplasm. Cats with sunburn exhibit erythema without destructive ulcerative lesions.
25. **e** Unlike dogs, cats rarely develop lipomas.

NOTES

SECTION

5

Hematology

S.M. Cotter, W.J. Dodds

Recommended Reading

Cowell RL, Tyler RD: *Diagnostic cytology of the dog and cat,* ed 2, St. Louis, 1998, Mosby.

Duncan JR et al: *Veterinary laboratory medicine,* ed 3, Ames, Iowa, 1994, Iowa State University Press.

Jain NC: *Essentials of veterinary hematology,* Baltimore, 1993, Williams & Wilkins.

Meyer DJ et al: *Veterinary laboratory medicine: interpretation and diagnosis,* Philadelphia, 1992, WB Saunders.

Willard MD et al: *Small animal clinical diagnosis by laboratory methods,* ed 2, Philadelphia, 1994, WB Saunders.

Practice answer sheet is on page 291.

Questions

1. *Smears of blood from dogs with autoimmune hemolytic anemia often show:*
   a. rouleaux formation
   b. spherocytosis
   c. Heinz bodies
   d. elliptocytosis
   e. hypochromasia

2. *The red blood cells of animals with iron-deficiency anemia are classically:*
   a. hyperchromic and normocytic
   b. polychromatophilic
   c. hypochromic and macrocytic
   d. hypochromic and microcytic
   e. hypochromic and normocytic

3. *The nonregenerative anemia that accompanies chronic renal failure is caused by:*
   a. chronic blood loss
   b. erythropoietin deficiency
   c. erythrophagocytosis
   d. elevated blood urea nitrogen
   e. hypoparathyroidism

4. *A common cause of chronic blood loss anemia in young animals is:*
   a. parasitism (fleas, hookworms)
   b. rodenticide toxicosis (warfarin)
   c. primary bleeding disorder
   d. immune-mediated hemolytic disease
   e. copper deficiency

Correct answers are on pages 26-27.

5. *Basophilic stippling of erythrocytes is characteristic of:*
   a. magnesium poisoning
   b. copper toxicosis
   c. lead poisoning
   d. hemobartonellosis
   e. babesiosis

6. *If a hemophiliac male is bred to an unrelated normal female, what proportion of offspring would show signs of bleeding?*
   a. one quarter
   b. none
   c. all the males
   d. all
   e. one half

7. *A 1-year-old collie was found lying on the porch after being outside unattended for 2 hours. The dog is pale and blood is obtained on abdominocentesis. The packed cell volume is 35%, platelet count is 150,000/μl (normal, 200,000 to 400,000/μl), prothrombin time (PT) is 12 seconds (control, 11 seconds), and activated partial thromboplastin time (APTT) is 17 seconds (control, 18 seconds). Fibrin split products are not detected. The most likely cause for the bleeding is:*
   a. warfarin toxicity
   b. immune-mediated thrombocytopenia
   c. von Willebrand's disease
   d. bleeding from trauma, with normal coagulation
   e. disseminated intravascular coagulation

8. *All of following signs may occur in cats with acetaminophen toxicity* ***except:***
   a. facial edema
   b. Heinz-body formation
   c. hepatic necrosis
   d. aplastic anemia
   e. hemolytic anemia

9. *A 5-year-old spayed poodle has petechiae on the gums and ventral abdomen. Following venipuncture, the dog bleeds for a prolonged period, but once bleeding ceases it does not recur. These findings suggest a defect in which component of the hemostatic mechanism?*
   a. extrinsic pathway factors
   b. plasminogen
   c. antithrombin III
   d. platelets
   e. fibrinogen

10. *To evaluate a patient's hemostatic mechanism, which anticoagulant is routinely used with blood samples?*
    a. citrate
    b. EDTA
    c. sodium heparin
    d. coumarin
    e. lithium heparin

11. *Which mechanism best explains interference with platelet function by aspirin?*
    a. prevention of adherence of platelets to collagen
    b. decreased synthesis of thromboxane (TXA_2)
    c. immune-mediated platelet lysis
    d. increased synthesis of prostacyclin (PGI_2)
    e. blocked binding of fibrin to platelet phospholipid

12. *Which hematopoietic growth factor has proven beneficial to patients with renal failure?*
    a. interleukin-3
    b. interleukin-2
    c. granulocyte-monocyte colony-stimulating factor
    d. thrombopoietin
    e. erythropoietin

13. *Which stain best demonstrates reticulocytes?*
    a. Wright's
    b. Giemsa
    c. new methylene blue
    d. hematoxylin
    e. any Romanowsky stain

14. *When the mean corpuscular volume (MCV) is decreased in an anemic animal, what is the most likely cause?*
    a. immune-mediated hemolytic anemia
    b. nonregenerative anemia from any cause
    c. iron deficiency
    d. myelodysplasia
    e. Heinz-body anemia

15. *Which of the following is **not** likely to be found in urine described as dark or red?*
    a. unconjugated bilirubin
    b. conjugated bilirubin
    c. urobilinogen
    d. hemoglobin
    e. red blood cells

16. *A complete blood count in a dog shows packed cell volume 35%, white blood cell count 1800/μl, 10% neutrophils, 50% lymphocytes, 20% monocytes, and 20% eosinophils. What is the most significant abnormality in this hemogram?*
    a. eosinophilia
    b. neutropenia
    c. lymphocytosis
    d. monocytosis
    e. anemia

17. *Addison's disease (hypoadrenocorticism) is a condition in which the adrenal cortex is unable to produce sufficient glucocorticoids and mineralocorticoids. Considering the effects of corticosteroids on the hemogram, what would you expect to see in an animal with Addison's disease?*
    a. neutrophilia
    b. lymphopenia
    c. eosinophilia
    d. monocytosis
    e. thrombocytopenia

18. *What is the stimulus for movement of granulocytes from the marginal pool to the circulating pool?*
    a. granulocyte colony-stimulating factor
    b. complement
    c. immunoglobulin
    d. corticosteroid
    e. epinephrine

19. *A 4-month-old male dachshund is presented because of lameness and swollen joints. Joint aspiration produces bloody fluid. You order a coagulation screen, the results of which are normal except for prolonged prothrombin time (PT), and activated partial thromboplastin time (APTT). Which of the following is **not** ruled out by these findings?*
    a. von Willebrand's disease
    b. hemophilia A
    c. hemophilia B
    d. factor VII deficiency
    e. factor V deficiency

20. *Hemoglobinuria in an anemic animal indicates:*
    a. IgM on red cells
    b. circulating immune complexes
    c. renal glomerular damage
    d. intravascular hemolysis
    e. decreased hepatic conjugation of bilirubin

21. *What is the mechanism of action of corticosteroids in treatment of autoimmune hemolytic anemia?*
    a. They suppress erythrophagocytosis and antibody binding.
    b. They bind to antibodies to block binding sites.
    c. They suppress chemotaxis and neutrophil function.
    d. They suppress release of IgG from plasma cells.
    e. They bind to macrophages to prevent attachment to antibodies.

Correct answers are on pages 26-27.

22. *A dog given a blood transfusion 3 weeks ago now needs another transfusion. Concerning a major crossmatch, which statement is most accurate?*
   a. Lack of reactivity indicates that the donor and recipient have the same blood type.
   b. Lack of reactivity indicates that the recipient does not have antibodies against donor red blood cell antigens.
   c. Lack of reactivity indicates that the recipient will not form antibodies against donor red blood cells.
   d. Crossmatching involves mixing donor plasma with recipient red blood cells and checking for agglutination.
   e. Crossmatching is not necessary if the donor is negative for DEA-1 (i.e., if the donor is A-negative).

23. *A 7-year-old male Airedale with weakness, pale mucous membranes, and splenomegaly has a packed cell volume of 12% and a reticulocyte count of 3%. The white blood cell count is 3800/μl, with 25% neutrophils, 68% lymphocytes (many atypical), and 7% monocytes. The platelet count is 72,000/μl. The procedure most likely to confirm the diagnosis is:*
   a. direct antiglobulin test
   b. cytologic examination of a bone marrow aspirate
   c. serum iron level
   d. serum creatinine level
   e. antiplatelet antibody test

24. *In cats, what is the best indication of regenerative anemia?*
   a. punctate reticulocytes
   b. aggregate reticulocytes
   c. circulating nucleated red blood cells
   d. increased mean corpuscular volume
   e. *Hemobartonella* on red blood cells

25. *A stray dog is presented to you after it was found in a collapsed state. Before you examine the dog, your technician collects a blood sample and tells you the packed cell volume is 52% and the total plasma protein level is 9.5 g/dl. The most appropriate initial interpretation of these findings is:*
   a. dehydration
   b. hyperglobulinemia
   c. hyperalbuminemia
   d. polycythemia
   e. laboratory error

Answers

1. **b** Affected dogs often show spherocytosis.
2. **d** The anemia of iron deficiency is hypochromic and microcytic.
3. **b** Patients with chronic renal disease are often anemic because of erythropoietin deficiency.
4. **a** Young animals with a heavy flea infestation or hookworm infection are often anemic because of blood loss.
5. **c** Lead poisoning can cause basophilic stippling of red blood cells.
6. **b** All female offspring would be normal carriers; all males would be normal (X-linked inheritance).
7. **d** Bleeding from thrombocytopenia is unlikely with a platelet count greater than 100,000/μl.
8. **d** The marrow is not affected.
9. **d** Platelet abnormalities are characterized by petechiae, mucosal bleeding, and sometimes bleeding from venipuncture.
10. **a** Citrate loosely binds calcium.
11. **b** Thromboxane is important in platelet aggregation.
12. **e** Erythropoietin is deficient in renal failure, resulting in anemia.
13. **c** The stain shows residual ribonucleic acid (RNA) as a weblike reticulum.
14. **c** Iron-deficiency anemia is microcytic hypochromic.
15. **a** Unconjugated bilirubin in not water soluble, so it is not passed into the urine.
16. **b** Absolute neutropenia is present. Numbers of the other white blood cells are only relatively (not absolutely) increased.

17. **c** Corticosteroids cause eosinopenia and lymphopenia, and insufficiency of endogenous corticosteroids is likely to cause the converse.
18. **e** Physiologic neutrophilia can occur with excitement (epinephrine release).
19. **e** Because both PT and APTT are prolonged, the defect must involve the common pathway (fibrinogen, prothrombin, factor V or X) or multiple factors (vitamin K antagonists).
20. **d** Destruction of circulating red blood cells releases hemoglobin.
21. **a** Corticosteroids do not directly suppress antibody production but tend to suppress antibody binding and macrophage function.
22. **b** The major crossmatch (donor cells with recipient plasma) detects only antibodies already present to any of several antigens on red blood cells.
23. **b** Nonregenerative anemia, neutropenia, and thrombocytopenia often indicate bone marrow disease. Abnormal lymphocytes could indicate malignancy in the bone marrow.
24. **b** Aggregate reticulocytes indicate active production of red blood cells by the bone marrow.
25. **a** Both the packed cell volume and total plasma protein level increase in dehydration.

NOTES

NOTES

SECTION

6

Medical Diseases

S.K. Fooshee, D.W. Macy, S. Merchant, F.W. Scott, R.G. Sherding, J. Taboada, J.P. Thompson, C.B. Waters, M.D. Willard

Recommended Reading

Bonagura JD: *Kirk's current veterinary therapy XII,* Philadelphia, 1995, WB Saunders.

Ettinger SJ, Feldman EC: *Textbook of veterinary internal medicine,* ed 4, Philadelphia, 1995, WB Saunders.

Feldman EC, Nelson RW: *Canine and feline endocrinology and reproduction,* ed 2, Philadelphia, 1996, WB Saunders.

Greene CE: *Infectious diseases of the dog and cat,* Philadelphia, 1990, WB Saunders.

Guilford WG et al: *Strombeck's small animal gastroenterology,* Philadelphia, 1996, WB Saunders.

Leib MS, Monroe WE: *Small animal internal medicine,* Philadelphia, 1997, WB Saunders.

Nelson RW, Couto CG: *Essentials of small animal internal medicine,* St. Louis, 1992, Mosby.

Practice answer sheets are on pages 293-298.

Questions

DOGS

S.R. Merchant and J. Taboada

1. *Which condition is **least** likely to result in syncope or intermittent weakness?*
   a. sick sinus syndrome
   b. Doberman cardiomyopathy
   c. chronic renal disease
   d. hypoadrenocorticism
   e. myasthenia gravis

2. *Cough is a likely clinical sign in all the following disorders **except:***
   a. tracheal collapse
   b. right-sided congestive heart failure
   c. *Bordetella bronchiseptica* infection
   d. blastomycosis
   e. acute bacterial bronchitis

3. *A dog with severe heartworm disease would most likely have which electrocardiographic or radiographic abnormality?*
   a. a tall R wave on lead II of the electrocardiogram (ECG)
   b. a wide P wave on lead II of the ECG
   c. a bulge at the 3-o'clock position on a ventrodorsal radiograph of the heart
   d. small, volume-depleted pulmonary arteries on a lateral thoracic radiograph
   e. deep S waves in leads II, III, and aV_F of the ECG

4. *What is the most common nasal fungal infection in dogs?*
   a. sporotrichosis
   b. cryptococcosis
   c. aspergillosis
   d. blastomycosis
   e. histoplasmosis

5. *What is the most common nasal tumor of dogs?*
   a. adenocarcinoma + fibrosarcoma
   b. mast-cell tumor
   c. chondrosarcoma
   d. osteosarcoma
   e. turbinatoma

6. *What is the treatment of choice for nasal tumors in dogs?*
   a. surgical removal
   b. chemotherapy
   c. radiation therapy
   d. combination therapy with surgery and chemotherapy
   e. topical nasal decongestants

7. *Which disorder is **least** likely to cause epistaxis?*
   a. nasal neoplasia
   b. blastomycosis
   c. *Ehrlichia canis* infection
   d. polycythemia
   e. canine distemper

8. *Which disorder is **least** likely to cause inspiratory distress?*
   a. laryngeal paralysis
   b. pharyngeal abscess
   c. elongated soft palate
   d. proximal tracheal collapse
   e. acute bronchitis

9. *Which tissues are most likely to be affected by pythiosis (phycomycosis)?*
   a. kidneys and gastrointestinal tract
   b. liver and pancreas
   c. prostate and testes
   d. gastrointestinal tract and skin
   e. skin and nasal cavity

10. *During bronchoscopic examination of a dog in sternal recumbency, what is the most cranial major bronchus leaving a main-stem bronchus ventrally?*
    a. right cranial bronchus
    b. right middle bronchus
    c. right caudal bronchus
    d. left cranial bronchus
    e. left caudal bronchus

11. *Which disorder is **least** likely to cause acidemia?*
    a. renal disease
    b. diabetes mellitus
    c. hypoadrenocorticism
    d. hyperventilation
    e. severe anemia

12. *Which drug is a bronchodilator that acts by β_2-receptor stimulation?*
    a. aminophylline
    b. terbutaline
    c. oxtriphylline
    d. atropine
    e. atenolol

13. *Which of the following most accurately lists the tissues most commonly affected by blastomycosis?*
    a. lungs, skin, and eyes
    b. lungs, gastrointestinal tract, and bone
    c. lungs, prostate, and central nervous system
    d. nasal cavity and central nervous system
    e. skin, nasal cavity, and mucocutaneous junctions

14. *Which of the following most accurately lists the tissues most commonly affected by histoplasmosis?*
    a. lungs, skin, and eyes
    b. lungs, gastrointestinal tract, and bone
    c. lungs, prostate, and central nervous system
    d. nasal cavity and central nervous system
    e. skin, nasal cavity, and mucocutaneous junctions

15. *Which disorder is **least** likely to cause regenerative anemia?*
    a. babesiosis
    b. autoimmune hemolytic anemia
    c. chronic gastrointestinal blood loss
    d. hemangiosarcoma
    e. hypothyroidism

16. *Which disorder is **least** likely to cause pulmonary thromboembolism?*
    a. hyperadrenocorticism
    b. renal amyloidosis
    c. dirofilariasis
    d. aortic valve vegetative endocarditis
    e. autoimmune hemolytic anemia

17. *Which disorder is most likely to cause transudative ascites?*
    a. nephrotic syndrome
    b. dirofilariasis
    c. hemangiosarcoma
    d. carcinomatosis
    e. pancreatitis

18. *Which antimicrobial is **least** appropriate for treating a dog with a bacterial urinary tract infection and decreased tear production?*
    a. amoxicillin
    b. cephalexin
    c. trimethoprim-potentiated sulfonamide
    d. enrofloxacin
    e. amoxicillin-clavulanate

19. *All the following would be useful in differentiating vomiting from regurgitation **except:***
    a. retching
    b. prodromal nausea
    c. observing bile within the material produced
    d. time of occurrence relative to eating
    e. abdominal contractions

20. *Megaesophagus may be associated with all the following disorders **except:***
    a. myasthenia gravis
    b. lead toxicity
    c. hypothyroidism
    d. severe esophagitis
    e. hyperadrenocorticism

21. *Which laboratory finding is **least** likely to indicate abnormal liver function?*
    a. alkaline phosphatase 1437 IU/L (normal 0 to 90 IU/L)
    b. albumin 1.3 mg/dl (normal 2.9 to 4.0 mg/dl)
    c. blood urea nitrogen (BUN) 5 mg/dl (normal 10 to 28 mg/dl)
    d. glucose 40 mg/dl (normal 80 to 120 mg/dl)
    e. partial thromboplastin time 25 seconds (normal 7 to 14 seconds)

Correct answers are on pages 140-171.

22. *A 2-year-old female Yorkshire terrier has been depressed and lethargic for the past 2 weeks. The owners have noticed some behavioral changes, including head pressing, especially after eating. Laboratory tests show slightly increased activity of liver enzymes, low serum albumin level, increased bile acid and ammonia levels, and microcytosis. What is the most likely cause of these findings?*

a. toxic hepatopathy
b. chronic active hepatitis
c. familial copper-associated chronic hepatitis
d. portosystemic vascular anomaly
e. corticosteroid hepatopathy

23. *Which of the following is **least** indicated in medical management of a dog with hepatoencephalopathy?*

a. lactulose
b. neomycin
c. metronidazole
d. low-protein diet
e. diazepam

24. *Which breed is **not** predisposed to familial chronic hepatitis caused by hepatic copper toxicosis?*

a. West Highland white terrier
b. Doberman pinscher
c. Bedlington terrier
d. cocker spaniel
e. Skye terrier

25. *You suspect fulminant hepatic failure and hepatoencephalopathy in a 1-year-old female poodle with severe neurologic signs. Two hours before admission the dog had lapsed into a coma. Which of the following would be **least** useful in management of this dog?*

a. 0.9% saline solution
b. dextrose
c. warm-water enema
d. methionine
e. lactulose

26. *Which diagnostic finding would be **least** useful in diagnosing pancreatitis?*

a. increased BUN level
b. increased trypsinlike immunoreactivity
c. increased serum lipase activity
d. increased serum amylase activity
e. characteristic findings on abdominal sonograms

27. *Which drug does **not** have an antacid effect?*

a. aluminum hydroxide
b. sulfasalazine
c. famotidine
d. omeprazole
e. cimetidine

28. *Against which parasitic infection is fenbendazole **not** effective?*

a. ancylostomiasis
b. trichuriasis
c. ascariasis
d. giardiasis
e. coccidiosis

29. *Which finding is most consistent with a diagnosis of hemorrhagic gastroenteritis in a dog with acute onset of vomiting and bloody diarrhea?*

a. coronavirus particles on electron microscopy of the stool
b. neutrophilic leukocytosis with a pronounced left shift
c. increased packed cell volume (PCV) (above 55%) with increased total plasma protein level
d. increased PCV (above 55%) with normal total plasma protein level
e. hypokalemia with metabolic alkalosis

30. *What is the most common cause of gastric ulcers in dogs?*

a. use of nonsteroidal antiinflammatory drugs
b. gastric adenocarcinoma
c. mast-cell tumor
d. viral gastritis
e. chronic active hepatitis

31. *What is the diagnostic test of choice for exocrine pancreatic insufficiency?*
    a. trypsinlike immunoreactivity
    b. fecal proteolytic activity by x-ray film digestion
    c. Sudan staining of feces for fat
    d. evaluation for plasma turbidity following oral administration of corn oil
    e. intestinal biopsy

32. *Which infiltrative intestinal disease of dogs generally has the best prognosis?*
    a. lymphocytic-plasmacytic enteritis
    b. granulomatous enteritis
    c. eosinophilic gastroenteritis
    d. gastrointestinal lymphosarcoma
    e. immunoproliferative enteritis of basenjis

33. *Blood studies in an anorectic dog reveal a serum albumin level of 1.9 g/dl (normal 2.5 to 4.0 g/dl), a total plasma protein level of 3.0 g/dl (normal 5.5 to 7.5 g/dl), and a PCV of 38% (normal 35% to 50%). What is the most likely cause of these findings?*
    a. glomerulonephritis
    b. chronic gastrointestinal blood loss
    c. cirrhosis
    d. Rocky Mountain spotted fever
    e. lymphangiectasia

34. *Which of the following would be **least** effective in treating idiopathic colitis?*
    a. sulfasalazine
    b. prednisone
    c. metronidazole
    d. increased dietary fiber
    e. isopropamide with prochlorperazine

35. *Chronic active hepatitis of Doberman pinschers (familial chronic inflammatory hepatitis) is most likely to occur in:*
    a. young male Dobermans
    b. young female Dobermans
    c. middle-aged male Dobermans
    d. middle-aged female Dobermans
    e. very old male or female Dobermans

For Questions 36 through 40, select the correct answers from the five choices below.

a. blastomycosis
b. histoplasmosis
c. sporotrichosis
d. coccidioidomycosis
e. aspergillosis

36. *Fungal infection that commonly affects the gastrointestinal tract, causing chronic diarrhea*

37. *Infections occuring in the desert southwest and west coast of the United States*

38. *Fungal infection that typically causes chronic nasal discharge*

39. *Infection caused by a thick-walled yeast that buds from a broad base; the organism is commonly observed on impression smears of cutaneous lesions or vitreal aspirates from affected eyes*

40. *Fungal infection that typically affects the skin but rarely causes systemic disease*

41. *A 2-year-old male mongrel with epistaxis has a prolonged partial thromboplastin time (PTT), but the prothrombin time (PT) and platelet count are normal. What is the most likely cause of these findings?*
    a. hemophilia A
    b. ehrlichiosis
    c. warfarin toxicity
    d. chronic liver disease
    e. disseminated intravascular coagulation

42. *On ultrasound examination of a dog with polycystic kidney disease, a fluid-filled cyst in the kidney would:*
    a. appear hyperechoic relative to the surrounding renal parenchyma
    b. appear of the same echogenicity as the surrounding renal parenchyma
    c. appear hypoechoic relative to the surrounding renal parenchyma
    d. appear of variable echogenicity relative to the surrounding renal parenchyma
    e. not be apparent on the sonogram

Correct answers are on pages 140-171.

43. *Urinary protein/creatinine ratio would be useful in monitoring urinary protein loss in all the following conditions* ***except:***

a. urinary tract infection
b. glomerulonephritis
c. renal amyloidosis
d. hyperadrenocorticism
e. systemic lupus erythematosus

44. *Which disorder is* ***least*** *likely to cause systemic hypertension?*

a. hyperadrenocorticism
b. glomerulonephritis
c. chronic interstitial nephritis
d. idiopathic dilative cardiomyopathy
e. hyperthyroidism

45. *Which of the following is* ***least*** *likely to produce nephrotoxicity?*

a. amikacin
b. amphotericin B
c. *cis*-platinum
d. ethylene glycol
e. primidone

46. *The rate of intravenous infusion of potassium solution should* ***not*** *exceed:*

a. 2 mEq/kg/hr
b. 0.5 mEq/kg/hr
c. 5 mEq/kg/hr
d. 0.05 mEq/kg/hr
e. 10 mEq/kg/hr

47. *Which disorder is most likely to be associated with hypocalcemia?*

a. pancreatitis
b. lymphosarcoma
c. primary hyperparathyroidism
d. hypoadrenocorticism
e. vitamin D toxicity

48. *What is the most common cause of urinary tract infections in dogs?*

a. *Pseudomonas aeruginosa*
b. *Klebsiella pneumoniae*
c. *Bacteroides nodosus*
d. *Escherichia coli*
e. *Streptococcus viridans*

49. *You have treated a 10-year-old female Labrador retriever for a bacterial urinary tract infection using 3-week courses of cephalexin on three separate occasions, but the infection has recurred each time. A recent urinalysis revealed hematuria, pyuria, a pH of 7.5, and a specific gravity of 1.030. Urine culture yields* Escherichia coli *that is sensitive to cephalexin, using the Kirby-Bauer technique. What is the* ***least*** *likely reason for recurrence of the infection?*

a. The dog has a cystic urolith.
b. The dog has a transitional-cell carcinoma of the bladder.
c. The owners have failed to give the antibiotic for the entire course of therapy.
d. The *E. coli* is not sensitive to cephalexin if a minimum inhibitory concentration technique is used.
e. The dog has pyelonephritis and should be treated longer.

50. *A male dog has two 2-cm–diameter oxalate uroliths in its bladder. Which of the following is the most appropriate treatment?*

a. cystotomy for removal of the uroliths
b. allopurinol use for 2 months, followed by reevaluation
c. antibiotic treatment to control infection, followed by dietary acidification of the urine
d. dietary acidification of the urine using a low-protein diet
e. D-penicillamine use for 1 month, followed by reevaluation

51. *Concerning diabetes mellitus in dogs, which statement is most accurate?*

a. Polyuria is a common finding because affected dogs lack antidiuretic hormone.
b. NPH insulin should be given once daily because this type of insulin is effective for longer than 24 hours in most dogs.
c. Most dogs have non–insulin-dependent diabetes and therefore do not require insulin; these dogs should be treated with a high-fiber diet and oral hypoglycemic drugs.
d. Prednisone administration improves control in about one third of diabetic dogs.
e. Chronic pancreatitis may predispose to diabetes mellitus.

52. *Which of the following is most likely to be observed in a dog with a functional pancreatic β-cell tumor?*

a. hypertension
b. increased serum lipase activity
c. hypoglycemia
d. hyperkalemia
e. bradycardia

53. *Which drug is **least** appropriate in management of hyperkalemia in a dog with hypoadrenocorticism?*

a. desoxycorticosterone pivalate
b. dexamethasone
c. insulin and dextrose
d. sodium bicarbonate
e. fludrocortisone acetate

54. *Which of the following would be most appropriate in management of an epileptic dog that has been having seizures every other day despite receiving phenobarbital at a dosage that produces serum phenobarbital concentrations well within the therapeutic range?*

a. Increase the phenobarbital dosage.
b. Change the antiepileptic therapy to primidone.
c. Add oral diazepam to the treatment regime.
d. Have the owners administer diazepam per rectum during the seizures.
e. Add potassium bromide to the treatment regimen.

55. *You are presented with a 9-year-old boxer with acute onset of ataxia, head tilt to the right, and falling to the right. On examination you note horizontal nystagmus, with the fast phase to the left. The right pupil is miotic, as compared with the left. The right eye shows slight ptosis and enophthalmos. Other findings of the neurologic and physical examination are normal. What is the most likely cause of these findings?*

a. a tumor affecting the right cerebral cortex
b. distemper affecting multifocal areas of white matter in the brain
c. a tumor affecting the right midbrain
d. right-sided otitis externa
e. right-sided otitis interna and otitis media

56. *A 7-year-old cocker spaniel has a drooping lip and ear on the left side and cannot blink the left eye. There are no other abnormalities. What is the most likely cause of these findings?*

a. facial nerve paralysis
b. right-sided ear disease
c. hypothyroidism
d. myasthenia gravis
e. central nervous system infection

57. *Concerning corticosteroid-responsive meningitis, which statement is **least** accurate?*

a. Large-breed dogs are affected more commonly than small-breed dogs.
b. Young dogs (less than 2 years old) are affected most commonly.
c. Cervical pain is the most common clinical sign.
d. Neurologic deficits are common.
e. The prognosis for survival and complete resolution is excellent with treatment.

58. *Which diagnostic finding is most consistent with a diagnosis of toxoplasmosis in a dog with caudal paresis?*

a. a single positive immunoglobulin G (IgG) titer
b. a single positive IgM titer
c. granulomatous inflammation observed on muscle biopsy
d. increased protein content and high mononuclear cell numbers in cerebrospinal fluid
e. coccidia observed on fecal examination

Correct answers are on pages 140-171.

59. *A 7-year-old male German shorthaired pointer has had difficulty with prehension of food; the mouth has hung open for the past 3 days. You note atrophy of the muscles of mastication. Other findings of the physical and neurologic examination are normal. What is the most likely cause of these findings?*

a. myositis of the masticatory muscles
b. granulomatous meningoencephalitis
c. corticosteroid-responsive meningitis
d. trigeminal nerve paralysis
e. acute polyradiculoneuritis

60. *Which chemotherapeutic agent is most likely to cause cardiotoxicity?*

a. cyclophosphamide
b. vincristine
c. doxorubicin
d. *cis*-platinum
e. L-asparaginase

61. *All the following may be seen in dogs with obstructive pharyngeal disease* ***except:***

a. inspiratory stridor
b. stertor (snoring noises) while sleeping
c. gagging and hypersalivation
d. pulmonary edema
e. coughing

62. *A complete blood count on a canine blood sample shows markedly regenerative anemia, spherocytosis, and neutrophilia, with a left shift back to metamyelocytes. What is the most likely cause of these findings?*

a. autoimmune hemolytic anemia
b. babesiosis
c. ehrlichiosis
d. gram-negative septicemia
e. gastrointestinal blood loss

63. *Thoracentesis on a dog with pleural effusion yields a modified transudate (protein 3 g/dl, 1000 cells/µl, with 85% small lymphocytes and 15% nondegenerate neutrophils). The cholesterol level in the effusion is lower than that found in the serum, but the triglyceride level is much higher. What is the most likely cause of these findings?*

a. left-sided heart failure
b. lymphosarcoma
c. chylothorax
d. diaphragmatic hernia
e. pyothorax

64. *Which drug is most appropriate for treatment of a dog with chronic renal disease and nonregenerative anemia (PCV 18%)?*

a. stanozolol
b. prednisone
c. human recombinant epoetin alfa
d. testosterone
e. estrogen

65. *Hematologic examination of a canine blood sample shows a PCV of 70% and a normal total plasma protein level. Other hematologic findings are normal. What is the* ***least*** *likely cause of these findings?*

a. hemorrhagic gastroenteritis
b. renal adenocarcinoma
c. chronic pulmonary disease
d. dehydration
e. polycythemia vera

66. *What is the most likely cause of severe bloody diarrhea, vomiting, and leukopenia in a dog?*

a. parvoviral enteritis
b. coronaviral enteritis
c. mercury toxicity
d. protothecosis
e. hemorrhagic gastroenteritis

67. *You diagnose severe adult-onset pustular generalized demodectic mange in a 6-year-old intact female poodle. What is the most appropriate course of action?*

 a. Begin treatment with amitraz (Mitaban) and continue treatment until the mite infestation is resolved.
 b. Search for an underlying cause; administer appropriate antibiotics; begin treatment with a miticide, and continue treatment until the mite infestation is resolved; spay the dog when the skin disease is improved.
 c. Administer antiinflammatory doses of prednisone for 1 or 2 weeks before treating with a miticide.
 d. Administer antiinflammatory doses of prednisone and large doses of estrogen for 1 or 2 weeks.
 e. Begin immunostimulation therapy with levamisole or thiabendazole.

68. *Clinical signs of hypothyroidism include all the following* ***except:***

 a. lethargy
 b. dry, brittle, lusterless hair coat
 c. infertility
 d. heat seeking
 e. polyphagia

69. *What is the most common cause of hypothyroidism in dogs?*

 a. thyroid gland atrophy
 b. overuse of methimazole (Tapazole) to treat hyperthyroidism
 c. iodine deficiency from feeding of generic dog foods
 d. thyroid destruction by a tumor
 e. congenital hypothyroidism

70. *Concerning use of a baseline T_4 level to evaluate hypothyroidism in dogs, which statement is most accurate?*

 a. Systemically ill dogs with a borderline (marginally normal) value should be evaluated with a free T_4 level and/or TSH blood level.
 b. Exogenous corticosteroids do not affect the baseline T_4 value.
 c. A T_3 value is a better predictor of thyroid disease but is technically too difficult to determine.
 d. Human and veterinary reference laboratories can perform a T_4 assay because thyroid values in people and dogs are virtually identical.
 e. Anticonvulsant therapy with phenobarbital can elevate the baseline T_4 level.

71. *Which abnormalities are most likely to be observed in dogs with hyperadrenocorticism?*

 a. polyuria, polydipsia, hepatomegaly, eosinopenia, and elevated serum alkaline phosphatase activity
 b. polyuria, polydipsia, hepatomegaly, neutropenia, and elevated serum alanine transferase activity
 c. polyuria, polydipsia, eosinopenia, elevated serum alkaline phosphatase activity, and splenomegaly
 d. hepatomegaly, neutropenia, elevated serum aspartate transferase activity, and partial anorexia
 e. partial anorexia, splenomegaly, eosinopenia, and elevated serum alkaline phosphatase activity

72. *What is the test of choice in diagnosing iatrogenic (exogenous) Cushing's syndrome?*

 a. low-dosage dexamethasone test
 b. adrenocorticotropic hormone (ACTH) stimulation test
 c. assay for blood ACTH level
 d. glucagon tolerance test
 e. high-dosage dexamethasone test

73. *Which drugs are most effective in treatment of pituitary-dependent hyperadrenocorticism?*

 a. fluconazole, itraconazole, and ketoconazole
 b. ketoconazole, mitotane, and deprenyl
 c. cyproheptadine, fluconazole, and bromocriptine
 d. griseofulvin, mitotane, and bromocriptine
 e. itraconazole, deprenyl, and cyproheptadine

Correct answers are on pages 140-171.

74. *Which of the following is considered a screening test (not a differentiating test) for hyperadrenocorticism in dogs?*

a. ACTH stimulation test
b. high-dosage dexamethasone suppression test
c. assay for blood ACTH level
d. glucose tolerance test
e. cortisol suppression test

75. *Which glucocorticoid is **least** likely to be effective for mineralocorticoid replacement in a dog with hypoadrenocorticism?*

a. hydrocortisone
b. dexamethasone
c. deoxycorticosterone pivalate
d. fludrocortisone acetate
e. prednisolone acetate

76. *Which cutaneous lesion does **not** support a diagnosis of hypothyroidism in dogs?*

a. bilateral symmetric alopecia
b. seborrhea sicca
c. calcinosis cutis
d. hyperpigmentation
e. myxedema

77. *The polydipsia and polyuria of diabetes mellitus are caused by:*

a. primary polydipsia from effects on the central nervous system
b. antidiuretic hormone resistance
c. osmotic diuresis caused by glycosuria
d. renal medullary washout
e. increased need for fluids because of polyphagia

78. *How much water do normal dogs consume daily?*

a. 5 to 10 ml/lb
b. 60 to 70 ml/lb
c. 20 to 40 ml/lb
d. more than 80 ml/lb
e. 10 to 70 ml/lb, depending on activity and ambient temperature

79. *Resistance to large doses of exogenous insulin is **least** likely to occur in dogs with:*

a. hyperadrenocorticism
b. diestrus
c. insulinoma
d. obesity
e. septicemia

80. *What are the clinical signs of uveodermatologic (Vogt-Koyanagi-Harada) syndrome?*

a. bilateral anterior uveitis and cutaneous depigmentation
b. retinal detachment and cutaneous depigmentation
c. bilateral anterior uveitis and pustules and papules on the trunk
d. retinal detachment and ulcerations of the foot pads
e. lens luxation and ulcerations of the foot pads

81. *In uveodermatologic (Vogt-Koyanagi-Harada) syndrome, against what substances is the primary inflammatory reaction directed?*

a. basement membrane zone protein
b. cement between epithelial cells
c. fibroblasts and collagen
d. melanin and melanocytes
e. elastin and reticulin fibers

82. *Aside from iatrogenic causes, what is the most common cause of hyperadrenocorticism?*

a. pituitary tumor
b. unilateral adrenal tumor
c. bilateral adrenal tumor
d. hypothalamic disorder
e. adrenocortical hyperplasia

83. *During surgical exploration of the abdomen in a dog with classic clinical signs of Cushing's disease, you note that one adrenal gland is large and the other is atrophied. What is the most likely explanation for these findings?*

 a. Unilateral congenital adrenal hypoplasia has caused one gland to appear larger.
 b. This is a normal phenomenon; one adrenal gland is normally larger than the other.
 c. The larger gland is affected by a tumor; the other gland is atrophied because of decreased ACTH secretion from the pituitary gland.
 d. Decreased vascular circulation has caused atrophy of the smaller gland.
 e. Pituitary-dependent hyperadrenocorticism has caused hypertrophy of one gland.

84. *Panting is a common clinical sign of hyperadrenocorticism. What are the most likely underlying causes of panting in affected dogs?*

 a. pulmonary thromboembolism, weakness of respiratory muscles, and increased pressure on the diaphragm from hepatomegaly
 b. interstitial pulmonary calcification, discomfort from an enlarged bladder (secondary to polyuria), and increased fat deposition over the thorax
 c. pulmonary thromboembolism, discomfort from an enlarged stomach (secondary to polyphagia), and ketoacidosis secondary to concurrent diabetes mellitus
 d. increased fat deposition over the thorax, interstitial calcification, and weakness of respiratory muscles
 e. ketoacidosis secondary to concurrent diabetes mellitus, discomfort from an enlarged bladder (secondary to polyuria), and increased pressure on the diaphragm from hepatomegaly

85. *What are potential complications of hyperadrenocorticism?*

 a. hypothyroidism, congestive heart failure, and pyelonephritis
 b. diabetes mellitus, congestive heart failure, and pulmonary thromboembolism
 c. anemia, diabetes mellitus, and pyelonephritis
 d. pulmonary thromboembolism, pyelonephritis, and hypothyroidism
 e. anemia, thrombocytopenia, and diabetes mellitus

86. *For the past several years you have been treating a diabetic dog with insulin. The dog now develops hyperadrenocorticism and you institute mitotane (Lysodren) therapy. How will this new development likely affect the regimen of insulin treatment?*

 a. Insulin requirement will remain the same.
 b. Insulin requirement will most likely decrease with time.
 c. Insulin requirement will most likely increase with time.
 d. Insulin therapy will be discontinued during mitotane therapy because of possible toxicity from drug interaction.
 e. Insulin will be changed from long-acting insulin to shorter-acting insulin.

87. *Causes of hypercholesterolemia/hyperlipidemia include all the following* ***except:***

 a. hypothyroidism
 b. hyperadrenocorticism
 c. hypoglycemia
 d. nephrotic syndrome
 e. pancreatitis

88. *Causes of polyuria and polydipsia include all the following* ***except:***

 a. diabetes mellitus
 b. chronic renal failure
 c. pyometra
 d. hyperadrenocorticism
 e. hypocalcemia

89. *A dog with hair loss, polydipsia, and polyuria has a high urine cortisol/creatinine ratio. What is the most likely explanation for these findings?*

 a. The dog has hyperadrenocorticism.
 b. The dog has hypoadrenocorticism.
 c. The dog has glomerular disease.
 d. The dog does not have hyperadrenocorticism.
 e. The dog may have hyperadrenocorticism but further testing is needed.

Correct answers are on pages 140-171.

Questions 90 and 91

90. *Urinalysis reveals the following results: specific gravity 1.010, pH 6.5, glucose negative, ketones negative, protein 4+, blood 2+, white blood cells too numerous to count, bacteria 3+, and urine protein/creatinine ratio of 6. What is the most likely cause of these findings?*

   a. acute glomerulonephritis
   b. chronic renal failure
   c. urinary tract infection
   d. diabetes mellitus
   e. diabetes insipidus

91. *What does the urine protein/creatinine ratio of 6 indicate?*

   a. glomerular protein loss
   b. glomerulonephritis
   c. tubular protein loss
   d. pyelonephritis
   e. no specific renal disease

92. *What would be the effect of giving sodium bicarbonate to a dog with hypercalcemia?*

   a. decrease the serum total calcium level
   b. increase the serum total calcium level
   c. decrease the serum ionized calcium level
   d. increase the serum ionized calcium level
   e. no change in the serum total or ionized calcium levels

93. *Administration of 0.9% saline solution to a dog with hypercalcemia would decrease the serum calcium level because of:*

   a. increased resorption of calcium from the distal collecting ducts in the kidney
   b. decreased gastrointestinal absorption of calcium
   c. decreased osteoclastic activity in bone
   d. decreased resorption of calcium from the ascending limb of the loop of Henle in the kidney
   e. decreased parathyroid hormone release in response to fluid-induced diuresis

94. *What is the significance of bilirubinuria in dogs?*

   a. nonspecific finding of no particular clinical significance
   b. indicative of icterus
   c. indicative of glomerular disease
   d. usually indicative of liver disease
   e. usually indicative of renal failure

95. *Increased fasting and postprandial serum bile acid levels are indicative of:*

   a. liver disease
   b. exocrine pancreatic insufficiency
   c. chronic renal disease
   d. hyperadrenocorticism
   e. pancreatitis

96. *Decreased trypsinlike immunoreactivity is indicative of:*

   a. liver disease
   b. exocrine pancreatic insufficiency
   c. chronic renal disease
   d. hyperadrenocorticism
   e. pancreatitis

97. *Which clinical pathologic finding is **least** likely to be observed in a dog that has been treated with prednisone for the past 2 months?*

   a. neutrophilia
   b. lymphocytosis
   c. eosinopenia
   d. monocytosis
   e. increased serum alkaline phosphatase activity

98. *Which clinical pathologic finding is **least** likely to be observed in a dog with babesiosis?*

   a. anemia
   b. reticulocytosis
   c. hemoglobinuria
   d. thrombocytosis
   e. neutrophilia

99. *A dog that you vaccinated for rabies 3 months previously is bitten by an unvaccinated stray dog. The stray dog runs off and cannot be found. What is the most appropriate course of action?*
    a. Immediately euthanize the bitten dog, and have the brain examined for rabies.
    b. Quarantine the bitten dog for 10 days, and observe for signs of rabies.
    c. Quarantine the bitten dog for 30 days, and observe for signs of rabies.
    d. Revaccinate the bitten dog against rabies, and send it home.
    e. Collect blood from the bitten dog to check for rabies antigen.

100. *What is the drug of choice for treatment of* Ehrlichia canis *infection?*
    a. ampicillin
    b. penicillin G
    c. tetracycline
    d. enrofloxacin
    e. gentamicin

DOGS

M.D. Willard

101. *The most common and most severe side effect of amphotericin B therapy is:*
    a. hepatic failure
    b. renal failure
    c. thrombocytopenia
    d. phlebitis caused by extravasation of the drug
    e. cardiac failure

102. *A 57-kg, male, mixed-breed dog has acute, severe hypovolemic shock. There is a large amount of blood in the abdomen, but you are uncertain of its origin. The most appropriate course of action is to:*
    a. infuse 1 unit of packed red blood cells intravenously and given an injection of vitamin K_3
    b. apply a compression bandage to the abdomen
    c. infuse large volumes of physiologic saline solution intravenously
    d. immediately perform an exploratory laparotomy
    e. perform autotransfusion of blood withdrawn from the abdomen until the patient's condition is stabilized

103. *Concerning blastomycosis in dogs, which statement is* ***least*** *accurate?*
    a. Commonly used serologic tests have poor sensitivity and specificity.
    b. Pulmonary miliary interstitial patterns are commonly found on radiographs of animals with disseminated blastomycosis.
    c. Cytologic examination of cutaneous lesions and material aspirated from enlarged lymph nodes is often diagnostic.
    d. Culture of the yeast is rarely needed for diagnosis.
    e. On radiographs, osseous blastomycosis may closely resemble osseous neoplasia.

104. *In a dog with severe hepatic cirrhosis of unknown origin and associated encephalopathy and ascites, treatment should* ***not*** *include:*
    a. dexamethasone
    b. lactulose
    c. oral neomycin
    d. a low-protein diet
    e. a low-salt diet

Correct answers are on pages 140-171.

105. *Concerning barium enemas in dogs with lymphocytic-plasmacytic colitis, which statement is most accurate?*

a. Iodide contrast agents provide better detail and are safer than other contrast agents.
b. You can expect to see an "apple-core" lesion in many affected dogs.
c. You can expect to see thickening of the colonic wall in many affected dogs.
d. This procedure is not sensitive in detecting mucosal disease.
e. This procedure is best done immediately after colonoscopy and biopsy of the colon (assuming there are no gross lesions), while the dog is still anesthetized.

106. *A dog has a large wound on the medial aspect of the right rear leg. The owner noticed the wound 3 days previously, at which time he removed a large wooden splinter from it. Now the wound is discolored blue-black and has obvious crepitus in the surrounding tissues. What is the most appropriate treatment for this animal?*

a. enrofloxacin plus gentamicin
b. amikacin
c. metronidazole plus cefazolin
d. oxytetracycline
e. trimethoprim with sulfadiazine

107. *Which of the following is* **not** *a likely reason why a dog with exocrine pancreatic insufficiency may fail to respond to therapy with oral pancreatic enzyme supplementation?*

a. failure to preincubate the food with the supplemental pancreatic enzymes
b. small intestinal bacterial overgrowth
c. poor-quality supplemental pancreatic enzymes
d. use of an enteric-coated supplemental pancreatic enzyme preparation
e. use of a high-fat diet

108. *What is the most likely cause of chronic hematemesis in a middle-aged dog?*

a. *ollulanus* infection
b. coagulopathy
c. gastric ulceration
d. *helicobacter* infection
e. *Physaloptera* infection

109. *A dog has a large wound on its side. The wound shows dark discoloration, a malodorous exudate, and crepitus. The pathogens most likely to be isolated from this wound are:*

a. *Pseudomonas aeruginosa, Proteus*
b. *Blastomyces dermatitidis, Escherichia coli*
c. *Bacteriodes, Clostridium*
d. *Actinomyces, Nocardia*
e. *E. coli, Mycobacterium toetuitum*

110. *A 9-year-old intact male bull mastiff has had dyschezia and tenesmus for 5 months. The problem has not worsened. The feces are normal in consistency and appearance, but it takes the dog 2 to 5 minutes to defecate. The dog appears normal on physical examination, but you cannot adequately perform an abdominal or rectal examination because of the dog's large size (69 kg). What is the most likely cause of these signs?*

a. anal sac carcinoma
b. perineal hernia
c. perianal fistulae
d. anal sacculitis
e. prostatomegaly

111. *A mature castrated dog has had a fever (39.3° to 40.1° C) of unknown origin for 3 days but otherwise is in good condition. The dog lives in a kennel in the northern midwestern United States. The client requests that you initiate antibiotic therapy for a suspected bacterial infection, rather than perform any diagnostic tests. Which drug is the best choice for this animal?*

a. cefazolin
b. amikacin
c. lincomycin
d. tetracycline
e. trimethoprim

112. *A dog is clinically normal but then suddenly develops acute, fulminating hepatic failure. A finding that would* **not** *be expected in this dog after a 1-day illness is:*

a. vomiting
b. coagulopathy
c. hepatic encephalopathy
d. hypoglycemia
e. polyuria, polydipsia

113. *A 3-year-old hunting dog has a chronic pleural effusion. The fluid grossly resembles blood and contains small clots in the exudate; cytologic examination reveals many degenerate neutrophils. The dog has lost some weight and has a persistent fever (39.0° to 39.4° C). There is no evidence of pulmonary parenchymal involvement. The most likely cause of these signs is:*

a. tuberculosis
b. aspergillosis
c. blastomycosis
d. nocardiosis
e. pythiosis

114. *In a 2-year-old dog with abdominal distention, abdominocentesis yields fluid with the following characteristics: specific gravity 1.009, total protein concentration <1 g/dl, and nucleated cell count 450/μl. The most likely cause of this effusion is:*

a. renal disease
b. right-sided cardiac failure
c. left-sided cardiac failure
d. abdominal neoplasia
e. ruptured urinary tract

115. *A 3-year-old Shih Tzu is continually licking its anal region, and the owner has seen white "grains" on the hair of the perineal region, and on the feces. You find no abnormalities after a thorough physical examination. The most appropriate course of action is to:*

a. perform a fecal flotation
b. administer pyrantel
c. perform a proctoscopic examination
d. perform a direct fecal smear
e. administer praziquantel

116. *A dog has voluminous peritoneal effusion with the following characteristics: specific gravity 1.020, total protein concentration 2.1 g/dl, and nucleated cell count 2780/μl. Which procedure would be most useful in determining the cause of the effusion in this dog?*

a. urine protein/creatinine ratio
b. plain abdominal radiographs
c. endoscopic biopsy of the duodenum
d. culture of the peritoneal fluid
e. postprandial serum bile acid determination

117. *Concerning blastomycosis in dogs, which statement is most accurate?*

a. Ketoconazole should be used if there is substantial hepatic disease.
b. Itraconazole is an effective treatment.
c. Infected dogs pose a substantial human health risk.
d. Clotrimazole is a useful treatment.
e. Amphotericin B is the preferred treatment.

118. *A dog that has been depressed, anorectic, and vomiting bile for 2 days has a modest amount of peritoneal fluid with the following characteristics: specific gravity 1.035, total protein concentration 4.2 g/dl, and nucleated cell count 49,000/μl. Which procedure is* **not** *indicated in this dog at this time?*

a. abdominal ultrasonographic examination
b. plain abdominal radiographs
c. culture of the peritoneal fluid
d. preprandial and postprandial bile acid determinations
e. complete blood count and serum chemistry profile

119. *Which drug is* **least** *likely to cause iatrogenic hepatic disease, as detected by clinical signs or significantly altered liver-derived enzyme activity?*

a. chloramphenicol
b. betamethasone
c. phenobarbital
d. primidone
e. thiacetarsamide

Correct answers are on pages 140-171.

120. *A dog has a voluminous peritoneal effusion with the following characteristics: specific gravity 1.007, total protein concentration <1 g/dl, and nucleated cell count 100/µl. Which procedure is **least** likely to yield useful information?*

a. urine protein:creatinine ratio
b. thoracic radiography
c. endoscopic biopsy of the duodenum
d. preprandial and postprandial serum bile acid determinations
e. abdominal ultrasonography

121. *The drug most likely to cause gastrointestinal ulceration or erosion in a dog is:*

a. erythromycin
b. triamcinolone
c. ibuprofen
d. trimethoprim-sulfadiazine
e. quinacrine

122. *A 9-year-old dog that has been vomiting for 3 days has moderate amounts of straw-colored peritoneal effusion with the following characteristics: specific gravity 1.028, total protein concentration 3.4 g/dl, and nucleated cell count 20,000/µl. Most of the cells in the fluid are nondegenerate neutrophils. The dog exhibits discomfort on abdominal palpation. The most appropriate course of action is to:*

a. make a series of positive-contrast radiographs using barium sulfate to search for intestinal leakage
b. perform simultaneous bilirubin determinations on peritoneal fluid and serum
c. perform simultaneous creatinine determinations on peritoneal fluid and serum
d. make a series of positive-contrast radiographs using an iodide agent to search for intestinal leakage
e. perform an exploratory laparotomy as soon as possible

123. *Concerning liver biopsy in dogs with suspected hepatic disease, which statement is **least** accurate?*

a. Biopsy is often useful to detect metastatic malignancies.
b. Blood coagulation should be assessed before liver biopsy.
c. It may be useful to perform another biopsy during or after treatment to assess therapeutic efficacy.
d. Localized masses in the liver are an indication for biopsy.
e. There is little or no benefit in biopsying a liver that is clearly smaller than normal.

124. *A middle-aged dog that is kept outside on a large farm is found moribund and recumbent. The dog has a distended abdomen, but ballottement does not produce a fluid wave. After several attempts at abdominocentesis, you finally obtain 5 ml of bloody fluid containing three small blood clots. This dog most likely:*

a. has a hepatic rupture with subsequent bleeding
b. has a coagulopathy, possibly caused by rodenticide poisoning
c. has a chronically bleeding abdominal neoplasm
d. has a splenic rupture with subsequent bleeding
e. does not have evidence of hemoabdomen

125. *A 3-year-old dog with a dry, unproductive cough began coughing 3 days after returning home from a boarding kennel. The animal is otherwise normal. The most appropriate initial course of action is to:*

a. administer terbutaline for bronchodilation
b. administer prednisolone to reduce tracheal irritation
c. perform a complete blood count to seek evidence of tracheal infection
d. administer tetracycline to treat for *Bordetella bronchiseptica* infection
e. administer theophylline for bronchodilation

126. *A 4-year-old German shepherd that travels throughout the United States has numerous ticks attached to it. The dog has a fever of 39.5° C and has been depressed for 1 day. Which statement concerning this dog is the most accurate?*

a. A normal platelet count would make borreliosis very unlikely.
b. The dog could have a negative *Rickettsia rickettsii* titer and still have Rocky Mountain spotted fever.
c. A therapeutic trial with ampicillin and gentamicin is reasonable if a diagnostic workup is declined by the owner.
d. Absence of hyperglobulinemia would make ehrlichiosis a much less likely diagnosis.
e. A positive *Borrelia* titer would be excellent evidence of clinical borreliosis.

127. *A 3-year-old dog that is markedly depressed and anorectic has vomited bile hourly for the last 12 hours of the past day. The dog is hypothermic (36° C), has very injected sclerae, and has a peritoneal effusion with the following characteristics: specific gravity 1.032, total protein concentration 5.3 g/dl, and nucleated cell count 150,000/μl. The most likely cause of these signs is:*

a. alimentary tract leakage
b. severe hepatic cirrhosis
c. abdominal carcinomatosis
d. abdominal hemangiosarcoma
e. severe pancreatitis

128. *Concerning aspergillosis in dogs, which statement is most accurate?*

a. Cytologic examination of smears of nasal swabs or washes is a preferred method of diagnosis.
b. Nasal aspergillosis is best distinguished from nasal carcinoma by the fact that aspergillosis typically does not cause destruction of nasal turbinates, evident on radiographs.
c. A chronic nasal discharge, often containing blood, is the most common sign of nasal aspergillosis.
d. Amphotericin B is the treatment of choice for systemic aspergillosis.
e. Resection of lesions, with administration of ketoconazole is the treatment of choice for nasal aspergillosis.

129. *A 2-year-old male German shepherd that has traveled throughout the United States has had diarrhea for 5 months. The diarrhea occurs 1 to 3 times daily and is soft and brown, without mucus, blood, or straining. The dog has lost 6% of its body weight despite a good appetite. The animal is otherwise normal. A complete blood count and serum chemistry profile, including creatinine, blood urea nitrogen, total protein, albumin, glucose, alanine aminotransferase, alkaline phosphatase, calcium, and phosphorus determinations, are normal. The* ***least*** *likely cause of these signs is:*

a. giardiasis
b. lymphocytic-plasmacytic enteritis
c. alimentary lymphosarcoma
d. exocrine pancreatic insufficiency
e. colonic adenocarcicnoma

130. *A 7-year-old German wire-haired pointer has had diarrhea for 8 months. The diarrhea occurs 2 to 4 times daily and is soft and brown, without mucus, blood, or straining. The dog has lost 4% of its body weight despite a reasonable appetite. The animal is otherwise normal. Three fecal flotations have been negative. A complete blood count and serum chemistry profile are normal, except for hypoalbuminemia (1.3 g/dl; normal 2.5 to 4.5 g/dl) and hypoproteinemia (3.0 g/dl; normal 5.0 to 7.5 g/dl). The* ***least*** *likely cause of these signs is:*

a. exocrine pancreatic insufficiency
b. lymphocytic-plasmacytic enteritis
c. intestinal lymphangiectasia
d. alimentary lymphosarcoma
e. eosinophilic enteritis

131. *Concerning babesiosis in dogs in the United States, which statement is most accurate?*

a. A core bone marrow biopsy is the most practical method of diagnosis.
b. It can be differentiated from immune-mediated hemolytic anemia in that babesiosis is characterized by a negative Coombs' test and nonregenerative anemia.
c. Doxycycline is the preferred treatment.
d. Infected dogs are human health hazards.
e. Babesiosis may often be diagnosed by examining a peripheral blood smear.

Correct answers are on pages 140-171.

132. *Beginning 2 days previously, a 3-year-old dog suddenly began to regurgitate solid food but not liquids. There are no prodromal signs, and the dog consistently regurgitates within 5 minutes of eating. The animal seems otherwise normal. The most appropriate initial course of action is to:*

a. treat conservatively with a central-acting antiemetic
b. make plain thoracic radiographs
c. do a complete blood count and serum chemistry profile
d. make plain abdominal radiographs
e. treat with subcutaneous fluids and oral kaolin-pectin (Kaopectate)

133. *A 4-year-old spayed Doberman pinscher has become anorectic and has started drinking and urinating excessively over the past 6 days. Until that time the dog was normal. In addition, it has begun vomiting bile-stained fluid every 2 to 3 days. Laboratory findings include hypoalbuminemia (2.2 g/dl; normal 2.5 to 4.4 g/dl), hyperbilirubinemia (3.2 mg/dl; normal <1 mg/dl), decreased blood urea nitrogen level (2 mg/dl; normal 5 to 20 mg/dl), increased serum alanine aminotransferase activity (8 times normal), and increased serum alkaline phosphatase activity (8 times normal). The liver is smaller than normal on abdominal radiographs. The most likely cause of these abnormalities is:*

a. chronic pancreatitis causing obstruction of the common bile duct
b. steroid hepatopathy causing cirrhosis
c. hepatic lipidosis causing cirrhosis
d. hepatic lymphosarcoma
e. chronic hepatitis causing cirrhosis

134. *In dogs with blastomycosis, which body system is **least** often affected?*

a. lymph nodes
b. eyes
c. lungs
d. central nervous system
e. skin

135. *A mixed-breed dog has had a relatively severe, dry cough for at the past 10 days. The cough began 4 to 5 days after the animal was housed at a kennel. The most likely cause of this dog's disease is:*

a. herpesvirus
b. *Streptococcus pneumoniae*
c. *Klebsiella pneumoniae*
d. *Bartonella henselae*
e. *Bordetella bronchiseptica*

136. *A 6-week-old schnauzer recently began to regurgitate food at almost every meal. There is no bile or blood in the material, and there is no obvious retching associated with the act. The dog seems otherwise normal. Which statement concerning this dog is most accurate?*

a. Barium contrast radiographs of the stomach and intestines are indicated.
b. The dog is at increased risk of death from fluid and electrolyte abnormalities.
c. The dog is at increased risk of death from respiration pneumonia.
d. This problem is likely to spontaneously resolve within the next month.
e. Endoscopic examination should be performed as the next step.

137. *The most reasonable treatment for a dog that appears to be rapidly exsanguinating into the peritoneal cavity because of gastrointestinal ulceration is to:*

a. apply a tight bandage around the abdomen
b. administer vitamin K_1
c. resect the ulcer
d. administer large doses of cimetidine and sucralfate
e. autotransfuse blood

138. Concerning borreliosis in dogs, which statement is most accurate?

a. Renal failure is a common complication of chronic disease.
b. An indirect fluorescent antibody (IFA) titer >1:1000 has a high positive predictive value.
c. Thrombocytopenia is a common finding.
d. Recurrent, intermittent nonerosive arthritis is the major clinical sign of chronic disease.
e. Skin lesions at the site of the tick bite are often reported.

*139. The disease in which metronidazole treatment is **not** indicated is:*

a. giardiasis
b. salmon poisoning
c. inflammatory bowel disease
d. *Bacteroides* infection
e. small intestinal bacterial overgrowth

140. Concerning botulism in dogs, which statement is most accurate?

a. Antitoxin is most effective if administered within 3 days of the onset of clinical signs.
b. Diagnosis is best made by culturing the causative bacterium from the feces.
c. Progressive, ascending flaccid paralysis is the most common sign.
d. Affected dogs usually have markedly increased serum alanine aminotransferase and creatine phosphokinase activities.
e. Affected dogs usually have diminished pain perception, in addition to quadriplegia.

141. A 12-year-old German shepherd has been severely constipated for 1 week. The dog strains for several minutes without passing any stool. It has been fed only commercial dog food and has been kept indoors, except for a 35-minute leash walk daily. On abdominal palpation the colon is distended to 2 times its normal size throughout its length. The most appropriate initial course of action is to:

a. perform a digital rectal examination
b. obtain a complete blood count and serum chemistry profile
c. make plain abdominal radiographs
d. administer a warm-water enema and then urecholine parenterally
e. administer mineral oil per os and feed the dog a fiber-enriched diet

*142. In a 5-month-old dog with a moderately severe congenital portosystemic shunt, which laboratory finding would **not** be expected?*

a. markedly increased postprandial serum bile acid concentration
b. markedly increased serum alanine aminotransferase activity
c. moderate hypoalbuminemia
d. decreased blood urea nitrogen level
e. moderate hypocholesterolemia

143. Concerning brucellosis in dogs, which statement is most accurate?

a. Most infections with *Brucella canis* are inapparent.
b. The rapid slide agglutination test is sensitive and specific in dogs.
c. Aggressive therapy with tetracycline is relatively reliable for eliminating the infection.
d. *Brucella canis* infections in people are typically severe.
e. Infected male dogs typically only shed the organism for 2 to 3 weeks or less.

144. Four young dogs that are unrelated and owned by different clients have developed severe bloody diarrhea within the past 4 days in your clinic. The dogs are also anorectic and depressed. One of your kennel assistants develops acute gastroenteritis. The most likely cause of diarrhetic disease in these dogs, especially if the kennel person contracted the infection from the dogs, is:

a. *Escherichia coli* infection
b. *Salmonella* infection
c. *Campylobacter jejuni* infection
d. *Giardia* infection
e *Yersinia* infection

Correct answers are on pages 140-171.

145. *An 8-year-old male German shepherd that is constantly kept indoors has had a distended abdomen for at least 5 to 8 days. The oral mucosae are very pale, and there is a palpable fluid wave in the abdomen. Abdominocentesis yields frank blood. The dog is not in obvious distress but is weak. The clients say the dog has been like this for the past 9 days. The most appropriate initial course of action is to:*

a. autotransfuse blood withdrawn from the abdominal cavity
b. perform abdominal ultrasonography
c. perform an exploratory laparotomy
d. apply a compression bandage to the abdomen
e. transfuse 1 unit of fresh whole blood and observe the patient

146. *Concerning trypanosomiasis in dogs in the United States, which statement is most accurate?*

a. Clindamycin is the preferred treatment.
b. Stupor and somnolence are the most characteristic signs.
c. The most common means of diagnosing this disease is by finding the organism in a capillary blood smear.
d. Myocarditis and right-sided heart failure are the most common signs.
e. This disease is principally limited to the Pacific Northwest portion of the United States.

147. *The most appropriate treatment for a 5-month-old dog with mild, acute diarrhea of 2 days' duration and of unknown origin is:*

a. oral rehydration solution
b. a bland, easily digested diet
c. oral cefazolin
d. loperamide
e. methscopolamine

148. *Concerning coccidioidomycosis in dogs, which statement is most accurate?*

a. Osseous disease tends to occur within 1 to 3 weeks of exposure.
b. Disseminated coccidioidomycosis is usually preceded by an obvious respiratory phase.
c. Osseous coccidioidomycosis can be distinguished from neoplasia because it tends to exclusively cause osteolysis.
d. Acute, primary coccidioidomycosis is often self-limiting.
e. Infection is primarily via inoculation of cutaneous or oral lesions.

149. *A dog with hepatic cirrhosis of unknown origin has been successfully treated conservatively for 8 months. Over the past 24 hours, however, the dog has again begun having severe signs of encephalopathy. Which of the following is* ***not*** *a likely cause of this sudden relapse of clinical signs?*

a. bacterial infection
b. gastroduodenal ulceration
c. ingestion of a high-protein meal
d. administration of an inappropriate drug
e. accumulation of ascitic fluid

150. *Which type of enema should* ***not*** *be administered to a constipated Maltese dog?*

a. warm soapy water
b. warm water
c. hypertonic phosphate
d. mineral oil
e. warm water with dioctyl sodium sulfosuccinate

151. *A 3-year-old mixed-breed male hunting dog has been coughing for 3 months, has lost about 10% of its body weight, and has an intermittent fever (39.3° to 39.8° C). There is mild, generalized lymphadenopathy, and respiratory sounds are dry and harsh. The disease is slowly getting worse. The most likely cause of these signs is:*

a. bartonellosis
b. cryptococcosis
c. bordetellosis
d. blastomycosis
e. distemper

152. *A 3-year-old Bedlington terrier with congenital hepatic disease unrelated to a vascular anomaly would benefit most from treatment with:*
   a. lactulose
   b. prednisolone
   c. surgery
   d. trientine
   e. a low-protein diet

153. *Which symptomatic treatment is most likely to be effective for acute, severe hepatic encephalopathy causing coma in a dog?*
   a. nothing per os, systemic antibiotics, and intravenous fluid therapy with lactated Ringer's solution supplemented with potassium and dextrose
   b. nothing per os, warm-water enemas, and intravenous fluid therapy with half-strength saline solution supplemented with potassium and dextrose
   c. nothing per os, intravenous phenobarbital, and intravenous fluid therapy with 5% dextrose in water supplemented with potassium
   d. lipotropic agents (e.g., methionine), intramuscular amoxicillin, and intravenous fluid therapy with 5% dextrose in water supplemented with potassium
   e. diazepam, lactulose, and intravenous fluid therapy with lactated Ringer's solution supplemented with potassium and dextrose

154. *An 8-year-old male dog has had bright red blood on the surface of its stools for the past 3 weeks. The stool is otherwise normal. Blood is occasionally found on the floor where the dog has been lying. Grossly, the perineal region appears normal and there is no obvious evidence of a rectal mass or ulcer on digital rectal examination. Which statement concerning this dog is most accurate?*
   a. The dog should be fed a high-fiber diet.
   b. Coagulopathy is a likely cause of the hematochezia.
   c. Anal sac disease is a likely cause of the hematochezia.
   d. The dog should be treated with oral tylosin.
   e. The pelvic and anal areas should be radiographed.

155. *A 4-year-old, 17-kg male miniature schnauzer is presented for a routine checkup. You determine that the dog has marked lipemia, even after fasting for 29 hours. Which statement concerning this dog is most accurate?*
   a. This dog probably will soon develop diabetes mellitus.
   b. This dog probably has hypothyroidism.
   c. This dog probably has nephrotic syndrome.
   d. This dog probably has hyperadrenocorticism.
   e. This dog is at risk for developing acute pancreatitis.

156. *Concerning perineal hernia in dogs, which statement is* ***least*** *accurate?*
   a. Rectal examination is usually diagnostic.
   b. The most common presenting signs include difficulty in defecation and/or perianal swelling.
   c. It is primarily found in older, intact male dogs.
   d. German shepherds, boxers, and Labrador retrievers are commonly affected breeds.
   e. Dyschezia or fecal incontinence is an occasional presenting sign.

157. *Concerning salmonellosis in dogs, which statement is most accurate?*
   a. Gentamicin with amoxicillin is a preferred therapy for acute gastroenteritis caused by salmonellosis.
   b. Cytologic examination of feces is often diagnostic in animals with diarrhea.
   c. Acute salmonellosis typically causes high mortality.
   d. Most animals carrying *Salmonella* are asymptomatic.
   e. Infected dogs usually have a short period of fecal shedding of *Salmonella* organisms.

Correct answers are on pages 140-171.

158. *Concerning oral administration of a hypertonic water-soluble iodinated contrast solution for contrast radiography of canine intestines, which statement is **least** accurate?*

a. It can cause vomiting in some animals.
b. The medium is usually progressively diluted, resulting in poor contrast.
c. The medium can occasionally be seen entering the kidneys.
d. It is the preferred contrast agent for severely dehydrated animals.
e. The medium tends to move through the intestinal tract faster than barium sulfate.

159. *A 4-month-old puppy was obtained 10 days previously and has had diarrhea for the past 8 days. The stool is soft but does not contain mucus or blood. The problem has not worsened. The dog is otherwise normal and is fed a commercial brand of puppy chow. Which statement concerning this dog is most accurate?*

a. Dietary intolerance is a likely cause of the diarrhea.
b. A parasympatholytic drug is the preferred therapy.
c. Increased dietary fiber is the preferred therapy.
d. A barium contrast radiographic study of the intestines is indicated.
e. A first-generation cephalosporin should be given.

160. *A 2-year-old great Dane that has traveled throughout the United States is anorectic and acutely lame in its right rear leg. The dog has a slight fever (39.4° C) and a slightly swollen but painful stifle. The animal is otherwise normal. Which of the following would be most likely to cause the dog's disease?*

a. *Norcardia asteroides*
b. *Helicobacter pylori*
c. *Yersinia pestis*
d. *Borrelia burgdorferi*
e. *Neorickettsia helmithoeca*

161. *Concerning benign adenomatous polyps in dogs, which statement is most accurate?*

a. One may easily distinguish benign polyps from malignant growths by their gross appearance.
b. They principally cause hematochezia coupled with constipation.
c. They are often ameliorated by a hypoallergenic diet.
d. They principally occur in the rectum.
e. Most rectal polyps arise from chronically inflamed anal sacs.

162. *Concerning lymphocytic-plasmacytic colitis in dogs, which statement is most accurate?*

a. Untreated affected dogs often develop alimentary lymphosarcoma.
b. Prednisone in large doses is the preferred therapy.
c. The milder forms often respond to appropriate dietary therapy.
d. Most affected dogs have hematochezia despite otherwise normal stools.
e. Azathioprine is typically needed to control signs in mildly to moderately affected animals.

163. *In a 7-month-old dog with acute onset of fever, anorexia, and coughing, what is the best way to help confirm your presumptive diagnosis of acute distemper?*

a. finding enamel hypoplasia on oral examination
b. finding chorioretinitis on ophthalmoscopic examination
c. finding lymphopenia on the complete blood count
d. finding inclusion bodies in white blood cells
e. watching for development of "chewing gum" seizures

164. *A 3-year-old German shepherd has had diarrhea for 19 months. The diarrhea occurs 2 to 4 times daily and is soft and brown. No mucus, blood, or straining has been noted. The animal has lost 9% of its body weight despite a good appetite. The dog is otherwise normal. Three fecal flotations have been negative. A complete blood count and serum chemistry profile, including creatinine, urea nitrogen, total protein, albumin, glucose, alanine aminotransferase, and alkaline phosphatase, are normal. The most likely cause of these signs is:*

a. small intestinal bacterial overgrowth
b. granulomatous enteritis
c. enteric salmonellosis
d. intestinal lymphangiectasia
e. alimentary lymphosarcoma

165. *Concerning coccidioidomycosis in dogs, which statement is most accurate?*

a. Ketoconazole is the recommended therapy for dogs with central nervous system involvement.
b. Cytologic examination of lesions is often diagnostic because there are usually numerous organisms present.
c. Culture of exudates is recommended if cytologic and serologic examinations are not diagnostic.
d. Osseous coccidioidomycosis is usually cured with amphotericin B therapy.
e. Hilar lymphadenopathy is a common radiographic finding in pulmonary coccidioidomycosis.

166. *Concerning dogs that regurgitate or vomit, which statement is most accurate?*

a. Most dogs with esophageal disease regurgitate food in a tubular form.
b. Vigorous retching suggests vomiting and is uncommon in dogs with esophageal disease.
c. Most dogs that regurgitate have grossly evident dilations in their neck, caused by an enlarged cervical esophagus.
d. Most dogs that regurgitate expel food mixed with green or yellow foam.
e. Regurgitation caused by esophageal disease invariably occurs within 1 to 15 minutes of eating.

167. *Concerning protein-losing enteropathy in dogs, which statement is* ***least*** *accurate?*

a. Histoplasmosis can cause this syndrome.
b. Gastrointestinal ulceration can cause this syndrome.
c. The prognosis is very poor.
d. Affected dogs often have panhypoproteinemia.
e. A low-fat diet plus medium-chain triglycerides are often useful in treating one of the causes of this syndrome.

168. *Which of the following is* ***least*** *appropriate, either alone or combined with other therapy, for a dog with vomiting caused by gastrointestinal disease of unknown origin?*

a. intravenous physiologic saline
b. intravenous fluids with sodium bicarbonate added
c. abdominal radiography
d. intravenous fluids with dextrose added
e. intravenous Ringer's solution

169. *In a 7-year-old mixed-breed dog with intestinal lymphangiectasia of unknown origin, the most appropriate initial therapy is:*

a. a trial elimination (hypoallergenic diet)
b. prednisolone plus azathioprine
c. an ultralow-fat diet plus medium-chain triglycerides
d. oral tetracycline
e. a high-fiber diet plus sulfasalazine (Azulfidine)

170. *A 7-year-old German shepherd is obstipated. The dog has been obviously uncomfortable when defecating during the past 7 weeks. Now it cannot defecate at all. The colon is full of hard feces. The rectal area seems somewhat swollen, but you cannot examine the area well because the dog is extremely painful there. The dog refuses to allow you to perform a rectal examination. The most likely cause of these signs is:*

a. a chronic, healed pelvic fracture
b. perianal fistulae
c. ingestion of difficult-to-digest trash (popcorn, hair, plastic wrapping)
d. rectal polyps
e. a low-fiber diet

Correct answers are on pages 140-171.

171. *Which of the following best describes the radiographic appearance of diffuse infiltrative disease as seen on barium contrast radiographs of the intestines?*

a. flat mucosa, with small linear fissures
b. "feathering" of the mucosa
c. drastically decreased passage of barium through the intestines
d. "thumb printing" or scalloped margins
e. inconsistent width of the bowel lumen

172. *Concerning* Ehrlichia canis *infection in dogs, which statement is most accurate?*

a. Doxycycline is very effective in treating ehrlichiosis, but this drug is more nephrotoxic than tetracycline.
b. Epistaxis is expected in affected dogs.
c. A 7-day course of therapy with tetracycline is effective in acute ehrlichiosis.
d. Clinical signs of acute ehrlichiosis often include fever and anorexia.
e. Chronically infected dogs serve as an important reservoir of the disease for other dogs.

173. *Concerning esophageal foreign bodies in dogs, which statement is* ***least*** *accurate?*

a. Many foreign bodies can be removed endoscopically.
b. The cricopharyngeal sphincter is the most common site at which foreign bodies lodge.
c. Animals with a partial obstruction often regurgitate solids but not liquids.
d. Some animals with esophageal obstruction become anorectic and drool excessively.
e. Esophageal perforation is often accompanied by fever, depression, and anorexia.

174. *A 9-year-old dog has been straining on defecation for the past 3 weeks. The dog had bright red blood on the surface of the feces for 2 to 4 weeks before that time. At physical examination the anus seems constricted by a circumferential band of tissue. Which statement concerning this dog is most accurate?*

a. You should treat the dog with tylosin or amoxicillin.
b. You should perform surgery and try to resect this band of tissue.
c. You should perform proctoscopy and obtain a deep biopsy of this band of tissue.
d. The dog probably has benign adenomatous rectal polyps.
e. The dog probably has severe anal sac disease.

175. *Concerning acquired esophageal weakness in older dogs, which statement is most accurate?*

a. Myopathies, neuropathies, and junctionopathies are important causes.
b. The condition resolves in most affected dogs with conservative dietary management for 3 to 8 weeks.
c. Esophageal perforation is a major cause of death in affected dogs.
d. Cimetidine is often useful in alleviating clinical signs.
e. Affected dogs should receive prophylactic antibiotics as long as they have the condition.

176. *A 3-year-old miniature schnauzer began having bloody vomiting and bloody diarrhea 3 hours previously. The dog is now somewhat depressed and has a packed cell volume of 74% (normal 35 to 55%). The most likely cause of these signs is:*

a. gastrointestinal ulceration
b. hemorrhagic gastroenteritis
c. parvoviral enteritis
d. coagulopathy
e. heavy-metal intoxication

177. *Concerning distemper in dogs, which statement is most accurate?*

a. Distemper is one of the most common causes of convulsions in dogs less than 6 months of age.
b. The distemper virus's marked resistance to the environment is the reason this disease is so easily spread from animal to animal.
c. Definitive antemortem diagnosis of acute distemper is best accomplished with serologic testing.
d. Distemper may be differentiated from ehrlichiosis because the latter causes thrombocytopenia.
e. The fluorescent antibody test on conjunctival scrapings is most useful in dogs with chronic distemper encephalitis.

178. *A 9-month-old dog has* Toxocara *and* Ancylostoma *ova plus* Isospora *oocysts in the feces. The dog appears normal and has normal stools. The best treatment for this dog is:*

a. sulfadimethoxine
b. metronidazole
c. fenbendazole
d. piperazine
e. quinacrine

179. *What observation on a lateral radiograph can best indicate an increase or decrease in liver size?*

a. gastric silhouette
b. cranial extent of the duodenal silhouette
c. cranial extent of the left kidney silhouette
d. size of the fat pad under the liver
e. cranial extent of the jejunal silhouette

180. *Concerning diagnosis of gastric dilatation/ volvulus, which statement is most accurate?*

a. Successful passage of a stomach tube rules out volvulus as a diagnostic consideration.
b. Right lateral recumbency is the position of choice for radiographic diagnosis.
c. Contrast radiographs should be obtained to distinguish dilatation with torsion from dilatation without torsion.
d. Chronic, intermittent bloating rules out gastric torsion as a diagnostic consideration.
e. Torsion is usually diagnosed by observing the pylorus on the right side of the abdomen on the ventrodorsal radiographic projection.

181. *Concerning* Ehrlichia canis *infection in dogs, which statement is most accurate?*

a. *Ehrlichia* morulae are commonly found in peripheral white blood cells during the first 3 weeks of infection.
b. Antibody titers ≥1:128 are needed for a definitive diagnosis.
c. Thrombocytopenia is a common hematologic finding in acute and chronic ehrlichiosis.
d. Successful therapy is documented by an undetectable *Ehrlichia* titer 3 to 5 months after therapy.
e. Pancytopenia associated with ehrlichiosis is caused by replacement of the bone marrow with plasma cells.

182. *Concerning perianal fistulae in dogs, which statement is **least** accurate?*

a. Fecal incontinence is a concern after aggressive, wide resection of lesions.
b. Topical therapy with antibiotics and corticosteroids may be curative.
c. Recurrence after surgery is rare.
d. High tail amputation has been helpful in halting disease progression and eliminating the fistulae in some dogs.
e. Mild cases can be confused with anal sac abscesses.

183. *At weaning, a 5-month-old dog begins to regurgitate at every meal. There are no prodromal signs; the dog simply puts its head down and gags up food and mucus. The dog is otherwise normal. The most likely cause of these signs is:*

a. a vascular ring anomaly
b. pyloric stenosis
c. a portosystemic shunt
d. a gastric foreign body
e. food intolerance

184. *Which of the following drugs is most likely to control severe vomiting of unknown origin?*

a. metoclopramide
b. bismuth subsalicylate
c. misoprostol
d. diphenhydramine
e. methoscopolamine

Correct answers are on pages 140-171.

185. *A 7-year-old dog has had diarrhea consistently for the past 4 months. The diarrhea occurs 2 to 4 times per day, does not contain mucus or blood, and is not associated with straining. The dog has lost 4% of its body weight. Which statement concerning this dog is most accurate?*

a. The dog has signs of chronic large intestinal diarrhea.
b. The dog has signs of chronic small intestinal diarrhea.
c. The dog has signs of chronic large and small intestinal diarrhea.
d. One cannot reasonably predict whether the large or small intestine is involved.
e. The dog probably has a protein-losing enteropathy.

186. *Concerning initial (immediately after admission) management of a dog with gastric dilation/volvulus, which statement is most accurate?*

a. Shock should be treated with 7% saline solution at 30 to 40 ml/lb intravenously.
b. Large doses of flunixin meglumine and dexamethasone should be administered initially as part of treatment for shock.
c. Intravenous lidocaine or intramuscular quinidine should be used in initial management to prevent cardiac arrhythmias.
d. Potassium chloride (40 mEq/L) should be added to the fluids initially infused to treat shock.
e. Aggressive intravenous fluid therapy with isotonic crystalloids (administered through multiple catheters if needed) is indicated in initial management.

187. *A 5-year-old dog has been apparently normal at home and is normal on physical examination, but its serum alkaline phosphatase activity is 8 times normal. There are no significant abnormalities on a complete blood count. Serum glucose, alanine aminotransferase, total protein, albumin, bilirubin, calcium, sodium, and potassium values are within normal limits. These findings are most likely caused by the animal's exposure, in the past 2 to 3 weeks, to:*

a. a third-generation cephalosporin
b. furosemide
c. triamcinolone
d. fenbendazole
e. ivermectin

188. *A mature mixed-breed dog has become increasing depressed during the past 12 hours and is now moribund and vomiting repeatedly. The abdomen seems painful on palpation. A plain abdominal radiograph reveals poor serosal contrast and free gas in the peritoneal cavity. What is the most appropriate course of action?*

a. Perform an exploratory laparotomy as soon as symptomatic therapy improves the dog's condition for anesthesia.
b. Perform a positive-contrast radiographic study of the intestines, using iodide contrast medium.
c. Collect samples for a complete blood count, urinalysis, and serum chemistry profile, and administer intravenous fluids while awaiting these test results.
d. Perform abdominocentesis, and culture and fluid collected; treat with broad-spectrum antibiotics until culture results are known.
e. Administer flunixin meglumine, antibiotics, and intravenous fluids, and lavage the abdominal cavity with warm crystalloid solution via a multifenestrated catheter.

189. *Concerning infectious canine hepatitis, which statement is most accurate?*

a. Corneal edema is most commonly seen in the most severely affected dogs.
b. Icterus is common in dogs with acute disease.
c. Dogs can become ill and die within hours of the onset of signs.
d. Lack of thrombocytopenia helps differentiate this disease from ehrlichiosis.
e. The causative virus is very labile; most disinfectants readily destroy it.

190. *Which of the following is **least** likely to occur in a dog with severe septic peritonitis associated with spontaneous small intestinal rupture?*

a. metabolic acidosis
b. shock
c. regurgitation
d. disseminated intravascular coagulation
e. azotemia

191. *Concerning perineal hernia in dogs, which statement is most accurate?*
   a. Recurrence is uncommon in animals that have been treated surgically.
   b. Fecal softeners and occasional enemas are useless in controlling signs.
   c. Retroflexion of the urinary bladder into the hernia can cause acute postrenal uremia.
   d. Dogs with testicular tumors (interstitial-cell tumors, seminomas) have a much lower likelihood of developing perineal hernia.
   e. Ultrasonography or positive-contrast radiographs are often needed for definitive diagnosis.

192. *Concerning hepatozoonosis in dogs, which statement is most accurate?*
   a. Acute right-sided heart failure is the main cause of death in affected animals.
   b. Most affected dogs have mild to moderate thrombocytopenia.
   c. Radiography of the lumbar vertebrae and pelvis is the best method of diagnosing this disease.
   d. Intermittent fever and emaciation are the most common presenting complaints.
   e. Marked eosinophilia is the most common and most suggestive hematologic abnormality in affected dogs.

193. *Which of the following would you expect to find in a dog with an acquired hepatic portosystemic shunt caused by severe cirrhosis but only rarely find in a dog with congenital portosystemic shunt?*
   a. vomiting
   b. hypoalbuminemia
   c. ascites
   d. microhepatia
   e. decreased blood urea nitrogen level

194. *A 10-year-old dog has been vomiting yellow phlegm and material resembling coffee grounds 2 to 4 times per week for the past 3 weeks. On physical examination the dog appears normal. Which statement concerning this dog is most accurate?*
   a. The dog should be treated with intravenous fluids.
   b. The dog may have gastric mucosal hyperplasia.
   c. The dog should be treated with metoclopramide.
   d. The dog may have a gastric malignancy.
   e. The dog should be treated with a β-lactam antibiotic.

195. *Concerning herpesvirus infection in dogs, which statement is most accurate?*
   a. Hepatomegaly is the primary gross necropsy finding in fatally affected animals.
   b. Viral inclusions may often be found in circulating white blood cells.
   c. Most puppies are infected via the dam's milk.
   d. Chloramphenicol is the preferred therapy for affected puppies.
   e. Affected puppies often die between 1 and 3 weeks of age.

196. *The drug that most effectively prevents motion sickness in dogs is:*
   a. kaolin-pectin (Kaopectate)
   b. atropine
   c. acepromazine
   d. cimetidine
   e. misoprostol

197. *Concerning histoplasmosis in dogs, which statement is most accurate?*
   a. Subclinical infections are rare in dogs.
   b. Skin testing is inaccurate, but serologic examination is useful in diagnosing disseminated histoplasmosis.
   c. Dogs with disseminated histoplasmosis often have concurrent ocular and osseous lesions.
   d. Large bowel diarrhea is common in dogs with disseminated histoplasmosis.
   e. Cytologically, it is difficult to distinguish *Histoplasma capsulatum* from *Cryptococcus neoformans*.

Correct answers are on pages 140-171.

198. *An 8-year-old West Highland white terrier has been vomiting for 4 months. On exploratory laparotomy the distal gastric antrum is filled with enlarged folds of gastric mucosa that are not ulcerated. The wall of the antrum and the pylorus are not involved. There are no other abnormalities. The most likely cause of these signs is:*

a. partial gastric torsion
b. gastric adenocarcinoma
c. gastric lymphosarcoma
d. hypertrophic mucosal hypertrophy
e. *Physaloptera* infection

199. *On a plain abdominal radiograph of a constipated dog, you note that the colon is filled with feces and appears to be displaced dorsally at the pelvic inlet. The most likely cause of these findings is:*

a. colonic foreign body
b. enlarged sublumbar lymph nodes
c. rectal tumor
d. megacolon
e. prostatomegaly

200. *You are presented with a dog that has been depressed and febrile (39.4° to 40° C) for the past 3 days. The dog also has marked lymphadenopathy (all lymph nodes are 4 to 5 times normal size) and severe bilateral uveitis. The most likely cause of these signs is:*

a. coccidioidomycosis
b. blastomycosis
c. cryptococcosis
d. sporotrichosis
e. histoplasmosis

201. *The drug that is* ***least*** *useful to treat gastrointestinal ulceration in dogs is:*

a. chlorpromazine
b. cimetidine
c. sucralfate
d. omeprazole
e. ranitidine

202. *It is the middle of summer, and you are presented with a 3-year-old mixed-breed hunting dog that travels throughout the southern United States. The dog has been sick for 2 days. It is febrile (39.2° to 39.4° C), depressed, and anorectic and has a dry cough, moderate generalized lymphadenopathy, and some pitting edema of the extremities. The most likely cause of these signs is:*

a. coccidioidomycosis
b. blastomycosis
c. histoplasmosis
d. borreliosis
e. Rocky Mountain spotted fever

203. *Which signs are most common in dogs with acute ileocolic intussusception?*

a. profuse watery diarrhea, abdominal distension
b. hematochezia, vomiting
c. vomiting, bowel mucosa protruding from the anus
d. abdominal pain, abdominal distention
e. hypoproteinemia, diarrhea

204. *Which findings are most suggestive of a congenital portosystemic shunt in a 15-month-old dog?*

a. microhepatia, hypoalbuminemia, and increased postprandial serum bile acid levels
b. hepatomegaly, hypoalbuminemia, and hypocholesterolemia
c. increased serum alkaline phosphatase and γ-glutamyltransferase activity and increased preprandial serum bile acid levels
d. hyperbilirubinemia, decreased blood urea nitrogen level, and increased postprandial serum bile acid levels
e. hypoproteinemia, decreased serum alanine aminotransferase activity, and decreased serum bilirubin level

205. *The most common side effect of ketoconazole use in dogs is:*

a. renal disease
b. hepatic disease
c. fever
d. gastric ulceration
e. cardiac disease

206. *Concerning gastrointestinal ulceration in dogs, which statement is most accurate?*
   a. A positive-contrast barium radiographic study is insensitive for diagnosis.
   b. Ultrasonographic examination is a sensitive diagnostic method.
   c. Most affected dogs die from this disease.
   d. Almost all affected dogs have very low serum, total iron concentrations.
   e. Almost all affected dogs have markedly increased white blood cell counts.

207. *On a plain lateral radiograph of a dog with abdominal distention, you see excellent serosal detail, and the intestines are pushed into the dorsal aspect of the abdominal cavity. Radiographic findings are otherwise normal. Which statement concerning this dog is most accurate?*
   a. The dog probably has hepatic failure.
   b. A peritoneal effusion is probably displacing the intestines dorsally.
   c. Mesenteric lymphadenopathy is probably displacing the intestines dorsally.
   d. There is probably a lot of fat in the abdomen.
   e. The dog probably has an intestinal foreign body.

208. *Concerning leptospirosis in dogs, which statement is most accurate?*
   a. Most cases are acute or peracute.
   b. Peracute leptospirosis is usually manifested as renal failure and icterus.
   c. The most reliable way to diagnose acute leptospirosis is by culturing urine on blood agar plates.
   d. Renal biopsy is the most sensitive and specific means of diagnosing acute leptospirosis.
   e. Treatment with penicillin followed by doxycycline offers a good chance of a cure.

209. *Concerning a dog with its first episode of moderate anal sacculitis (no abscessation), which statement is most accurate?*
   a. The gland should be expressed and an antibiotic-corticosteroid solution instilled.
   b. Systemic antibiotic therapy is typically needed.
   c. Anal sac ablation is the most practical and desirable way to treat this problem.
   d. Systemic corticosteroids are typically needed.
   e. Dietary therapy is of no benefit.

210. *Concerning use of sulfasalazine (Azulfidine) in dogs, which statement is most accurate?*
   a. It is probably effective because of its sulfa moiety.
   b. It may cause keratoconjunctivitis sicca as a side effect.
   c. It is most useful for chronic small bowel diarrhea.
   d. It should be used concurrently with corticosteroids.
   e. It should never be used in cats.

211. *Concerning treatment and/or prevention of gastrointestinal ulceration in dogs, which statement is most accurate?*
   a. Feeding bland foods significantly aids healing.
   b. Injectable histamine-2 antagonists are effective in preventing ulceration.
   c. Oral kaolin-pectin (Kaopectate) is an effective treatment for most ulcers.
   d. Oral sucralfate is an effective treatment for most ulcers.
   e. Metoclopramide aids healing of ulcers by increasing gastric blood flow.

Correct answers are on pages 140-171.

212. *A 2-month-old dog has had episodes of behavioral change for the past 6 months. These episodes occur at any time and tend to develop gradually. Typically, the dog becomes anorectic and unaware of its surroundings, walking into walls, and furniture. The episodes usually last 12 to 96 hours and then slowly resolve spontaneously. On physical examination the dog is normal except that it is noticeably small as compared with its litter mates. A complete blood count, urinalysis, and serum chemistry profile are normal, except that the blood urea nitrogen level is 3 mg/dl (normal 6 to 20 mg/dl). The most appropriate course of action is to:*

a. obtain preprandial and postprandial serum bile acid determinations.
b. perform and electroencephalographic examination and cerebrospinal fluid analysis
c. determine the serum glucose/insulin ratio during periods of hypoglycemia
d. perform an intravenous glucose tolerance test and serum insulin determination
e. perform an 8-hour fasting serum glucose determination

213. *The treatment that is **least** likely to benefit a dog with gastric ulceration of unknown origin is:*

a. omeprazole and chlorpromazine
b. sucralfate and metoclopramide
c. nothing per os, intravenous fluids, and famotidine
d. aminopentamide and flunixin meglumine
e. cimetidine and chlorpromazine

214. *A young male mixed-breed dog has had a fever (39.5° C) and has been vomiting bile for 3 days. Today the dog is slightly icteric. The most likely cause of these signs is:*

a. chronic active hepatitis
b. distemper
c. blastomycosis
d. leptospirosis
e. bacterial endocarditis

215. *A 5-year-old obese miniature schnauzer has been anorectic and vomiting food and/or phlegm for 1 day. These signs began after the dog got loose and roamed the neighborhood for 2 days. Today the dog seems to have cranial abdominal pain when palpated. The sclerae are bright yellow, but the mucous membranes are obviously pink. The most likely cause of these signs is:*

a. hepatic cirrhosis
b. chronic hepatitis
c. extrahepatic bile duct obstruction
d. steroid hepatopathy
e. hemolytic anemia

216. *A 5-year-old female Shih Tzu has a painful, inflamed, swollen area to the left of the anus, with a small amount of exudate over the area. The dog has a rectal temperature of 39.7° C. The most appropriate course of action is to:*

a. make plain radiographs of the perineal area
b. perform a proctoscopic examination to look for neoplasia and/or fistulous tracts
c. immediately resect the affected anal sac
d. widely resect the perianal fistulae causing these signs
e. give systemic antibiotics, apply warm compresses to the area, and eventually lance and flush the anal sac abscess

217. *Concerning* Neospora caninum *infection in dogs, which statement is most accurate?*

a. Most clinically evident infections are self-limiting and do not require therapy.
b. Chronic fever of unknown origin is the most common presenting complaint.
c. The diagnosis is best made by multiple fecal examinations.
d. Doxycycline is the preferred therapy.
e. Clinical findings may mimic those seen with toxoplasmosis.

218. *Concerning vascular ring anomalies in dogs, which statement is most accurate?*
   a. German shepherds seem to be predisposed to these anomalies.
   b. Congenital esophageal weakness is usually also identified.
   c. Aspiration pneumonia is rare in affected animals.
   d. Most affected dogs recover completely after appropriate surgery.
   e. Most affected dogs have significant concurrent congenital cardiac anomalies.

219. *Which of the following is **not** a recognized potential side effect of trimethoprim-sulfa administration in dogs?*
   a. prostatic disease
   b. thrombocytopenia
   c. keratoconjunctivitis sicca
   d. hepatic disease
   e. nonseptic arthritis

220. *Which set of laboratory findings is most suggestive of complete gastric outlet obstruction?*
   a. hypochloremia, hypokalemia, metabolic alkalosis
   b. hyponatremia, hypochloremia, metabolic acidosis
   c. hyponatremia, hyperkalemia, metabolic alkalosis
   d. hypokalemia, metabolic acidosis
   e. hyperchloremia, metabolic acidosis

221. *Concerning nocardiosis in dogs, which statement is most accurate?*
   a. Infected animals with a copious effusion are a human health hazard.
   b. Culture of material for *Nocardia* requires anaerobic transport and culture conditions.
   c. Not all *Nocardia* species produce so-called sulfur granules.
   d. Penicillin and enrofloxacin are the drugs of choice.
   e. Culture of infected material typically produces growth of the organism within 2 to 4 days.

222. *A plain lateral abdominal radiograph reveals that the small intestines are in the cranial abdomen, crowded against the liver and stomach. This finding is most likely related to extreme enlargement of the:*
   a. mesenteric lymph nodes
   b. left kidney
   c. spleen
   d. urinary bladder
   e. right adrenal gland

223. *A 5-year-old schnauzer that is kept in the house or a fenced backyard has been anorectic and vomiting bile for 2 days. The dog shows discomfort on palpation of the cranial abdomen. Laboratory findings include a packed cell volume of 57% (normal 35% to 55%), white blood cell count of 27,690/μl (normal 6000 to 14,000/μl), and urine specific gravity of 1.045. The dogs serum is too lipemic for blood chemistry assays. Which statement concerning this dog is **least** accurate?*
   a. Intravenous fluids are warranted at this time.
   b. Abdominal surgery is inappropriate at this time.
   c. Abdominal ultrasonography is indicated.
   d. Exocrine pancreatic insufficiency is a likely diagnosis.
   e. The dog should not be given food or water per os for at least the next 24 to 72 hours.

224. *Concerning paragonimiasis in dogs, which statement is most accurate?*
   a. A Baermann concentration technique is required to demonstrate larvae in the feces.
   b. Thiabendazole is the treatment of choice.
   c. Thoracic radiographs often demonstrate air-filled cysts or small masses in the lungs.
   d. This parasite has a direct life cycle and can be spread from animal to animal within a kennel.
   e. The most common result of infection is sudden collapse.

Correct answers are on pages 140-171.

225. *Concerning dogs with esophageal disease causing regurgitation, which statement is most accurate?*

a. Esophagitis is a common cause of symptomatic esophageal disease.
b. Aspiration pneumonia is a common cause of death.
c. Distal esophageal myotomy is often useful if there is acquired esophageal weakness.
d. Surgical plication of redundant esophageal tissue is reasonable therapy if the esophagus is greatly dilated.
e. Histamine-2 antagonists are recommended to alleviate clinical signs.

226. *The best treatment for moderately severe, symptomatic, biopsy-confirmed, chronic hepatitis in a dog is:*

a. neomycin
b. lactulose
c. a low-protein diet
d. prednisolone
e. trientine

227. *Concerning parvoviral infection in dogs, which statement is most accurate?*

a. A positive-contrast barium radiographic study usually reveals intestinal ulcers.
b. Myocarditis is common in animals affected before 14 weeks of age.
c. Severe lymphopenia is a sensitive and specific indicator of this disease.
d. Fecal enzyme-linked immunosorbent assay is a sensitive test for 15 to 21 days after the onset of signs.
e. Many infections probably are clinically mild or inapparent.

228. *Concerning gastrointestinal ulceration in dogs, which statement is most accurate?*

a. Pure-bred dogs are more commonly affected than mixed breeds.
b. Severe pancreatitis often causes it.
c. Severe hepatic failure may cause it.
d. Athletic or working dogs are more commonly affected than nonworking dogs.
e. Dogs that chew bones are more often affected than those that do not.

229. *What is the best antimicrobial treatment for a dog with fulminating abdominal sepsis associated with leakage of colonic contents?*

a. cephalothin and amoxicillin
b. enrofloxacin and gentamicin
c. amikacin, ampicillin, and metronidazole
d. clindamycin
e. enrofloxacin, amikacin, and trimethoprimsulfadiazine

230. *Concerning pythiosis in dogs, which statement is most accurate?*

a. Most animals with disseminated disease have marked monocytosis.
b. Serologic examination is useful for diagnosis.
c. The subcutaneous tissues of the legs are typically swollen.
d. The stomach and intestines are the most commonly affected sites.
e. Amphotericin B is an effective treatment in approximately 40% to 60% of cases.

231. *The **least** likely postoperative complication of surgery to correct gastric dilatation-volvulus in dogs is:*

a. disseminated intravascular coagulation
b. cardiac arrhythmias
c. gastric motility disorders
d. renal failure
e. gastric ulceration

232. *The drug that most effectively controls diarrhea in dogs is:*

a. loperamide
b. atropine
c. methscopalamine
d. kaolin-pectin (Kaopectate)
e. aminopentamide

233. *Concerning rabies in dogs, which statement is most accurate?*
   a. One of the first signs of the paralytic stage is incoordination.
   b. Death occurs from purulent meningoencephalitis, usually 11 to 14 days after clinical signs are first seen.
   c. Immunologic examination of skin biopsies (especially the sensory vibrissae) allows reliable antemortem diagnosis.
   d. Rabies virus is relatively resistant, and the area around an infected dog should be disinfected repeatedly with phenolic disinfectants.
   e. Rabies is invariably fatal within 2 to 3 weeks of infection.

234. *For the past 8 days, a 4-year-old female Bedlington terrier has been depressed, anorectic, and vomiting bile. The dog's serum alanine aminotransferase activity is 12 times normal, and serum alkaline phosphatase activity is 10 times normal. The most likely cause of these signs is:*
   a. cholangitis-cholangiohepatitis
   b. steroid hepatopathy
   c. leptospirosis
   d. hepatic lipidosis
   e. copper storage disorder

235. *Concerning Rocky Mountain spotted fever in dogs, which statement is most accurate?*
   a. The major vector in the United States is *Rhipicephalus sanguineus.*
   b. Rocky Mountain spotted fever rarely causes thrombocytopenia, while ehrlichiosis commonly causes thrombocytopenia.
   c. Tetracycline is clearly superior to chloramphenicol for treatment.
   d. Dogs with acute disease typically have a titer ≥1:128.
   e. Some infections in dogs probably are inapparent.

236. *A 3-year-old spayed miniature schnauzer that is kept in the house has been depressed, anorectic, and vomiting bile for 36 hours. The dog shows discomfort on palpation of the cranial abdomen. Laboratory findings include a packed cell volume of 58% (normal 35% to 55%), white blood cell count of 29,390/μl), and urine specific gravity of 1.055. The serum is moderately lipemic, and assays show a blood urea nitrogen level of 64 mg/dl (normal 6 to 20 mg/dl), serum creatinine level of 2.8 mg/dl (normal 0.1 to 1.9 mg/dl), serum alanine aminotransferase activity of 145 IU/L (normal <120 IU/L), serum alkaline phosphatase activity of 245 IU/L (normal <147 IU/L), and serum lipase activity of 145 IU/L (normal 30 to 150 IU/L). The most likely cause of these findings is:*
   a. pyelonephritis
   b. acute hepatitis
   c. acute pancreatitis
   d. inflammatory bowel disease
   e. gastroenteritis from ingestion of garbage

237. *The* ***least*** *effective treatment to decrease gastric acidity is:*
   a. famotidine administered once daily
   b. cimetidine administered 3 times daily
   c. ranitidine administered twice daily
   d. omeprazole administered once daily
   e. aluminum hydroxide administered twice daily

238. *Concerning salmon poisoning in dogs, which statement is most accurate?*
   a. Detection of *Nanophyetus salmincola* ova in the feces is diagnostic.
   b. Oxytetracycline and chloramphenicol are reasonable therapeutic choices.
   c. Diagnosis is best made by finding a titer for *Neorickettsia helminthoeca.*
   d. This disease does not cause lymphadenopathy as consistently as does ehrlichiosis.
   e. Most clinically affected dogs recover spontaneously.

Correct answers are on pages 140-171.

239. *A walker hound that has traveled throughout the United States has had diarrhea containing specks of red blood for the past 4 weeks. There is no straining at defecation, and the dog has not lost weight. The dog is normal on physical examination and rectal palpation. The complete blood count shows neutrophilic leukocytosis (14,500 segs/μl; normal 4000 to 14,000/μl). The serum chemistry profile and urinalysis findings are normal. No parasites or ova are noted on a single fecal flotation. The most likely cause of these signs is:*

a. coccidiosis
b. giardiasis
c. protothecosis
d. salmonellosis
e. trichuriasis

240. *Which radiographic technique is most preferred for diagnosing ileocolic intussusception?*

a. plain standing lateral radiograph of the abdomen
b. upper gastrointestinal radiographic contrast series
c. abdominal ultrasonography
d. pneumoperitoneography
e. plain abdominal radiographs

241. *Concerning sporotrichosis in dogs, which statement is most accurate?*

a. Serologic examination is the most reliable means of diagnosis.
b. Cytologic examination of material from lesions usually reveals numerous organisms.
c. Cutaneous and cutaneolymphatic lesions are the most common forms.
d. Griseofulvin is the treatment of choice for cutaneous sporotrichosis.
e. Amphotericin B is the treatment of choice for cutaneous sporotrichosis.

242. *A 2-year-old German shepherd has had diarrhea for 8 months. The diarrhea occurs 1 to 3 times daily and is soft and brown. No mucus, blood, or straining has been noted. The dog has lost 8% of its body weight despite a good appetite. Five fecal flotations performed with zinc sulfate solution have been negative. The dog is otherwise normal. The most appropriate course of action is to:*

a. examine a direct fecal smear and perform another fecal flotation
b. perform a serum trypsinlike immunoreactivity determination
c. obtain plain abdominal radiographs
d. perform gastroduodenoscopy and obtain an intestinal biopsy
e. perform abdominal ultrasonography

243. *Concerning tetanus in dogs, which statement is most accurate?*

a. The incubation period ranges from days to months, in part depending on how far the wound is from the central nervous system.
b. Definitive diagnosis requires electromyographic analysis.
c. As compared with other animals and people, dogs are relatively susceptible to tetanus.
d. Such drugs as diazepam and methocarbamol are ideal for treatment, whereas phenobarbital and acepromazine are not useful.
e. Large does of antitoxin are effective in neutralizing toxin that has reached peripheral nerve fibers or passed through the blood-brain barrier.

244. *At weaning a 5-month-old dog begins regurgitating at every meal. There are no prodromal signs; the dog simply puts its head down and gags up food and mucus. The dog is otherwise normal. The most appropriate course of action is to:*

a. obtain plain thoracic radiographs
b. perform a complete blood count and serum chemistry profile
c. obtain plain abdominal radiographs
d. perform a positive-contrast barium study of the intestines
e. perform liver function tests

245. *Concerning tuberculosis in dogs, which statement is most accurate?*
    a. Dogs are more likely to acquire the infection from people than people are to acquire the infection from dogs.
    b. Affected dogs usually have gastrointestinal signs.
    c. Dogs usually are infected with *Mycobacterium bovis.*
    d. Affected dogs should be treated with a combination of gentamicin, ampicillin, and isoniazid.
    e. Intradermal testing is the preferred method of diagnosis.

246. *A 2-year-old dog has been vomiting digested blood daily for 1 week. The dog is also somewhat anorectic. The most likely cause of these signs is:*
    a. gastric foreign body
    b. use of corticosteroids
    c. acute pancreatitis
    d. salmonellosis
    e. use of nonsteroidal antiinflammatory drugs

247. *Concerning cryptococcosis in dogs, which statement is most accurate?*
    a. On cytologic preparations, *Cryptococcus* is best distinguished from other yeasts by its small size and intracellular location.
    b. Dogs are generally affected more commonly than cats.
    c. It is the most common mycosis affecting the canine nasal cavity.
    d. The latex agglutination test for cryptococcal antigen is sensitive and specific.
    e. Ketoconazole is the treatment of choice for central nervous system involvement.

248. *Concerning congenital esophageal weakness in dogs, which statement is most accurate?*
    a. Most affected dogs can be successfully managed with conservative dietary therapy plus antiemetics.
    b. Endoscopic examination is the sensitive and most specific means of diagnosis.
    c. Metoclopramide routinely alleviates clinical signs.
    d. Cisapride therapy routinely alleviates clinical signs.
    e. Barium contrast radiographs are the most sensitive and specific diagnostic test.

249. *Which laboratory finding is **least** likely to be observed in a dog with severe acute pancreatitis?*
    a. hypercalcemia
    b. neutrophilic leukocytosis
    c. increased serum alkaline phosphatase and/or alanine aminotransferase activities
    d. azotemia
    e. hyperglycemia

250. *Of the following drugs, which is the most effective antiemetic for dogs with severe vomiting?*
    a. aminopentamide
    b. kaolin-pectin (Kaopectate)
    c. atropine
    d. chlorpromazine
    e. cimetidine

251. *Concerning chronic, complete jejunal obstruction in dogs, which statement is most accurate?*
    a. Dilated intestinal loops can often be seen on plain abdominal radiographs.
    b. Endoscopic examination is the most sensitive means of diagnosis.
    c. Contrast radiographs are indicated if you suspect such an obstruction.
    d. Abdominal palpation is usually all that is required for diagnosis.
    e. If a positive-contrast radiographic study is performed, an iodide contrast agent is preferred.

Correct answers are on pages 140-171.

252. *A 9-month-old boxer has had diarrhea for 4 months. The problem waxes and wanes but has persisted. The stool is soft, without mucus or blood, and is passed 2 to 4 times per day without straining. The dog has lost 3 to 4 lb in the past 4 weeks and is fed a high-quality commercial diet. A direct fecal examination reveals numerous, rapidly motile, pear-shaped protozoa. Which statement concerning this dog is most accurate?*

a. The dog should be treated with loperamide.
b. The dog should be treated with sulfadimethoxine.
c. The dog should be treated with fenbendazole.
d. The protozoa are probably not significant; you should recommend a dietary change.
e. The dog should be treated with sulfasalazine (Azulfidine).

253. *A 9-year-old mixed-breed dog suddenly begins to regurgitate its food without warning up to 3 times daily. The dog has also developed a soft, moist cough that began 2 weeks before the regurgitation was noted. The dog is otherwise normal, except that the moist cough can easily be elicited by rubbing the trachea. Which statement concerning this dog is most accurate?*

a. Neuromuscular disease may be causing the signs in this dog.
b. Gastric neoplasia may be causing the signs in this dog.
c. A positive-contrast barium radiographic series of the stomach and intestines should next be performed.
d. A complete blood count and serum chemistry profile should next be performed.
e. Abdominal ultrasonography should next be performed.

254. *A 4-year-old basenji is emaciated and has hypoalbuminemia (1.3 g/dl; normal 2.5 to 4.4 g/dl) and hyperproteinemia (8.7 g/dl; normal 5.5 to 7.0 g/dl). The most likely cause of these findings is:*

a. hepatic insufficiency
b. alimentary lymphosarcoma
c. protein-losing nephropathy
d. immunoproliferative enteropathy
e. intestinal lymphangiectasia

255. *On cytologic preparations of lymph node aspirates from dogs with histoplasmosis,* Histoplasma *organisms appear as:*

a. small (2 to 4 μm), round organisms with a basophilic center, often found within the host's cells
b. large (10 to 80 μm), round organisms containing numerous smaller structures
c. moderate-sized round yeast bodies with an obvious capsule around them
d. pleomorphic, cigar-shaped organisms
e. nonseptate hyphae without obvious spores

256. *Gastric outlet obstruction caused by benign pyloric stenosis associated with hypertrophy of the circular muscle fibers of the pylorus principally occurs in:*

a. young Doberman pinschers and old great Danes
b. old dogs of giant breeds
c. young dogs of brachycephalic breeds
d. old miniature schnauzers and young Yorkshire terriers
e. deep-chested dogs of any age

257. *A dog with moderately severe chronic large intestinal diarrhea for 6 weeks has traveled throughout the United States and has been in Montana for the past 2 months. The client has declined any diagnostic tests. Given this dog's history, the most appropriate treatment is with:*

a. prednisolone
b. a trial elimination diet with added fiber
c. praziquantel
d. pyrantel pamoate
e. sulfasalazine (Azulfidine)

258. *A 7-year-old dachshund has had diarrhea for 4 weeks. The problem waxes and wanes but has persisted. The stool is soft, without blood or mucus, and is passed 2 to 4 times per day without straining. The dog has lost 5% of its body weight in the past week and is fed a high-quality commercial diet. Three fecal flotations reveal a few oocysts. Which statement concerning this dog is most accurate?*
   a. A barium contrast radiographic study of the intestines is warranted.
   b. The dog should be treated with fenbendazole.
   c. The dog should be treated with trimethoprim-sulfadiazine.
   d. The dog should be treated with loperamide.
   e. The parasite represented by the oocysts is probably not responsible for the diarrhea.

259. *A 7-year-old mixed-breed dog has had marked hepatomegaly but is otherwise normal on physical examination. Serum alkaline phosphatase activity is 13 times normal, and serum alanine aminotransferase activity is normal. Serum glucose, total protein, albumin, urea nitrogen, creatinine, and electrolyte values are normal. A complete blood count reveals lymphopenia. The urine specific gravity is 1.028. The most likely cause of these findings is:*
   a. copper storage disease
   b. disseminated histoplasmosis
   c. hepatic cirrhosis
   d. steroid hepatopathy
   e. portosystemic shunt

260. *An undersized 8-month-old Yorkshire terrier that was the "runt of the litter" is presented for ovariohysterectomy. The surgery goes without problems, but the dog does not awaken from anesthesia for 28 hours. The most likely cause of delayed recovery from anesthesia in this dog is:*
   a. mild hydrocephalus
   b. anesthetic overdose
   c. a congenital portosystemic shunt
   d. hypoglycemia
   e. congenital renal amyloidosis

261. *Shortly after you give a dog several swallows of a liquid barium suspension, you note barium pooling in the pyloric antrum on the first radiograph made in the series. This observation indicates that the dog probably:*
   a. is in left lateral recumbency
   b. is in right lateral recumbency
   c. has significant gastric outflow obstruction
   d. has significant gastric paresis
   e. is normal

262. *The drug most likely to be effective in treating acute diarrhea in a dog is:*
   a. sucralfate
   b. bismuth subsalicylate
   c. barium sulfate
   d. atropine
   e. cimetidine

263. *Five mature dogs in your clinic have developed diarrhea in the past 6 days. Each dog acutely develops profuse, bloody diarrhea but is otherwise normal. You have treated each dog with some combination of kaolin-pectate, aminopentamide, amoxicillin, and/or loperamide. The diarrhea usually resolves within 2 to 4 days, regardless of which treatment you use. The most likely cause of this outbreak of diarrhea is:*
   a. salmonellosis
   b. clostridial enteritis
   c. parvoviral enteritis
   d. coronaviral enteritis
   e. giardiasis

264. *You perform a positive-contrast barium gastrogram in a dog with history of vomiting bile. The next day, radiographs reveal that all the barium is in the colon, except for two small, discrete "spots" in the gastric antrum, in which barium is retained. Which statement concerning this dog is most accurate?*
   a. The dog probably has gastric ulcers.
   b. The dog probably has a gastric foreign body.
   c. The dog should be treated with metoclopramide.
   d. The dog should be treated with chlorpromazine.
   e. The dog probably has pancreatitis.

Correct answers are on pages 140-171.

265. *Concerning exocrine pancreatic insufficiency in dogs, which statement is most accurate?*

a. It can be reliably diagnosed by fecal film digestion test.
b. It is often accompanied by small intestinal bacterial overgrowth.
c. It is usually caused by chronic or relapsing pancreatitis.
d. It reliably responds to pancreatic enzyme supplementation.
e. It typically causes moderate to marked hypoproteinemia.

266. *You are presented with a dog that has recently ingested a noncorrosive toxic substance. The most reliable emetic for use in this dog is:*

a. apomorphine
b. xylazine
c. syrup of ipecac
d. salt water
e. hydrogen peroxide

267. *A litter of 2-week-old Corgi puppies suddenly becomes ill. The dogs are weak and have very pale oral mucosae and scant, dark diarrhea. These dogs:*

a. should immediately be treated with pyrantel pamoate
b. should immediately be treated with metronidazole
c. should be examined by direct fecal smears and fecal flotation
d. should be tested by enzyme-linked immunosorbent assay for parvoviral enteritis
e. should immediately be treated with sulfadimethoxine

268. *A 4-year-old female great Dane has had diarrhea for 6 weeks. The stools are soft (especially toward the end of defecation) and covered with mucus. There is no blood or straining associated with defecation, but the animal occasionally defecates in the house when it cannot get outside quickly enough. The dog is otherwise normal. Which statement concerning this dog is most accurate?*

a. The dog should be treated with loperamide.
b. The dog should be treated with pyrantel pamoate.
c. The dog probably has chronic large intestinal diarrhea.
d. The dog probably has protein-losing enteropathy.
e. The dog probably has a chronic helminth infection.

269. *Concerning* Ehrlichia platys *infection in dogs, which statement is most accurate?*

a. Concurrent infections with *Ehrlichia canis* are probably rare.
b. Finding inclusion bodies in platelets during periods of severe thrombocytopenia is the easiest and most reliable means of diagnosis.
c. Infected animals typically are ill with fever and epistaxis.
d. The pancytopenia caused by this rickettsia tends to be more severe than that caused by *Ehrlichia canis.*
e. The serologic test for antibodies to *Ehrlichia canis* does not cross react with antibodies of *Ehrlichia platys.*

270. *Concerning radiographic demonstration of esophageal foreign bodies, which statement is most accurate?*

a. If a foreign body is seen on plain thoracic radiographs, one should perform contrast esophagography to determine if perforation has occurred.
b. Use of barium sulfate is generally contraindicated if a foreign body may be present.
c. Metoclopramide should be administered during a barium esophagography to ensure even distribution of the contrast agent.
d. Most foreign bodies can be seen on plain radiographs of the thorax.
e. Parasympatholytics may be given to reduce esophageal spasm and facilitate contrast radiographs.

271. *A 9-month-old mixed-breed dog has had episodes of abnormal behavior during the past 5 months. These episodes principally occur after meals and tend to develop and resolve gradually. The dog becomes ataxic and stumbles into walls and furniture. In addition, the dog seems to drink and urinate excessive amounts and is much smaller than its litter mates. The urine specific gravity is 1.011, serum phosphorus concentration is 7.7 mg/dl (normal 2.5 to 5.5 mg/dl), serum alkaline phosphatase activity is 201 IU/L (normal <145 IU/L), and serum albumin concentration is 2.0 g/dl (normal 2.5 to 4.4 g/dl). The most likely cause of these findings is:*

    a. hyperkalemic periodic paralysis
    b. idiopathic epilepsy
    c. renal failure
    d. intermittent hypoglycemia
    e. hepatic insufficiency

272. *A 3-month-old mixed-breed dog has peracute onset of severe depression, fever, anorexia, vomiting, and diarrhea. The vomitus consists of food and yellow phlegm, and the diarrhea is dark brown and watery. The most likely cause of these signs is:*

    a. salmonellosis
    b. coronaviral diarrhea
    c. parvoviral diarrhea
    d. gastrointestinal foreign body
    e. gastroenteritis from ingestion of garbage

273. *The finding most indicative of hemorrhagic gastroenteritis in dogs is:*

    a. degenerative left shift in peripheral white blood cells on a complete blood count
    b. platelet count <100,000/µl
    c. dilated small intestinal loops on abdominal radiographs
    d. packed cell volume of ≥70%
    e. bacterial spores in feces

274. *An obese 62-kg mixed-breed dog is retching unproductively and has had a painful cranial abdomen for 2 hours. Findings of the physical examination are otherwise unremarkable except that the dog is clearly depressed. The most appropriate course of action is to:*

    a. perform a complete blood count and serum chemistry profile
    b. administer metoclopramide
    c. perform a positive-contrast barium radiographic study of the abdomen
    d. administer flunixin meglumine
    e. make plain abdominal radiographs

275. *A 1-year-old male boxer has severe large intestinal diarrhea unrelated to parasites or diet. Considering the dog's age and breed, the most likely cause of diarrhea is:*

    a. cecocolic intussusception
    b. eosinophilic enteritis
    c. intestinal adenocarcinoma
    d. pythiosis
    e. histiocytic ulcerative colitis

276. *A sign **rarely** observed in dogs with congenital portosystemic shunt is:*

    a. seizures
    b. ascites
    c. stunted growth
    d. polyuria/polydipsia
    e. vomiting

277. *Concerning tapeworm infection in young dogs, which statement is most accurate?*

    a. *Taenia* species are the most common tapeworms in dogs in the United States.
    b. Most affected animals have soft stools and show a decline in physical condition.
    c. Vomiting of proglottids is often the first sign of infection with *Spirometra.*
    d. Large doses of fenbendazole are effective as treatment for infection with the types of tapeworms found in the United States.
    e. Fleas and lice are intermediate hosts for the most common species.

Correct answers are on pages 140-171.

278. *Concerning viral enteritis in dogs, which statement is most accurate?*

a. Severe coronaviral infections cause intestinal crypt necrosis.
b. Severe parvoviral infections cause widespread destruction of villi.
c. Severe rotaviral infections cause intestinal crypt necrosis.
d. Coronavirus is very resistant to the environment and most disinfectants.
e. Rotaviral infections often result in concurrent aspiration pneumonia.

279. *A 4-year-old dog has been sick for the past 2 weeks. It vomits food every 2 to 3 days and has a diminished appetite. Yesterday it began passing black, tarry diarrhea. The dog has lost about 5% of its body weight and has pale mucous membranes. The most likely cause of these signs is:*

a. chronic large intestinal diarrhea
b. chronic pancreatitis
c. exocrine pancreatic insufficiency
d. gastroduodenal ulceration
e. large intestinal neoplasia

280. *During a positive-contrast barium radiographic study of the esophagus, which drug would probably cause significant artifacts on the esophagogram and make it appear that a normal dog had generalized esophageal weakness?*

a. xylazine
b. glycopyrrolate
c. metoclopramide
d. cimetidine
e. sucralfate

281. *After a normal dog is given liquid barium sulfate per os, the barium solution typically reaches the area of the ileocolic valve within:*

a. 15 to 45 minutes
b. 30 to 90 minutes
c. 90 to 120 minutes
d. 180 to 240 minutes
e. 240 to 300 minutes

282. *You examine a 23-week-old mixed-breed dog that appears to have 2 to 3 inches of bowel mucosa protruding from its anus. The dog has been somewhat depressed and losing weight for the past week, and the protruding segment of bowel was noticed 4 days previously. The most appropriate course of action is:*

a. resect the prolapsed tissue
b. replace the mucosa and keep it in place with a purse-string suture
c. perform a rectal examination to see if there is a cul-de-sac between the mucosa and rectal wall
d. perform a colonopexy
e. replace the mucosa and administer a lidocaine enema before placing a purse-string suture

283. *A 3-year old German shepherd has severe flatulence. Which statement concerning this dog is most accurate?*

a. The gas is probably caused by malabsorbed carbohydrates reaching the colon.
b. The gas is probably caused by aerophagia.
c. A dietary fiber supplement should be fed.
d. Metoclopramide should be given.
e. Endoscopic biopsy of the colon is indicated as the next step.

284. *Which of the following is **least** likely to cause vomiting in a dog?*

a. uremia
b. hypercalcemia
c. diabetic ketoacidosis
d. hepatic failure
e. hyperadrenocorticism

285. *A 4-month-old Doberman pinscher puppy developed acute diarrhea this morning. This afternoon, the puppy is severely depressed, anorectic, and febrile (40.2° C) and has profuse, odiferous diarrhea, with occasional vomiting of bile. A complete blood count shows a packed cell volume of 32% (normal 35% to 53%) and a white blood cell count of 6000/µl (normal 5000 to 14,000/µl), with 94% neutrophils and 5% lymphocytes. A direct fecal examination reveals numerous hookworm and roundworm eggs, plus motile pentatrichomonad trophozoites. The most likely cause of these signs is:*

a. bacterial infection
b. food intolerance
c. endoparasitism
d. viral infection
e. reaction to ingestion of garbage

286. *In a dog with suspected acute ehrlichiosis, the most appropriate course of action is to:*

a. examine a peripheral blood smear for morulae
b. treat the dog with gentamicin for 10 days
c. aspirate and examine a bone marrow sample
d. treat the dog with chloramphenicol for 21 days
e. perform an ophthalmologic examination

287. *Which radiographic finding is **least** likely to be observed in a dog with acute pancreatitis?*

a. profuse ascites
b. poor serosal detail in the cranial right quadrant
c. displacement of the descending duodenum to the right
d. widening of the angle between the pyloric antrum and proximal duodenum
e. an air-filled duodenum that is somewhat dilated relative to the rest of the intestinal tract

288. *Which dog is **least** likely to have gastric intestinal disease?*

a. 1-year-old dog that vomits food, mucus, and what appears to be "coffee grounds" 1 to 3 hours after eating
b. 3-year-old dog that looks obviously sick and salivates for 5 to 10 minutes before vomiting apparently undigested food
c. 5-year-old dog that throws up copious amounts of yellow foam daily, especially in the morning
d. 2-year-old dog with vigorous retching and then projectile vomiting of food, shortly after eating
e. 4-year-old dog that unexpectedly gags up food and mucus, not associated with eating

289. *Concerning hyperbilirubinemia of 4 mg/dl (normal <1.0 mg/dl) and icterus in dogs, which statement is most accurate?*

a. Exocrine pancreatic insufficiency is a relatively common cause.
b. Icterus of this magnitude is to be expected in nearly every case of significant hepatic disease.
c. Hemolysis is a relatively common cause.
d. Gallstones commonly cause extrahepatic obstruction with this magnitude of bilirubinemia.
e. Steroid hepatopathy is a relatively common cause.

290. *Which statement best describes the position and course of the canine duodenum as seen in a ventrodorsal projection on a positive-contrast barium radiograph of the abdomen?*

a. It originates at the pylorus, courses caudally to the root of the mesentery, turns cranially, and then ascends.
b. It originates at the pylorus and then crosses to the left side of the abdomen and courses caudally to the root of the mesentery.
c. It originates at the pylorus, courses caudally to about the level of the seventh lumbar vertebra, and then crosses to the other side of the abdomen.
d. It originates at the pylorus, courses caudally to about the level of the seventh lumbar vertebra, turns cranially, and ascends on the left side.
e. It originates at the pylorus, courses caudally to about the level of the sacrum, and then turns cranially.

Correct answers are on pages 140-171.

291. *Concerning serum γ-glutamyltransferase activity in dogs, which statement is most accurate?*

a. It is a more sensitive indicator than serum bile acid levels for detecting portosystemic shunts.
b. Serum γ-glutamyltransferase activity does not increase in response to corticosteroid administration.
c. γ-Glutamyltransferase is a "leakage" enzyme.
d. It is a less sensitive indicator than serum alkaline phosphatase activity for detecting hepatic disease.
e. It is sensitive and specific in distinguishing hepatocellular disease from biliary obstruction.

292. *A 3-year-old Yorkshire terrier has had repeated bouts of ataxia and depression. The episodes began 14 months previously and have gradually gotten worse. The episodes principally occur after the dog is fed and can last hours to days. On physical examination (including rectal and ophthalmologic examinations), the dog seems normal except that it is clearly smaller than expected for its age and breed. The owner declines a diagnostic workup. Considering the dog's history and clinical signs, the most appropriate empiric treatment is with:*

a. oral primidone
b. a trial period of several small feedings per day of a hypoallergenic diet
c. lactulose, a low-protein diet, and oral neomycin
d. oral phenobarbital
e. oral potassium bromide

293. *What is the best treatment for a dog with moderately severe, acute pancreatitis?*

a. intravenous balanced crystalloid fluids plus sodium bicarbonate, analgesics, and small amounts of a bland diet
b. intravenous balanced crystalloid fluids, and small amounts of a low-fat diet
c. nothing per os and intravenous balanced crystalloid fluids
d. antibiotics, plasma transfusion, and nothing per os
e. intravenous balanced electrolyte fluids, corticosteroids, antibiotics, and small amounts of a low-fat diet

294. *The expected location of the cecum on a ventrodorsal radiograph of a dog's abdomen is in the:*

a. cranial half, to the right of midline, near the sixth lumbar vertebra
b. cranial half, to the left of midline, near the second lumbar vertebra
c. cranial half, to the right of midline, near the second lumbar vertebra
d. cranial half, to the left of midline, near the sixth lumbar vertebra
e. cranial half, on the midline, near the fourth lumbar vertebra

295. *A 4-month-old mixed-breed dog has a fever (40° C), diarrhea, anorexia, and depression that began 1 day previously. It is now vomiting bile-stained fluid, even when fasting. The most likely cause of these signs is:*

a. gastric ulceration
b. intestinal intussusception
c. gastrointestinal parasitism
d. parvoviral enteritis
e. food intolerance

296. *A plain ventrodorsal radiograph of a dog's abdomen reveals that the pylorus is markedly displaced caudally and medially. No other abnormalities are noted radiographically. The most likely cause of this finding is:*

a. nonlinear alimentary foreign body
b. alimentary lymphosarcoma
c. hemangiosarcoma
d. hepatoma
e. linear alimentary foreign body

297. *During the past 3 days, a 5-year-old dog has been anorectic and vomiting green phlegm 4 to 6 times per day. Initial (first day) management of this dog should include all the following* ***except:***

a. ultrasonographic examination of the abdomen
b. a serum chemistry profile
c. plain abdominal radiographs
d. intravenous fluids
e. endoscopic examination of the stomach and duodenum

298. *After a normal dog is given liquid barium sulfate per os, the barium solution typically begins to pass from the stomach into the duodenum within:*

a. 0 to 30 minutes
b. 30 to 45 minutes
c. 45 to 60 minutes
d. 60 to 90 minutes
e. 90 to 120 minutes

299. *Which clinical sign is **least** likely to be observed in a dog with severe, acute pancreatitis?*

a. vomiting
b. abdominal pain
c. fever
d. marked ascites
e. dehydration

300. *You inject an iodinated contrast agent into a jejunal vein and immediately make abdominal radiographs. Which radiographic observation is most suggestive of a congenital portosystemic shunt?*

a. several small vessels exiting the portal vein and coursing cranially, anastomosing with vessels near the esophagus
b. several small vessels exiting the portal vein before entering the liver, anastomosing with the azygos vein or caudal vena cava
c. a single vessel exiting the portal vein before entering the liver and coursing caudally, anastomosing with the renal vein or caudal celiac vein
d. the portal vein entering the liver and branching into many smaller vessels within the hepatic parenchyma
e. a single vessel exiting the portal vein before entering the liver, anastomosing with the azygos vein or caudal vena cava

CATS

S.K. Fooshee

301. *Hypokalemic polymyopathy is a neuromuscular disorder of cats that appears related to decreased dietary intake of potassium, as well as excessive renal wasting of potassium. The classic presenting sign for this polymyopathy is:*

a. urinary incontinence
b. nystagmus
c. ventroflexion of the neck
d. opisthotonos
e. hypalgesia of the extremities

302. *A common biochemical finding in cats with hypokalemic polymyopathy is:*

a. increased serum alkaline phosphatase activity
b. decreased serum alkaline phosphatase activity
c. decreased serum creatine phosphokinase activity
d. increased serum creatine phosphokinase
e. increased serum alanine aminotransferase activity

303. *β-Blockers, such as propranolol, are potentially indicated in treatment of all the following **except:***

a. systemic hypertension
b. asthmatic bronchitis
c. hypertrophic cardiomyopathy
d. cardiac arrhythmias
e. tachycardia

304. *Which breed is well recognized for a familial predisposition to renal amyloidosis?*

a. Abyssinian
b. domestic short hair
c. Siamese
d. Burmese
e. Himalayan

Correct answers are on pages 140-171.

305. *How do the pathologic findings of renal amyloidosis in cats differ from those of renal amyloidosis in dogs?*

a. In cats the amyloid deposits are more severe than in dogs.
b. In cats the proteinuria is more marked than in dogs.
c. In cats the amyloid deposits are medullary, whereas in dogs the deposits are glomerular.
d. In cats the prognosis is better than for dogs.
e. In cats renal amyloidosis is usually subclinical, whereas in dogs it is usually clinical.

306. *A geriatric cat has moderate azotemia, unilateral renomegaly, abdominal effusion, and vomiting. The cat tests negative for feline leukemia virus (FeLV) by serum enzyme-linked immunosorbent assay (ELISA) and has essentially normal urine. The most likely cause of these findings is:*

a. feline immunodeficiency virus infection
b. hemangiosarcoma
c. pancreatic adenocarcinoma
d. metastatic prostatic adenocarcinoma
e. lymphosarcoma

307. *Which clinicopathologic finding is consistent with feline infectious peritonitis (FIP)?*

a. increased serum globulin level
b. decreased serum globulin level
c. monoclonal gammopathy
d. Bence Jones proteinuria
e. decreased serum albumin level

308. *Cats are immunologically distinct from dogs. What immunoglobulin has been recognized in dogs but has **not** yet been identified in cats?*

a. IgA
b. IgD
c. IgM
d. IgE
e. IgG

309. *Both cats and dogs are frequently treated for hypovolemic shock as a result of trauma. Intravenous fluids must be more cautiously administered to cats than dogs, however, because cats have a smaller blood volume. The blood volume of cats (as a percentage of body weight) is approximately:*

a. 1% to 2%
b. 2% to 3%
c. 3% to 4%
d. 4% to 5%
e. 5% to 6%

310. *Which disease causes ventroflexion of the neck?*

a. spinal cord lymphoma
b. thiamin deficiency
c. hepatic lipidosis
d. ischemic encephalopathy
e. cerebellar hypoplasia

311. *Concerning the biologic behavior of osteosarcoma in cats, which statement is **least** accurate?*

a. It most commonly occurs in the hind limbs.
b. Pulmonary metastasis is less common in cats than in dogs.
c. It is the most common bone tumor of cats.
d. Affected cats generally have a shorter survival time than affected dogs.
e. It tends to occur in older, female, domestic, short-hair cats.

312. *Which test is most specific for evaluation of liver function in cats:*

a. fasting and postprandial serum bile acid levels
b. serum albumin level
c. BSP (bromsulfphalein) clearance
d. indocyanine green clearance
e. serum alanine aminotransferase activity

313. *The most common primary brain tumor of cats is:*

a. neuroglioblastoma
b. meningioma
c. astrocytoma
d. lymphoma
e. malignant melanosarcoma

314. *A thin, 15-year-old cat is presented to your clinic with acute onset of hind limb paresis. The owner is hysterical because the cat appears to be in a great deal of pain. You cannot elicit spinal reflexes in the rear limbs and do not feel any pulses in the femoral arteries. The foot pads appear cyanotic. The most likely cause of these signs is:*
   a. trauma
   b. spinal cord tumor, with vascular disruption
   c. coagulation disorder associated with hypertrophic cardiomyopathy
   d. bleeding into the spinal cord associated with an anticoagulant rodenticide
   e. intervertebral disk rupture

315. *Anisocoria is commonly associated with a spinal cord lesion at the level of:*
   a. C1
   b. C5
   c. T1
   d. T10
   e. L1

316. *A cat that has just been struck by an automobile is in extreme respiratory distress. On thoracic auscultation you cannot discern heart sounds or lung sounds. The most likely cause of these findings is:*
   a. diaphragmatic hernia
   b. peritoneopericardial hernia
   c. chylothorax
   d. pericardial tamponade
   e. pulmonary contusions

317. *Prolonged urethral obstruction in male cats can cause life-threatening metabolic derangements. These cats require immediate medical treatment to correct:*
   a. increased serum urea nitrogen and potassium levels, with metabolic alkalosis
   b. increased serum urea nitrogen and potassium levels, with metabolic acidosis
   c. increased serum urea nitrogen and decreased potassium levels, with metabolic alkalosis
   d. increased serum urea nitrogen and decreased potassium levels, with metabolic acidosis
   e. increased serum urea nitrogen and decreased potassium levels, with normal acid-base balance

318. *In cats a deficiency of which coagulation factor is commonly recognized yet rarely causes clinical bleeding?*
   a. factor III
   b. factor VII
   c. factor VII
   d. factor X
   e. factor XII

319. *Transfusion reactions are rare in cats. What is the most common manifestation of transfusion with incompatible blood?*
   a. hemolytic anemia
   b. respiratory arrest
   c. vomiting
   d. hemoglobinuria
   e. seizures

320. *Deficiency of which essential amino acid may lead to hepatic encephalopathy?*
   a. methionine
   b. leucine
   c. tryptophan
   d. arginine
   e. valine

321. *Which drug is* ***contraindicated*** *for treatment of hypertrophic cardiomyopathy in cats?*
   a. furosemide
   b. captopril
   c. digoxin
   d. diltiazem
   e. propranolol

Correct answers are on pages 140-171.

322. *The worldwide distribution of various feline blood groups appears to vary with geographic locale. For this reason, reactions to initial blood transfusion are uncommon in some regions. However, severe transfusion reactions almost invariably occur when a:*

a. type-A recipient receives type-B blood
b. type-B recipient receives type-A blood
c. type-A recipient receives type-C blood
d. type-B recipient receives type-C blood
e. type-C recipient receives type-B blood

323. *Giardiasis may cause chronic or acute diarrhea in cats. The life cycle of this parasite may involve all parts of the gastrointestinal tract* **except** *the:*

a. stomach
b. ileum
c. duodenum
d. jejunum
e. large intestine

324. *The cause of leprosy in cats is:*

a. *Mycobacterium lepraemurium*
b. *Mycobacterium fortuitum*
c. *Mycobacterium stenti*
d. *Mycobacterium paratuberculosis*
e. *Mycobacterium avium*

325. *In cats, mast-cell tumors most frequently involve the:*

a. brain and eyes
b. conjunctivae and gingivae
c. mucous membranes and heart base
d. abdominal viscera and skin
e. lymph nodes and lung

326. *One of the more commonly recognized clinical manifestations of acromegaly in cats is:*

a. dwarfism
b. blindness
c. severe insulin-resistant diabetes mellitus
d. hyperadrenocorticism
e. nephrogenic diabetes insipidus

327. *What is the most common systemic fungal infection of cats?*

a. coccidioidomycosis
b. cryptococcosis
c. histoplasmosis
d. blastomycosis
e. mycosis fungoides

328. *Latent infections with feline leukemia virus can only be detected by:*

a. radioallergosorbent testing (RAST) of serum
b. enzyme-linked immunosorbent assay (ELISA) of serum
c. indirect fluorescent antibody (IFA) testing of bone marrow
d. bone marrow culture and cell reactivation
e. enzyme-linked immunosorbent assay (ELISA) of tears

329. *In cats, bradycardia is generally defined as a heart rate less than:*

a. 250 beats/min
b. 200 beats/min
c. 160 beats/min
d. 120 beats/min
e. 80 beats/min

330. *Benzocaine is a topical anesthetic frequently sprayed into the larynx during endotracheal intubation of cats. Why should this practice be avoided in cats?*

a. The force of the spray aggravates laryngospasm.
b. The drug can cause methemoglobinemia.
c. The drug can cause cardiac arrhythmias.
d. The drug lowers the seizure threshold.
e. The spray can cause irreversible reflex apnea.

331. *Which drug is most useful in treatment of acetaminophen toxicosis?*

a. xylazine
b. diazepam
c. aspirin
d. acetylcysteine
e. ketoconazole

332. *Neuromuscular blockade and respiratory failure may occur with use of:*
   a. chloramphenicol
   b. enrofloxacin
   c. amoxicillin
   d. gentamicin
   e. metronidazole

Questions 333 and 334

333. *The most common dermatophyte isolated from cats is:*
   a. *Microsporum gypseum*
   b. *Microsporum canis*
   c. *Trichophyton mentagrophytes*
   d. *Candida albicans*
   e. *Pseudoallescheria boydii*

334. *Cats infected with the dermatophyte described in question 333 can be effectively treated with any of the following* ***except:***
   a. lime-sulfur dip
   b. captan rinse
   c. chlorhexidine shampoo
   d. amitraz dip
   e. chlorhexidine dip

335. *The cause of acromegaly in cats differs from that in dogs. Essentially all reported cases of acromegaly in cats have been attributed to:*
   a. progestagen induction of growth hormone–mediated insulin resistance
   b. primary brain tumor
   c. adrenal tumor
   d. pituitary tumor
   e. fluctuating progestagen levels caused by the reproductive cycle

336. *The renal threshold for glucose in cats is approximately:*
   a. 120 mg/dl
   b. 180 mg/dl
   c. 200 mg/dl
   d. 240 mg/dl
   e. 290 mg/dl

337. *In cats the term* walking dandruff *refers to infestation with:*
   a. *Notoedres cati*
   b. *Ctenocephalides felis*
   c. *Rhipicephalus sanguineus*
   d. *Cheyletiella blakei*
   e. *Otodectes cynotis*

338. *Cerebellar hypoplasia in kittens maybe caused by in utero infection with:*
   a. feline leukemia virus
   b. feline infectious peritonitis virus
   c. feline panleukopenia virus
   d. feline rhinotracheitis virus
   e. feline immunodeficiency virus

Questions 339 and 340

You are presented with a mature adult cat with severe facial excoriations. The cat appears intensely pruritic and is constantly clawing itself about the face, neck, and ears. The cat was previously seen by another veterinarian and given glucocorticoids, with no apparent response.

339. *What is the most likely cause of this pruritus?*
   a. flea-allergy dermatitis
   b. otitis interna
   c. food allergy
   d. sarcoptic mange
   e. contact hypersensitivity

340. *How can the cause of pruritus be definitively diagnosed?*
   a. skin biopsy
   b. trial feeding of a hypoallergenic diet
   c. necropsy
   d. trial course of antihistamine therapy
   e. isolation of the cat for 2 weeks in your clinic

Correct answers are on pages 140-171.

341. *Which of the following is an exceedingly rare (some say even nonexistent) intestinal parasite of cats?*
   a. *Trichuris* species
   b. *Ancylostoma tubaeformae*
   c. *Toxoplasma gondii*
   d. *Dipylidium caninum*
   e. *Taenia taeniaeformis*

342. *Which cardiovascular drug should* ***not*** *be used in cats:*
   a. propranolol
   b. diltiazem
   c. digoxin
   d. digitoxin
   e. nitroglycerin

343. *All the following are useful in management of constipated cats* ***except:***
   a. dioctyl sodium sulfosuccinate
   b. canned pumpkin pie filling
   c. psyllium
   d. providing fresh water and a clean litter box
   e. phosphate-containing enemas (e.g., Fleet)

344. *All the following can cause polyphagia and weight loss in cats* ***except:***
   a. hyperthyroidism
   b. exocrine pancreatic insufficiency
   c. diabetes mellitus
   d. inflammatory bowel disease
   e. hepatic lipidosis

Questions 345 and 346

345. *In a white cat that spends time indoors and outdoors, ulcerated lesions on the nasal planum and ear margins are most likely associated with:*
   a. dermatophytosis
   b. eosinophilic granuloma complex
   c. squamous-cell carcinoma
   d. pemphigus foliaceus
   e. mast-cell tumor

346. *If the cat in question 345 were a strictly indoor cat and, in addition to the aforementioned lesions, also had thick, hardened foot pads and a low-grade fever, what would be the most likely cause?*
   a. dermatophytosis
   b. eosinophilic granuloma complex
   c. squamous-cell carcinoma
   d. pemphigus foliaceus
   e. mast-cell tumor

347. *In cats, basophilic stippling of erythrocytes is pathognomonic for:*
   a. lead poisoning
   b. regenerative anemia
   c. disseminated intravascular coagulation
   d. feline leukemia virus infection of bone marrow
   e. no particular disease

348. *In a living cat, how is feline infectious peritonitis best diagnosed?*
   a. serologic testing for coronavirus
   b. detailed history and careful physical examination
   c. indirect antibody testing of conjunctival scrapings
   d. histopathologic examination of organ biopsies
   e. analysis of pleural or peritoneal fluid

349. *Cats are renowned for their sensitivity to many chemical compounds. Which of the following can produce profound neurologic disturbances that frequently result in death of the animal?*
   a. benzyl alcohol
   b. fenbendazole
   c. pyrethrin-based flea products
   d. third-generation cephalosporins
   e. gentamicin

350. *Effusion from cats with feline infectious peritonitis are characterized by their:*

a. high protein content, lack of bacteria, and relatively high cellularity
b. high protein content, large numbers of bacteria, and relatively low cellularity
c. low protein content, lack of bacteria, and relatively low cellularity
d. low protein content, large numbers of bacteria, and relatively high cellularity
e. high protein content, lack of bacteria, and relatively low cellularity

351. *The most important source of feline leukemia virus in transmission to susceptible uninfected cats is:*

a. urine from an infected cat
b. saliva from an infected cat
c. contaminated food and water bowls used by an infected cat
d. bites of infected fleas
e. sexual contact with an infected cat

352. *Hyperthyroidism is common in older cats and is frequently accompanied by several characteristic electrocardiographic changes. These include all the following* ***except:***

a. sinus tachycardia
b. increased R wave amplitude
c. electrical alternans
d. atrial premature complexes
e. ventricular tachycardia

353. *In cats, bacterial endocarditis most commonly affects:*

a. the mitral valve
b. the pulmonic valve
c. the aortic valve
d. the tricuspid valve
e. all valves equally

354. *Pleural effusion is not normally detectable on radiographs until the fluid volume reaches approximately:*

a. 10 ml
b. 25 ml
c. 50 ml
d. 100 ml
e. 200 ml

355. *A cat is presented to your clinic for evaluation of a lesion on the toe. Histopathologic examination identifies the mass as a squamous-cell carcinoma. Of the following statements, which is* ***least*** *appropriate for educating the client about this lesion?*

a. This tumor is likely to respond to a combined chemotherapy protocol.
b. This tumor is likely to respond to local irradiation.
c. This tumor is likely to manifest invasive behavior.
d. In the absence of clinically demonstrable metastasis, local excision or limb amputation may be warranted to prolong life.
e. Squamous-cell carcinoma of the digit has a tendency to metastasize early.

356. *Concerning the insulin molecule of cats, which statement is most accurate?*

a. It is nearly identical to the insulin of cattle.
b. It is nearly identical to the insulin of pigs.
c. It is nearly identical to the insulin of fish.
d. It is nearly identical to the insulin of people.
e. Its structure has not been defined.

357. *Heartworm infection may go undiagnosed in cats because of vague, nonspecific signs. Which of the following is considered a useful test for feline heartworm infection?*

a. profound eosinophilia on a complete blood count
b. concentrating techniques, such as the Knott's test
c. diagnostic imaging (radiography, ultrasonography, nonselective angiography)
d. serologic tests for heartworm antibody
e. response to thiacetarsamide therapy

Correct answers are on pages 140-171.

358. *Concerning neoplasia in cats, which statement is **least** accurate?*

a. Lymphoma is the most common tumor of cats of all ages.
b. Lymphoma is a common hepatic neoplasm in cats of any age, regardless of feline leukemia virus status.
c. Squamous-cell carcinoma is the most common oral neoplasm of cats.
d. Colonic adenocarcinoma is the most common gastrointestinal neoplasm of cats.
e. Mammary tumors in cats are usually malignant.

359. *You work in a small animal practice in the midwestern United States and are presented with an adult indoor/outdoor intact male cat. The cat is in profound shock and has a low-grade fever. The cat soon dies despite your efforts. On necropsy you find blood pooled in the abdomen and petechial hemorrhages on the serosal surfaces of the organs. Some mesenteric vessels contain small thrombi. You evaluate a cytologic specimen obtained from the spleen and find small ringlike parasites in virtually all the macrophages. The most likely cause of disease in this cat is infection with:*

a. *Ehrlichia platys*
b. *Hemobartonella felis*
c. *Histoplasma capsulatum*
d. *Trypanosoma cruzi*
e. *Cytauxzoon felis*

360. *In cats, infectious conjunctivitis is **least** likely to be caused by:*

a. feline rhinotracheitis virus
b. feline calicivirus
c. *Mycoplasma*
d. *Chlamydia*
e. *Mycobacterium lepraemurium*

361. *Propylthiouracil had traditionally been the drug of choice for treatment of hyperthyroidism in cats. It has fallen into disfavor because of increasing recognition of its association with:*

a. immune-mediated hemolytic anemia
b. hypocalcemia
c. urolithiasis
d. congestive heart failure
e. diabetes insipidus

362. *The most common cause of lymphadenomegaly in cats is:*

a. lymphosarcoma
b. feline leukemia virus infection
c. extramedullary hematopoiesis in response to anemia
d. lymphoid hyperplasia
e. metastatic adenocarcinoma

363. *An apparently healthy young adult cat is brought to your clinic for ovariohysterectomy. Preoperative clinicopathologic screening tests reveal hyperglycemia and glucosuria. The most likely cause of these finding is:*

a. diabetes mellitus
b. Fanconi syndrome (proximal tubular resorptive defect)
c. hypoadrenocorticism
d. hyperadrenocorticism
e. stress

364. *Which viral antigen of the feline leukemia virus is associated with glomerulonephritis in some infected cats?*

a. gp70
b. p27
c. feline oncornavirus–associated cell membrane antigen (FOCMA)
d. p15e
e. reverse transcriptase enzyme

365. *Concerning feline immunodeficiency virus (FIV), which statement is most accurate?*

a. It is most common in the cattery setting.
b. It is more common in older cats.
c. It is known for rapid and aggressive tumor induction.
d. It is transmitted to people and can cause AIDS in people.
e. It is transmitted to kittens in utero or through the milk.

*366. Concerning the teeth of cats, which statement is **least** accurate?*

a. The deciduous incisors are the first teeth to erupt and are usually present in kittens by 2 weeks of age.
b. Full deciduous dentition is present by 7 to 8 weeks of age.
c. Full permanent dentition is present by 7 months of age.
d. Cats are diphyodont animals.
e. The upper carnassial tooth is the first molar.

367. Exocrine pancreatic insufficiency is not commonly recognized in cats. However, practitioners should be aware that the best means of diagnosis is:

a. serum trypsinlike immunoreactivity
b. 24-hour total fecal fat passage
c. para-aminobenzoic acid (PABA) absorption
d. fecal proteolytic enzyme activity
e. x-ray film digestion

368. Which drug is most likely to cause ototoxicity in cats?

a. tetracycline
b. erythromycin
c. acetaminophen
d. gentamicin
e. cefazolin

Questions 369 and 370

A cat is presented to you for evaluation of a coagulation defect. You find that the prothrombin time and partial thromboplastin time are about 2.5 times longer than in control samples. Serum fibrin degradation product values are normal.

369. This coagulopathy is most likely related to:

a. disseminated intravascular coagulation
b. deficiency of factor XII
c. deficiency of factor VIII
d. deficiency of factors, II, VII, IX, and X
e. von Willebrand's disease

370. The most likely underlying cause for the hemostatic defect in this cat is:

a. toxicity from an anticoagulant rodenticide
b. toxicity from a cholecalciferol rodenticide
c. aspirin intoxication
d. thrombotic disease caused by antithrombin III deficiency
e. a hereditary defect

371. You suspect cryptococcosis in a cat but cannot isolate the organisms. What is the best test to confirm your diagnosis?

a. agar-gel immunodiffusion
b. indirect fluorescent antibody test
c. electrophoresis of cerebrospinal fluid
d. latex agglutination
e. trypsinlike immunoreactivity

372. A colleague asks you for advice concerning a problem in a cattery. During the previous 6 months, three adult cats in the cattery have died. Histopathologic examination identified the cause of death as feline infectious peritonitis. Of 18 cats remaining in the cattery, six have positive titers for coronavirus. What is the most appropriate interpretation of this situation?

a. The seropositive cats probably have feline infectious peritonitis and should be euthanized.
b. The seropositive cats have been exposed to feline infectious peritonitis virus and should be isolated for 6 weeks and then retested.
c. The seropositive cats probably are infected with feline leukemia virus in addition to feline infectious peritonitis virus.
d. The antibodies in the seropositive cats are not necessarily antibodies to the coronavirus of feline infectious peritonitis.
e. Feline infectious peritonitis is enzootic in this cattery, and the establishment should be closed.

Correct answers are on pages 140-171.

373. *Which of the following represents the formula for permanent dentition in adults cats?*

a. $\frac{(3I\ 1C\ 3P\ 1M) \times 2}{(3I\ 1C\ 2P\ 1M) \times 2}$ = 30 total teeth

b. $\frac{(3I\ 1C\ 2P\ 2M) \times 2}{(3I\ 1C\ 2P\ 2M) \times 2}$ = 36 total teeth

c. $\frac{(3I\ 1C\ 3P\ 2M) \times 2}{(3I\ 1C\ 3P\ 2M) \times 2}$ = 36 total teeth

d. $\frac{(4I\ 1C\ 3P\ 1M) \times 2}{(4I\ 1C\ 3P\ 1M) \times 2}$ = 36 total teeth

e. $\frac{(3I\ 1C\ 2P\ 1M) \times 2}{(3I\ 1C\ 3P\ 1M) \times 2}$ = 30 total teeth

374. *Which of the following should* **not** *be used in cats with heart failure associated with decompensated hypertrophic cardiomyopathy?*

a. oxygen
b. intravenous fluids
c. nitroglycerin
d. aspirin
e. diltiazem

375. *Which of the following is the* **least** *likely clinical finding in a cat with lymphoma?*

a. cranial mediastinal mass
b. unilateral renomegaly
c. small-bowel diarrhea with weight loss
d. multicentric (generalized) lymphadenopathy
e. mesenteric lymphadenopathy

376. *Giardiasis in cats is effectively treated with:*

a. metronidazole, quinacrine, or furazolidone
b. ketoconazole, methylene blue, or polymixin B
c. methimazole, fenbendazole, or ivermectin
d. quinidine, atipamezole, or diltiazem
e. sucralfate, cimetidine, or ceftiofur

377. *What is the most common clinical sign of overly rapid intravenous infusion of blood products to cats?*

a. ataxia
b. bradycardia
c. vomiting
d. opisthotonos
e. diarrhea

378. *Acute blindness with bilateral retinal hemorrhage and detachment in a geriatric cat is most likely to be caused by:*

a. chronic renal disease
b. toxoplasmosis
c. coagulopathy
d. acute hepatitis
e. snake bite

379. *The most commonly reported arrhythmia in cats is:*

a. sinus bradycardia
b. ventricular tachycardia
c. atrial tachycardia
d. sinus tachycardia
e. sinus arrest or block

380. *Recognized forms of feline cardiomyopathy include all the following* ***except:***

a. excessive moderator band cardiomyopathy
b. hypertrophic cardiomyopathy
c. dilative cardiomyopathy
d. excessive chordae tendinae/papillary muscle cardiomyopathy
e. restrictive cardiomyopathy

381. *The most common cause of death in feline leukemia virus–infected cats with persistent viremia is:*

a. lymphosarcoma
b. myeloproliferative disease
c. nonregenerative anemia
d. immunosuppression and secondary infectious disease
e. squamous-cell carcinoma

382. *Macular melanosis on the lips and nose of orange tabby cats is called:*

a. vitiligo
b. chromboblastosis
c. lentigo simplex
d. poliosis
e. melanosarcoma

383. *Which bacterial population is most likely to be found in a cat with septic pleural effusion (pyothorax)?*
   a. predominantly one species of gram-positive aerobes
   b. mixed population of gram-positive aerobes
   c. predominantly one species of gram-negative aerobes
   d. predominantly one species of gram-negative anaerobes
   e. mixed population of gram-negative anaerobes

384. *Which of the following is **not** an appropriate part of diagnosis and management of pyothorax?*
   a. culture (aerobic, anaerobic) of the effusion
   b. Gram stain of the effusion
   c. search for an underlying cause
   d. thoracic drainage and lavage
   e. intrathoracic instillation of antibiotics

385. *Which antibacterial is most appropriate for a cat with the typical microbial population found in pyothorax?*
   a. metronidazole
   b. gentamicin
   c. trimethoprim-sulfa
   d. enrofloxacin
   e. amikacin

386. *One of the more common causes of progressive forebrain dysfunction in cats is:*
   a. toxoplasmosis
   b. bacterial meningitis
   c. hydrocephalus
   d. intracranial neoplasia
   e. head trauma

387. *Which test is particularly useful in differentiating hyperthyroid cats from cats with nonthyroidal disease and basal serum thyroxine levels in the high-normal range?*
   a. thyroxine stimulation
   b. combined thyroxine stimulation/dexamethasone suppression test
   c. thyroxine suppression
   d. triiodothyronine suppression
   e. thyroid-stimulating hormone stimulation

388. *Which flea species most commonly infests cats:*
   a. *Pulex irritans*
   b. *Ctenocephalides felis*
   c. *Ctenocephalides canis*
   d. *Echidnophaga gallinacea*
   e. *Leptopsylla segnis*

389. *Which of the following is the **least** appropriate method of resolving hypothermia in the postoperative period?*
   a. recirculating warm-water blanket
   b. warm inspired air
   c. intravenous fluids at normal body temperature
   d. warm blankets
   e. electric heating pad

390. *Which feline viruses are most difficult to destroy by disinfection with chlorhexidine?*
   a. herpesvirus and leukemia virus
   b. sarcoma virus and immunodeficiency virus
   c. calicivirus and parvovirus
   d. rabies virus and infectious peritonitis virus
   e. immunodeficiency virus and herpesvirus

391. *What is the most efficient means of transmission of* Toxoplasma gondii *to cats?*
   a. congenital (in utero)
   b. predation on another host infected with cysts
   c. inhalation of aerosolized oocysts
   d. ingestion of feces
   e. contamination of a bite wound by oocysts

392. *What is the best available test to detect active toxoplasmosis in cats?*
   a. paired serum IgG titers
   b. single serum IgM titer
   c. indirect fluorescent antibody test of blood for *Toxoplasma* antibodies
   d. fecal examination for oocysts
   e. necropsy and histologic examination

Correct answers are on pages 140-171.

393. *Which drug is **not** appropriate for treatment of cats with toxoplasmosis?*

a. pyrimethamine
b. clindamycin
c. methylene blue
d. sulfamethazine
e. sulfadiazine

394. *One of your clients is pregnant and plans to get rid of her cat because her doctor has mentioned problems associated with toxoplasmosis. She did hear, however, that periodic cleaning of the litter box can minimize the risk of human infection. To prevent oocyst sporulation, how often must the litter box be cleaned?*

a. every 72 hours
b. every 24 hours
c. every 96 hours
d. every 48 hours
e. weekly

395. *Portosystemic shunts are being diagnosed with increasing frequency in cats. Surgical repair of these shunts is generally quite complicated and is usually a referral procedure. However, the practitioner should be aware that most portosystemic shunts in cats are:*

a. multiple, extrahepatic, and acquired
b. multiple, intrahepatic, and acquired
c. single, extrahepatic, and congenital
d. single, intrahepatic, and congenital
e. multiple, intrahepatic, and congenital

396. *Clinical signs associated with a portosystemic shunt may be exacerbated by any of the following **except:***

a. high-protein diet
b. benzodiazepine tranquilizers
c. gastrointestinal bleeding
d. increased dietary levels of branched-chain amino acids
e. increased dietary levels of aromatic amino acids

397. *What form of cardiomyopathy in cats is caused by a dietary deficiency of taurine?*

a. hypertrophic cardiomyopathy
b. restrictive cardiomyopathy
c. dilative cardiomyopathy
d. excessive moderator band cardiomyopathy
e. defective endocardial cushion cardiomyopathy

398. *Which drug is most likely to induce fever in cats?*

a. tetracycline
b. aspirin
c. clindamycin
d. gentamicin
e. vancomycin

399. *Ischemic encephalopathy is a well-defined neurologic syndrome in cats. Which of the following is **not** a common clinical finding in affected cats?*

a. seizures
b. personality change
c. crossed-extensor reflex
d. jumping in the air
e. circling

400. *Feline immunodeficiency virus is classified as:*

a. an oncornavirus
b. a lentivirus
c. a sarcomavirus
d. a syncytium-forming virus
e. a spumavirus

401. *Chloramphenicol is a very effective antibiotic in some circumstances but must be used with caution in cats because of the potential for:*

a. delayed hypersensitivity (type IV)
b. methemoglobinemia
c. bronchoconstriction
d. dose-dependent bone marrow suppression
e. uncontrollable fever

402. *The maximum rate for safe intravenous infusion of potassium to cats is:*
   a. 0.25 mEq/kg/hr
   b. 0.5 mEq/kg/hr
   c. 0.75 mEq/kg/hr
   d. 1 mEq/kg/hr
   e. 5 mEq/kg/hr

403. *Which of the following is the* ***least*** *common congenital heart defect in cats?*
   a. patent ductus arteriosus
   b. ventricular septal defect
   c. endocardial cushion defect
   d. pulmonic stenosis
   e. mitral valve dysplasia

404. *What is the predominant distribution of the feline liver fluke,* Platynosomum concinnum?
   a. northwestern United States
   b. southwestern United States
   c. Great Lakes area of the United States
   d. Puerto Rico and Florida
   e. northwestern United States

405. *What is the drug of choice for treatment of liver fluke infection in cats?*
   a. thiabendazole
   b. levamisole
   c. praziquantel
   d. mebendazole
   e. pyrantel pamoate

406. *All the following may cause insulin resistance in diabetic cats* ***except:***
   a. growth hormone–secreting pituitary tumor
   b. hyperadrenocorticism
   c. hypothyroidism
   d. obesity
   e. megestrol acetate

407. *Which pathogen is* ***least*** *likely to be isolated from abscesses caused by cat bites?*
   a. *Pasteurella multocida*
   b. β-hemolytic streptococci
   c. *Fusobacterium*
   d. coagulase-positive staphylococci
   e. *Clostridium tetani*

408. *What is the most appropriate antibacterial for treatment of an abscess caused by a cat bite?*
   a. amoxicillin
   b. chloramphenicol
   c. amikacin
   d. enrofloxacin
   e. trimethoprim-sulfa

409. *What is the most common hepatic neoplasm of cats?*
   a. hemangiosarcoma
   b. hepatocellular carcinoma
   c. bile duct carcinoma
   d. lymphoma
   e. mast-cell tumor

410. *The most common adverse reaction to griseofulvin is:*
   a. bone marrow disturbance
   b. fever
   c. diarrhea
   d. methemoglobinemia
   e. Heinz-body hemolytic anemia

Questions 411 and 412

An adult female cat is presented to you for examination and treatment. The owner has observed the cat attempting to urinate frequently for the past 3 or 4 days. The cat appears to be straining. On physical examination, the cat is alert and has normal vital signs. The urinary bladder is small and firm. On abdominal palpation the cat appears quite uncomfortable and immediately voids about 3 ml of serosanguineous urine.

411. *What is the most likely cause of these signs?*
   a. obstructive feline urologic syndrome
   b. bladder tumor
   c. renal tumor
   d. nonobstructive feline urologic syndrome
   e. bacterial vaginitis

Correct answers are on pages 140-171.

412. *You obtain a urine sample by cystocentesis and submit it for culture and sensitivity tests. What is most likely to be found on culture?*

a. *Staphylococcus aureus*
b. *Escherichia coli*
c. *Streptococcus epidermidis*
d. *Staphylococcus intermedius*
e. no growth

413. *In cats, stomatitis and gingivitis frequently indicate underlying:*

a. general immunosuppression
b. heartworm disease
c. nasopharyngeal polyps
d. pyelonephritis
e. oral cancer

414. *In 1982, five cases of an apparently "new" disease of cats were reported. The illness was characterized by weight loss, depression, persistent pupillary dilation, constipation, decreased tear production, prolapsed nictitating membranes, and megaesophagus. This disease is now recognized as:*

a. feline dysautonomia
b. feline AIDS
c. Chédiak-Higashi syndrome
d. Hashimoto syndrome
e. Maroteaux-Lamy syndrome (mucopolysaccharidosis VI)

Questions 415 and 416

Your practice is located in California near the coastline. You are presented with an adult male cat that is quite depressed. In obtaining the history, you learn that the cat is owned by a fisherman and eats primarily fresh fish, especially tuna. The cat is febrile and hyperesthetic and greatly resents handling. You find a large, painful subcutaneous nodule in the inguinal area.

415. *What is the most likely cause of these signs?*

a. hypokalemic myopathy
b. immune-mediated myositis
c. subcutaneous foreign body
d. steatitis
e. aberrant dirofilariasis

416. *The most appropriate treatment for this cat is:*

a. vitamin A
b. vitamin E
c. thiamin
d. potassium
e. taurine

417. *Normal cats no longer have any deciduous teeth by what age?*

a. 2 months
b. 3 months
c. 4 months
d. 6 months
e. 10 months

418. *Thromboembolism associated with hypertrophic cardiomyopathy:*

a. should be surgically treated (embolectomy) as soon as possible
b. may occur anywhere in the body and is nearly always fatal
c. should not be treated with propranolol, because it may cause vasoconstriction
d. responds well to heparin therapy
e. occurs in more than 75% of all cardiomyopathic cats

419. *Concerning gastrointestinal lymphoma in cats, which statement is **least** accurate?*

a. It is commonly a B cell lymphoma.
b. It is more commonly associated with negative feline leukemia virus status than positive status.
c. It may cause signs attributable to malabsorptive or obstructive disease.
d. It is commonly associated with peripheral eosinophilia.
e. It is generally seen in older cats.

420. *Hyperthyroidism in cats is most commonly associated with:*

a. thyroid carcinoma
b. thyroid adenoma
c. thyroid adenocarcinoma
d. thyroid and parathyroid adenoma
e. *Spirocerca lupi* infection

421. *Tyzzer's disease is caused by:*

a. *Francisella tularensis*
b. *Yersinia pestis*
c. *Dermatophilus congolensis*
d. *Mycobacterium avium*
e. *Bacillus piliformis*

422. *Which paraneoplastic syndrome may be associated with an aggressive mast-cell tumor in cats?*

a. hypercalcemia
b. hypoglycemia
c. hyponatremia
d. gastric ulceration caused by hyperacidity
e. insulin secretion by the tumor

423. *What is the most appropriate fluid to administer intravenously to a ketoacidotic diabetic cat?*

a. 5% dextrose in water
b. 2.5% dextrose in water
c. 0.9% saline
d. 0.45% saline
e. 7% saline

424. *One of the more commonly reported findings in cats with hepatic encephalopathy is:*

a. extensor rigidity
b. ptyalism
c. glucosuria
d. increased serum urea nitrogen level
e. weight gain

425. *Which antimetabolite chemotherapeutic agent is extremely dangerous to cats and should* ***never*** *be given under any circumstance?*

a. bleomycin
b. cyclophosphamide
c. cytosine arabinoside
d. methotrexate
e. 5-fluorouracil

426. *Cats differ significantly from most other mammals in their ability to metabolize certain compounds. In large part, this is a result of greatly diminished ability to conjugate drugs to make them more water soluble and thus more easily eliminated from the body. A relative deficiency of which enzyme is responsible for this?*

a. glucuronyl transferase
b. methemoglobin reductase
c. myeloperoxidase
d. hepatic phosphofructokinase
e. pyruvate kinase

427. *Concerning alkaline phosphatase in cats, which statement is* ***least*** *accurate?*

a. It has a shorter half-life than in dogs.
b. It may be induced by glucocorticoid administration.
c. It has a low sensitivity but relatively good specificity for liver disease in the cat.
d. It is found in relatively lower concentrations in the feline liver compared with the canine liver.
e. It may be induced by cholestatic disease.

428. *The anticonvulsant of choice for long-term control of seizures in cats is:*

a. phenobarbital
b. phenytoin
c. diazepam
d. acepromazine
e. valproic acid

429. *In the process of bile acid metabolism in cats, bile acids are conjugated with:*

a. valine
b. leucine
c. tryptophan
d. methionine
e. taurine

Correct answers are on pages 140-171.

430. *The most common cause of lower-lip swelling ("pouting cat") is:*

a. eosinophilic plaque
b. eosinophilic linear granuloma
c. eosinophilic ulcer
d. food allergy
e. squamous-cell carcinoma

431. *Which of the following is **least** likely to cause splenomegaly in cats?*

a. lymphoma
b. myeloproliferative disease
c. hemobartonellosis
d. mast-cell tumor
e. hemangioma

432. *The most common louse found on cats is:*

a. *Hematopinus eurysternus*
b. *Linognathus pedalis*
c. *Linognathus setosus*
d. *Heterodoxus spiniger*
e. *Felicola subrostrata*

433. *The underlying cause of acute conjunctivitis is best diagnosed by:*

a. detailed history and thorough physical examination
b. culture of conjunctival sac specimens
c. fluorescein staining of corneal specimens
d. cytologic examination of conjunctival scrapings
e. response to treatment

434. *Cats are less susceptible to urinary tract infections than dogs because:*

a. cats have a higher urinary pH than dogs
b. cats have a lower urinary pH than dogs
c. cats have a higher urine osmolality than dogs
d. cats have a lower urine osmolality than dogs
e. cats urinate more frequently than dogs

435. *The drug of choice for treating hemobartonellosis is:*

a. prednisone
b. tetracycline or oxytetracycline
c. ketoconazole
d. thiacetarsamide
e. chloramphenicol

436. *A classic sign of acetaminophen intoxication in cats is:*

a. pulmonary edema
b. icterus caused by acute hepatic necrosis
c. cyanosis
d. acute renal failure
e. heart failure caused by toxic myocardial damage

437. *Removal of the spleen in cats favors the appearance of which organism in the peripheral blood?*

a. *Eperythrozoon felis*
b. *Hemobartonella felis*
c. *Ehrlichia platys*
d. *Anaplasma marginale*
e. *Babesia microti*

438. *Use of megestrol acetate in cats is associated with all the following side effects **except:***

a. diabetes mellitus
b. hyperthyroidism
c. mammary hypertrophy
d. mammary tumors
e. cystic endometritis

439. *In cats there is a strong association between left ventricular hypertrophy and:*

a. diabetes mellitus
b. uremic pericarditis
c. inflammatory bowel disease
d. hyperthyroidism
e. multicentric lymphosarcoma

440. *Common clinical signs of dilative or hypertrophic cardiomyopathy in cats include all the following **except:***

a. gallop rhythm
b. ascites
c. pleural effusion
d. pulmonary edema
e. heart murmur

441. *Which tissue is most commonly affected by cryptococcosis?*

a. skin
b. nasal passages
c. cervical lymph nodes
d. lungs
e. central nervous system

442. *A positive indirect fluorescent antibody test for feline leukemia virus indicates:*

a. release of p15e from ruptured viral particles into the serum
b. p15e in the cytoplasm of bone marrow–derived cells
c. p27 in the cytoplasm of bone marrow–derived cells
d. FOCMA on the surface of bone marrow–derived cells
e. p27 on the surface of lymphoid-derived cells

443. *Concerning notoedric mange, which statement is **least** accurate?*

a. It is contagious to other cats.
b. It is caused by a mite of the Sarcoptidae family.
c. It is a nonpruritic skin condition.
d. It may be safely treated with lime-sulfur dips.
e. Early lesions appear mostly on the head, neck, and ears.

444. *Hepatic lipidosis is a common liver disorder in cats. What is a common predisposing cause?*

a. liver entrapment in a diaphragmatic hernia
b. acetaminophen administration
c. chemotherapy with alkylating agents
d. stress and anorexia in an obese cat
e. exposure to organophosphates

445. *Miliary dermatitis has been associated with all the following **except:***

a. flea-bite hypersensitivity
b. dermatophytosis
c. atopy
d. *Cheyletiella* infestation
e. mycosis fungoides

446. *Feline leukemia virus is classified as:*

a. an oncornavirus
b. a spumavirus
c. a lentivirus
d. a sarcoma virus
e. a syncytium-forming virus

447. *Which of the following is **least** appropriate for intravenous fluid therapy in a hypovolemic hypotensive cat?*

a. 0.9% sales
b. lactated Ringer's solution
c. Ringer's solution
d. 5% dextrose in water
e. citrated Ringer's solution

448. *The most common clinical sign in cats with inflammatory bowel disease is:*

a. vomiting
b. increased appetite
c. decreased appetite
d. weight loss
e. diarrhea

449. *External odontoclastic resorptive lesions (cervical line lesions or neck lesions) are found in the teeth of many cats. Concerning these lesions, which statement is most accurate?*

a. The lesion is painless when touched by a dental probe.
b. The lesion is treated by subgingival curettage.
c. The lesion may be treated by glass ionomer restoration, copal varnish applications, fluoride application, or tooth extraction.
d. Once the lesion has been located with the dental probe, dental radiographs are unnecessary.
e. The lesion is associated with chronic morbillivirus infection of the gingivae.

Correct answers are on pages 140-171.

450. *Which finding is always considered abnormal in feline urine?*

a. lipid droplets
b. bilirubinuria
c. proteinuria
d. glucosuria
e. urobilinogen

451. *Which antineoplastic drug is uniformly fatal when given to cats?*

a. doxorubicin
b. vincristine
c. cisplatin
d. cyclophosphamide
e. vinblastine

452. *A major postoperative complication of bilateral thyroidectomy is:*

a. hypercalcemia
b. hypocalcemia
c. hypermagnesemia
d. hyperbilirubinemia
e. hyponatremia

453. *Insecticide toxicity is relatively common in cats. Toxicity with which of the following is responsive to treatment with atropine?*

a. lindane
b. pyrethrin
c. carbamate
d. lime-sulfur
e. chlordane

Questions 454 and 455

454. *In cats, long-term ingestion of a diet consisting predominantly of organ meats may lead to:*

a. hyperphosphatemia
b. hypercalcemia
c. vitamin A toxicosis
d. vitamin D toxicosis
e. vitamin B_1 (thiamin) toxicosis

455. *Clinical signs of the condition described in question 454 include all the following* ***except:***

a. exostoses of the cervical vertebrae
b. steatitis
c. loss of the incisor teeth
d. lameness
e. pain in long bones

456. *Concerning pseudorabies, which statement is most accurate?*

a. In cats it begins with excitement and in dogs with depression.
b. In cats it begins with depression and in dogs with excitement.
c. Affected cats usually die much later in the course of the disease than dogs.
d. Affected cats are usually much less pruritic than dogs.
e. There is no variation between the clinical presentation in affected dogs and cats.

457. *Concerning rabies, which statement is most accurate?*

a. Rabid cats are usually very aggressive.
b. Rabid cats are less of a public health risk than rabid dogs.
c. It is definitely diagnosed by lack of response to supportive care.
d. Rabies is caused by a paramyxovirus.
e. Prodromal signs of miosis and subnormal body temperature last 10 to 12 days.

Questions 458 through 460

You are presented with an adult cat that is extremely anemic. You place a drop of blood on a slide for microscopic examination, but the blood agglutinates before you can make a smear.

458. *What is a likely cause of such agglutination?*

a. immune-mediated hemolytic anemia
b. hypoproteinemia
c. hemobartonellosis
d. hypereosinophilic syndrome
e. von Willebrand's disease

459. *What the most appropriate course of action?*
   a. Perform direct and indirect Coombs' tests for antibodies to red blood cells.
   b. Apply a drop of saline to look for clot dispersion.
   c. Obtain a bone marrow aspirate to evaluate the erythroid precursors.
   d. Administer a blood transfusion if the hematocrit is less than 20%.
   e. Perform an antithrombin III test.

460. *You apply a drop of saline to the slide, and the cells do not disperse. What is the most appropriate course of action?*
   a. Perform direct and indirect Coombs' tests for antibodies to red blood cells.
   b. Obtain a bone marrow aspirate to evaluate the erythroid precursors.
   c. Initiate heparin therapy.
   d. Initiate aspirin therapy.
   e. Initiate corticosteroid therapy.

461. *The anemia of chronic disease is usually:*
   a. macrocytic hypochromic
   b. microcytic hypochromic
   c. normochromic normocytic
   d. macrocytic hyperchromic
   e. microcytic hyperchromic

462. *Which of the following typifies iron metabolism in the anemia of chronic disease?*
   a. Serum iron levels and bone marrow iron stores are both decreased.
   b. Serum iron levels and bone marrow iron stores are both increased.
   c. Serum iron levels are increased, and bone marrow iron stores are decreased.
   d. Serum iron levels are decreased, and bone marrow iron stores are increased.
   e. Serum iron levels and bone marrow iron stores vary, depending on the particular disease.

463. *Which of the following is **least** likely to cause generalized seizures in a 2-year-old male cat?*
   a. idiopathic epilepsy
   b. feline infectious peritonitis
   c. trauma
   d. ischemic encephalopathy
   e. primary brain tumor

464. *In cats the most common cause of a pleural effusion containing neoplastic cells is:*
   a. metastatic pancreatic adenocarcinoma
   b. bronchoalveolar carcinoma
   c. chemodectoma
   d. cranial mediastinal lymphoma
   e. mesothelioma

465. *You are presented with a kitten that has been ataxic since birth. The kitten has a wide-based stance, and its head bobs up and down. What is the most likely site of the neurologic lesion causing these signs?*
   a. spinal cord segments C7-T3
   b. cerebellum
   c. cerebral ventricles
   d. forebrain
   e. spinal cord segments T4-T13

466. *How many pairs of mammary glands are normally found in cats?*
   a. 3
   b. 4
   c. 5
   d. 6
   e. 2

467. *Concerning mammary tumors in cats, which statement is **least** accurate?*
   a. They are usually malignant.
   b. They are best treated with early excision.
   c. Most cats with mammary tumors die from metastatic disease.
   d. They are responsive to hormonal treatment.
   e. Most feline mammary tumors are adenocarcinomas.

Correct answers are on pages 140-171.

468. *When the triiodothyronine (T_3) suppression test is performed on a normal cat, the serum thyroxine (T_4) level:*

a. increases
b. remains unchanged
c. decreases
d. may increase or decrease
e. first decreases, and then increases

469. *Which ocular disorder is associated with taurine deficiency in cats?*

a. retinal detachment
b. glaucoma
c. central retinal degeneration
d. anterior uveitis
e. iris bombe

470. *What is the drug of choice to manage a hyperthyroid cat until thyroidectomy or radiation therapy?*

a. propylthiouracil
b. methimazole
c. thyroxine
d. antithyroglobulin antiserum
e. cisplatin

471. *Which drug may be used to enhance bladder tone in a cat with bladder atony after lower urinary tract obstruction has been relieved?*

a. diazepam
b. phenylpropanolamine
c. phenoxybenzamine
d. bethanechol
e. acepromazine

472. *Which part of the eye is most likely to show a granulomatous response to feline infectious peritonitis virus?*

a. lens
b. sclera
c. conjunctiva
d. cornea
e. uvea

473. *The average life span of an adult heartworm in a cat is:*

a. 6 months
b. 1 year
c. 2 years
d. 3 years
e. 5 years

474. *Which type of aggression against a person is most likely to be exhibited by a cat in a single-cat household?*

a. play
b. territorial
c. epileptic
d. fear
e. sexual

475. *What is the most significant complicating factor of viral upper respiratory tract infection in kittens?*

a. pneumonia
b. ulcerations in the oral cavity
c. secondary bacterial infection
d. serous nasal discharge
e. sneezing

476. *The normal depth of the gingival sulcus in adult cats is:*

a. 0 to 1 mm
b. 1.5 to 3 mm
c. 3 to 4 mm
d. 4 to 4.5 mm
e. 5 to 5.5 mm

477. *What is the most common nutritional disorder of cats?*

a. vitamin A deficiency
b. thiamin deficiency
c. protein deficiency
d. obesity
e. calcium deficiency

478. *Concerning hypereosinophilic syndrome in cats, which statement is **least** accurate?*

a. Adult cats are usually affected.
b. The bone marrow is frequently involved.
c. Vomiting, diarrhea, and weight loss result from bowel infiltration.
d. Clinical signs are well controlled with long-term prednisone therapy.
e. The prognosis for recovery is guarded.

479. *The most common cause of death in cats falling from heights (high-rise syndrome) is:*

a. cranial trauma
b. spinal cord trauma
c. rupture of abdominal viscera
d. open fractures of long bones
e. thoracic trauma

480. *Of the following veins, which is **least** likely to be used for intravenous catheterization in cats?*

a. jugular vein and cephalic vein
b. cephalic vein
c. lateral saphenous vein
d. medial saphenous vein
e. jugular vein and medial saphenous vein

481. *In cats, which drug is teratogenic when used at any stage of pregnancy?*

a. cimetidine
b. propylene glycol
c. griseofulvin
d. pyrantel pamoate
e. fenbendazole

482. *Most cases of uveitis in cats are associated with:*

a. feline infectious peritonitis, cryptococcosis, rhinotracheitis viral infection, or pneumonitis
b. feline infectious peritonitis, toxoplasmosis, or feline immunodeficiency virus infection
c. rhinotracheitis, calicivirus infection, feline immunodeficiency virus infection, or feline leukemia virus infection
d. feline infectious peritonitis, toxoplasmosis, feline immunodeficiency virus infection, feline leukemia virus infection, cryptococcosis, histoplasmosis, or blastomycosis
e. feline infectious peritonitis, feline leukemia virus infection, feline immunodeficiency virus infection, or upper respiratory viral infection

483. *Hemobartonellosis is caused by* Hemobartonella felis. *To which order does this organism belong?*

a. Rickettsiales
b. Mycoplasmatales
c. Chlamydiales
d. Eubacteriales
e. Pseudomonales

484. *Which drug is **least** likely to exacerbate liver disease in a cat?*

a. diazepam
b. dioctyl sodium sulfylsuccinate
c. acepromazine
d. methionine
e. tetracycline

485. *Which nematode may inhabit the stomach and cause gastritis in cats?*

a. *Toxascaris leonina*
b. *Ollulanus tricuspis*
c. *Ancylostoma tubaeformae*
d. *Strongyloides stercoralis*
e. *Trichinella spiralis*

486. *Adequate urine-concentrating ability is signified by a urine specific gravity greater than:*

a. 1.025
b. 1.030
c. 1.010
d. 1.020
e. 1.035

Correct answers are on pages 140-171.

487. *An adult male cat has a peculiar plantigrade stance of the pelvic limbs. The hocks are dropped down, and the cat appears to be walking flat footed. The owner reports that the cat has a healthy appetite but continues to lose weight and has been drinking a bit more water than as a young adult. What is the most likely cause of these signs?*

a. hyperthyroidism
b. hypothyroidism
c. diabetes insipidus
d. diabetes mellitus
e. myasthenia gravis

488. *You are presented with a 5-month-old kitten found near a garbage container. The kitten appears malnourished and debilitated. Physical examination reveal two small holes in the skin, one behind the ear and the other under the neck. The holes are well circumscribed and exude a small amount of serosanguineous fluid. You see a small brown speck in the middle of each hole. What is the likely cause of this peculiar finding?*

a. wasp or bee sting
b. bite wounds that have abscessed and drained
c. cuterebriasis
d. aberrant migration of heartworm microfilariae
e. paragonimiasis

489. *Which of the following is* ***least*** *likely to produce icterus in cats?*

a. toxoplasmosis
b. feline infectious peritonitis
c. diabetes mellitus
d. hepatic lipidosis
e. cholangiohepatitis complex

490. *The "fading kitten" syndrome is generally attributed to:*

a. T lymphocyte hyperplasia
b. B lymphocyte deficiency
c. acute lymphoblastic leukemia
d. thymic atrophy
e. neutrophil function defect

491. *The drug of choice for treatment of nocardiosis in cats is:*

a. trimethoprim-sulfa
b. chloramphenicol
c. ampicillin
d. enrofloxacin
e. dexamethasone

492. *All the following are normal findings on the hemogram of cats* ***except:***

a. Heinz bodies
b. Howell-Jolly bodies
c. spherocytes
d. smaller mean corpuscular volume than in dogs
e. platelet numbers equal to those in dogs

493. *The most common tapeworm in cats is:*

a. *Echinococcus granulosus*
b. *Echinococcus multilocularis*
c. *Dipylidium caninum*
d. *Taenia taeniaeformis*
e. *Anoplocephala perfoliata*

494. *The cause of feline viral rhinotracheitis is a :*

a. herpesvirus
b. calicivirus
c. retrovirus
d. parvovirus
e. paramyxovirus

495. *Which organism is most commonly isolated from the uterus of cats with pyometra?*

a. *Escherichia coli*
b. *Pseudomonas aeruginosa*
c. *Pasteurella multocida*
d. *Proteus vulgaris*
e. *Fusobacterium necrophorum*

496. *What is the most common oral tumor in cats?*

a. squamous-cell carcinoma
b. malignant melanoma
c. lymphoma
d. fibrosarcoma
e. mast-cell tumor

497. *Accumulation of oily exudate over the tail head and on the tail of cats is termed:*

a. brushy tail
b. feline acne
c. stud tail
d. grease tail
e. comedone equinus

498. *Which drug combats the adverse metabolic effects of hyperkalemia but does **not** reduce serum potassium levels?*

a. sodium bicarbonate
b. glucose
c. insulin
d. calcium gluconate
e. prednisolone

Questions 499 and 500

499. *A blue smoke Persian cat has green irides, red fundic reflections, a propensity to bleed after venipuncture, and intracytoplasmic inclusions in neutrophils. This combination of findings comprises the:*

a. Pelger-Hüet anomaly
b. Chédiak-Higashi syndrome
c. Hashimoto syndrome
d. Klinefelter's syndrome
e. lentigo simplex syndrome

500. *Concerning the Persian cat in question 499, which statement is most accurate?*

a. The cat is likely to die of unregulated diabetes mellitus.
b. The cat is likely to be positive for feline leukemia virus on indirect fluorescent antibody testing of bone marrow.
c. The cat is likely to be sterile.
d. The cat is prone to recurrent infections.
e. The cat is likely to develop irreversible blindness.

R.G. Sherding

501. *Which infection is characterized by large intracytoplasmic inclusion bodies within epithelial cells from a conjunctival scraping of a cat?*

a. herpesviral infection
b. coronaviral infection
c. chlamydial infection
d. mycoplasmal infection
e. caliciviral infection

502. *Ulcerative keratitis is most likely to occur in a cat infected with:*

a. feline herpesvirus
b. feline coronavirus
c. *Chlamydia*
d. *Bordetella*
e. feline calicivirus

503. *Tongue ulceration in cats is most characteristic of infection with:*

a. *Mycoplasma*
b. *Bordetella*
c. feline calicivirus
d. *Chlamydia*
e. feline herpesvirus

504. *Concerning respiratory infections in cats, which statement is most accurate?*

a. Feline calicivirus has a predilection for the epithelium of the upper respiratory tract.
b. Feline caliciviral infection often causes ulceration of the cornea.
c. Chlamydial infection (pneumonitis) typically causes severe pneumonia.
d. Virulent strains of feline calicivirus have an affinity for the lung and often produce primary viral pneumonia.
e. Conjunctival involvement is unlikely in herpesviral infection.

Correct answers are on pages 140-171.

505. *A 4-month-old male domestic short-hair kitten has anorexia, a fever (103.8° F), marked mucopurulent oculonasal discharge, paroxysmal sneezing, a hacking cough, and excessive salivation. The most likely cause of these signs is infection with:*

a. feline calicivirus
b. *Mycoplasma*
c. feline herpesvirus
d. *Chlamydia*
e. feline reovirus

506. *Which feline virus, when latent, can be reactivated by stress in chronic carriers?*

a. panleukopenia virus
b. calicivirus
c. feline infectious peritonitis (FIP) virus
d. herpesvirus
e. enteric coronavirus

507. *Which drug is most effective for topical treatment of chlamydial conjunctivitis in cats:*

a. idoxuridine
b. gentamicin
c. polymixin B
d. tetracycline
e. prednisolone

508. *Which drug is a specific treatment for herpesviral keratitis in cats?*

a. idoxuridine
b. levamisole
c. chloramphenicol
d. tetracycline
e. prednisolone

509. *Which form of lymphoma is relatively uncommon in cats as compared with dogs?*

a. peripheral lymph node
b. mediastinal
c. hepatic
d. splenic
e. intestinal

510. *A cat tests positive for feline leukemia virus (FeLV) infection by enzyme-linked immunosorbent assay (ELISA) but tests negative by indirect fluorescent antibody (IFA) testing. Which of the following is **not** a possible explanation of these results?*

a. early transient FeLV infection
b. compartmentalized lymphoid infection
c. FeLV infection without active replication in bone marrow
d. laboratory error
e. latent (nonreplicating) FeLV infection

511. *Which of the following is **least** likely to be found in a cat with anemia related to feline leukemia virus infection?*

a. hematocrit below 12%
b. concurrent hemobartonellosis
c. positive Coombs' test
d. microcytic erythrocytes
e. hypoplastic bone marrow

512. *The principal cause of false-positive results of enzyme-linked immunosorbent assay for feline leukemia virus is:*

a. the virus's cross reactivity with feline calicivirus
b. use of serum instead of whole blood
c. use of outdated reagents
d. use of monoclonal antibody reagents
e. technical error in performing the test

513. *Feline leukemia virus is primarily transmitted via:*

a. fleas
b. feces
c. saliva
d. respiratory secretions
e. soil

514. *With which form of feline leukemia virus–induced neoplasia are cats* **least** *likely to be viremic?*

a. mediastinal lymphoma
b. intestinal lymphoma
c. multicentric lymphoma
d. nervous system lymphoma
e. myeloproliferative disorder

515. *In a small animal practice, which measure is* **least** *likely to reduce the rate of false-positive results of enzyme-linked immunosorbent assay (ELISA) for feline leukemia virus?*

a. use of the saliva test
b. use of serum instead of whole blood
c. use of the filter membrane format instead of the microwell format
d. use of very thorough washing steps in the procedure
e. use of ELISA kits with monoclonal instead of polyclonal antibody reagents

516. *Latent (nonreplicating) infection with feline leukemia virus is detected by:*

a. indirect fluorescent antibody (IFA) test
b. enzyme-lined immunosorbent assay (ELISA)
c. antibody titer against feline oncornavirus-associated cell membrane antigen
d. reactivation of virus from cultured bone marrow cells
e. virus-neutralizing antibody titer

517. *Veterinarians often confirm in-office results of enzyme-linked immunosorbent assay (ELISA) for feline leukemia virus by sending a serum sample to a diagnostic laboratory for indirect fluorescent antibody (IFA) testing. Which of the following is the most common discrepancy ("discordancy") between test results?*

a. microwell ELISA negative, IFA positive
b. microwell ELISA positive, IFA negative
c. membrane filter ELISA negative, IFA positive
d. membrane filter ELISA positive, IFA negative
e. saliva ELISA negative, IFA positive

518. *Assuming the tests are performed properly, which statement concerning testing for feline leukemia virus (FeLV) is* **least** *accurate?*

a. The indirect fluorescent antibody test detects cell-associated viremia.
b. The enzyme-linked immunosorbent assay detects viral antigen in blood, saliva, or tears.
c. The enzyme-linked immunosorbent assay is almost always positive if the direct fluorescent antibody test is positive.
d. The indirect fluorescent antibody test is almost always negative if the enzyme-linked immunosorbent assay is negative.
e. The indirect fluorescent antibody test usually becomes positive before the enzyme-linked immunosorbent assay becomes positive in the early stages of FeLV infection.

519. *Which form of lymphoma is most likely to occur in old cats?*

a. mediastinal
b. intestinal
c. peripheral lymph node
d. cutaneous
e. ocular

520. *Feline immunodeficiency virus is transmitted primarily via:*

a. urine
b. feces
c. saliva
d. milk
e. sexual contact

Correct answers are on pages 140-171.

521. *Concerning the routine enzyme-linked immunosorbent assay for feline immunodeficiency virus (FIV), which statement is most accurate?*

   a. It detects circulating FIV antigen in serum as an indication of current active infection.
   b. It detects FIV antigen in circulating lymphocytes as an indication of current active infection.
   c. It detects FIV antigen in saliva as an indication of current active infection and viral shedding.
   d. It detects circulating anti-FIV antibody as an indication of current and lifelong active infection.
   e. It detects circulating anti-FIV antibody as an indication of prior exposure and subsequent immune rejection of the virus.

522. *Infection with feline immunodeficiency virus is most commonly manifested as:*

   a. diarrhea
   b. gingivitis-stomatitis
   c. anterior uveitis
   d. jaundice
   e. urinary tract infection

523. *Which of the following is most compatible with the effusive ("wet") form of feline infectious peritonitis (FIP)?*

   a. suppurative exudate
   b. transudate
   c. serosanguineous effusion
   d. pyrogranulomatous exudate
   e. modified transudate

524. *The hallmark of feline infectious peritonitis is widespread vasculitis. Which of the following is most important in the pathogenesis of vasculitis in this disease?*

   a. deposition of antigen-antibody complexes in vessel walls
   b. direct viral attack on vascular endothelium
   c. formation of autoantibodies directed against vessel basement membranes
   d. fibrin deposition in the microcirculation, leading to vascular damage and disseminated intravascular coagulation
   e. vascular injury caused by toxins released from the virus

525. *The most common ocular manifestation of feline infectious peritonitis is:*

   a. ulcerative keratitis
   b. anterior uveitis
   c. conjunctivitis
   d. Horner's syndrome
   e. retrobulbar swelling

526. *Concerning feline coronaviral titers (so-called "feline infectious peritonitis antibody test"), which statement is most accurate?*

   a. It is rare for a healthy cat to have a positive titer on this test.
   b. Because a positive titer is highly specific for feline infectious peritonitis, this test is used to confirm the diagnosis.
   c. The major pitfall of this test is a high frequency of false-negative results, that is, negative titers in cats that are actually infected with the virus.
   d. This test should not be used to cull animals from a cattery on a "test and removal" basis.
   e. Intranasal vaccination with the commercial feline infectious peritonitis vaccine consistently produces high serum titers.

527. *Concerning feline coronaviral titers (so-called "feline infectious peritonitis antibody test"), which statement is **least** accurate?*

   a. The test also detects cross-reacting antibodies against feline enteric coronavirus, but this virus is very rare in the cat population.
   b. Evaluating paired serum samples for a rising antibody titer is not a reliable means of diagnosing feline infectious peritonitis.
   c. A few cats with documented feline infectious peritonitis may not have a coronaviral titer.
   d. The test should not be used in "test and cull" programs in catteries, because the test for feline leukemia virus is used.
   e. The feline infectious peritonitis virus antibody titer does not measure a protective immune response.

528. *What is the most common source of* Toxoplasma *infection in cats?*

a. raw meat
b. cat feces
c. soil
d. transplacental transmission
e. direct contact

529. *Concerning toxoplasmosis in cats, which statement is* ***least*** *accurate?*

a. Asymptomatic infection is more common than clinical infection.
b. Ingestion of raw meat containing *Toxoplasma* cysts is the most common source of infection in cats.
c. Shedding of fecal oocysts only occurs in cats.
d. Clindamycin is the drug of choice for treatment.
e. A single high serum IgG *Toxoplasma* antibody titer indicates active infection.

530. *The drug of choice for treating hemobartonellosis in cats is:*

a. ampicillin
b. cephalosporin
c. trimethoprim-sulfa
d. tetracycline
e. erythromycin

531. *Which fungal organism appears in feline cytologic specimens as a budding yeast with a distinctive thick, nonstaining, polysaccharide capsule?*

a. *Cryptococcus neoformans*
b. *Blastomyces dermatitidis*
c. *Coccidioides immitis*
d. *Histoplasma capsulatum*
e. *Aspergillus fumigatus*

532. *Which organism is* ***not*** *associated with anterior uveitis in cats?*

a. *Cryptococcus*
b. *Toxoplasma*
c. feline infectious peritonitis virus
d. *Chlamydia*
e. feline leukemia virus

533. *Cerebellar hypoplasia in kittens is caused by perinatal infection with:*

a. panleukopenia virus
b. herpesvirus
c. calicivirus
d. feline infectious peritonitis coronavirus
e. feline leukemia virus

534. *Feline enteric coronavirus is important because of the confusion it causes in laboratory testing for which other organism infecting cats?*

a. *Toxoplasma*
b. herpesvirus
c. feline infectious peritonitis virus
d. feline leukemia virus
e. *Chlamydia*

535. *Which oral antifungal drug is effective for treatment of histoplasmosis in cats?*

a. miconazole
b. amphotericin B
c. clotrimazole
d. 5-fluorocytosine
e. ketoconazole

536. *Hyperglobulinemia is a common clinical finding in cats with:*

a. herpesviral infection
b. cryptococcosis
c. panleukopenia
d. toxoplasmosis
e. feline infectious peritonitis

Correct answers are on pages 140-171.

537. *Concerning feline leukemia virus (FeLV) vaccination, which statement is most accurate?*

a. Vaccine side effects are mostly a reaction to the adjuvants used.
b. Most FeLV vaccines contain live virus, although the virus is attenuated for safety.
c. All FeLV vaccines induce anti-FOCMA (feline oncornavirus cell membrane antigen) antibody titers indicative of antitumor immunity.
d. FeLV testing before vaccination is recommended because vaccination of an FeLV-positive cat hastens progression of the disease.
e. Vaccine trials have shown consistently that nearly 100% of vaccinated cats are protected against FeLV challenge, regardless of the brand of vaccine used.

538. *In a cat with respiratory signs, a history of recent exposure to other cats in a multicat household environment is most important relative to increased risk of:*

a. thoracic trauma
b. exposure to fungi causing systemic mycoses
c. exposure to viruses
d. exposure to lungworm eggs or larvae
e. exposure to animal-derived allergens

539. *Concerning bronchial asthma in cats, which statement is* ***least*** *accurate?*

a. Typical presenting signs include chronic cough, wheezing, and dyspnea.
b. Air bronchograms are the most characteristic radiographic abnormality.
c. Hematologic examination sometimes reveals eosinophilia.
d. Effective treatment can include corticosteroids and bronchodilators.
e. The pathogenesis involves small-airway obstruction from bronchiolar smooth muscle contraction, bronchiolar inflammation, and intraluminal accumulation of mucus and exudate.

540. *Which drug is a sympathomimetic bronchodilator used in treatment of bronchial asthma in cats?*

a. theophylline
b. terbutaline
c. butorphanol
d. isopropamide
e. bethanecol

541. *Which drug is indicated for treatment of a cat with acute bronchial asthma?*

a. aminophylline
b. furosemide
c. propranolol
d. butorphanol
e. acepromazine

542. *In cats, polyps occur most often at which site?*

a. external nares
b. frontal sinus
c. nasopharynx
d. larynx
e. trachea

543. *Chronic granulomatous pulmonary disease with extensive fibrosis in cats is caused by:*

a. bacterial pneumonia
b. allergic pulmonary reaction
c. lungworm infection
d. mineral oil inhalation
e. smoke inhalation

544. *Cytologic examination of a transtracheal aspirate (airway washing) in a cat reveals predominantly eosinophils. The most likely cause of this finding is:*

a. bronchial asthma
b. nonspecific irritant bronchitis
c. pulmonary blastomycosis
d. aspiration pneumonia
e. bacterial bronchopneumonia

545. *Which bacteria are most consistently associated with pyothorax in cats?*

a. *Escherichia coli* and *Bacillus pisiformis*
b. streptococci and staphylococci
c. *Klebsiella* and *Rhodococcus*
d. *Pseudomonas* and *Corynebacterium*
e. anaerobic bacteria

546. *Radiographs of a cat reveal pleural effusion associated with a right middle lung lobe that is completely opaque. The most likely cause of these findings is:*

a. bronchopneumonia
b. aspiration pneumonia
c. chronic obstructive airway disease
d. lung lobe torsion
e. chylofibrosis

547. *In cats, thoracic lavage and drainage via chest tube are most appropriate for treatment of:*

a. pneumothorax
b. mediastinal lymphosarcoma
c. feline infectious peritonitis
d. pyothorax
e. chylothorax

548. *Most pleural effusions in cats are bilateral. Which disorder is most likely to cause unilateral pleural effusion?*

a. dilative cardiomyopathy
b. feline infectious peritonitis
c. mediastinal lymphoma
d. pyothorax
e. chylothorax

549. *In cats, decreased compliance of the cranial thorax on palpation is most commonly associated with:*

a. pneumomediastinum
b. pleural effusion
c. rib fracture
d. mediastinal lymphoma
e. rib tumor

550. *Increased resonance (increased tympany) on thoracic percussion of a cat typically indicates:*

a. pleural effusion
b. diaphragmatic hernia
c. consolidating pneumonia
d. intrathoracic neoplasia
e. pneumothorax

551. *In a cat, which clinical observation could be described as orthopnea?*

a. abnormal increase in the depth of respiration
b. abnormal increase in the rate of breathing
c. inability to breathe comfortably except in an upright (sitting or sternal) position, which allows maximal caudal excursion of the diaphragm
d. shallow, choppy restrictive breathing usually caused by painful breathing from rib fractures, pleuritis, etc.
e. difficult or labored breathing

552. *Aspiration pneumonia in cats is most often associated with:*

a. heartworm disease
b. esophageal disease
c. lungworm infection
d. thoracic trauma
e. tracheal collapse

553. *Which of the following is most effective in preventing retention of respiratory secretions and inspissation of airway mucus in an animal with severe pneumonia?*

a. antitussive drugs
b. fluid therapy to maintain systemic hydration
c. diuretics to reduce fluid retention
d. atropine to "dry up" secretions
e. cage rest to restrict exercise

554. *Which fungus has a predilection for the feline nasal cavity?*

a. *Histoplasma*
b. *Blastomyces*
c. *Coccidioides*
d. *Cryptococcus*
e. *Pythium (Hyphomyces)*

Correct answers are on pages 140-171.

555. *In cats, laryngeal paralysis is diagnosed by:*

a. radiography
b. blood gas analysis
c. auscultation
d. direct observation of the laryngeal orifice during breathing
e. cytologic examination of airway aspirates

556. *In a cat, a regimen consisting of a bronchodilator, a diuretic, and oxygen is most appropriate for treatment of:*

a. bronchial asthma
b. electrocution injury
c. pyothorax
d. traumatic hemothorax
e. bacterial pneumonia

557. *In which of the following would treatment with a bronchodilator alone be expected to produce the most rapid and pronounced improvement in a cat with respiratory disease?*

a. bronchial asthma
b. aelurostrongylosis
c. tracheobronchial foreign body
d. bacterial bronchopneumonia
e. noncardiogenic pulmonary edema

558. *Respiratory failure associated with paradoxic respirations is most likely to occur in a cat with:*

a. intercostal muscle avulsion
b. open pneumothorax
c. flail chest
d. tension pneumothorax
e. diaphragmatic hernia

559. *Which clinical manifestation is* ***least*** *likely in a cat with a lung tumor?*

a. pleural effusion
b. hemoptysis
c. dyspnea
d. stridor
e. cough

560. *A cat develops respiratory distress, subcutaneous emphysema, and pneumomediastinum after being hit by a car. The most likely injury underlying these signs is:*

a. tracheobronchial laceration
b. diaphragmatic hernia
c. rib fracture
d. flail chest
e. rupture of pulmonary alveoli

561. *Abrupt onset of unilateral nasal signs is most consistent with:*

a. viral rhinitis
b. allergic rhinitis
c. nasal tumor
d. nasal foreign body
e. nasal cryptococcosis

562. *Concerning* Campylobacter *infection, which statement is* ***least*** *accurate?*

a. Dogs and cats may carry *Campylobacter* asymptomatically.
b. Because *Campylobacter* is very species specific, there is minimal chance of animal-to-human transmission.
c. *Campylobacter* is difficult to isolate in culture and requires specialized selective media.
d. Microscopic examination of feces may be used for presumptive diagnosis of *Campylobacter* infection.
e. Erythromycin or neomycin is usually an effective treatment.

563. *For which feline diarrheal disease is metronidazole* ***not*** *an appropriate choice for therapy?*

a. giardiasis
b. salmonellosis
c. small intestinal bacterial overgrowth
d. chronic colitis
e. lymphocytic-plasmacytic inflammatory bowel disease

564. *Which disease of cats is best treated with sulfasalazine?*

a. salmonellosis
b. campylobacteriosis
c. giardiasis
d. chronic colitis
e. small intestinal bacterial overgrowth

565. *Which clinical sign is **least** likely to be associated with large-bowel diarrhea in a cat?*

a. urgency and frequency of defecation
b. melena
c. tenesmus (straining to defecate)
d. abundant mucus in the feces
e. frank red blood in the feces

566. *Duodenal ulcers caused by gastric hypersecretion of acid have been associated with which nonenteric neoplasm in cats?*

a. mastocytoma
b. thyroid adenoma
c. hemangiosarcoma
d. mammary adenocarcinoma
e. pulmonary adenocarcinoma

567. *The predominant inflammatory cell found in lesions of inflammatory bowel disease of cats is the:*

a. neutrophil
b. eosinophil
c. lymphocyte
d. macrophage
e. mast cell

568. *You find a fibrous, stricturelike stenotic lesion in the distal ileum of a 12-year-old cat with anorexia, chronic weight loss, and occasional vomiting. The most likely cause of this finding is:*

a. intestinal adenocarcinoma
b. intestinal lymphoma
c. intestinal histoplasmosis
d. eosinophilic enteritis
e. salmonellosis

569. *Severe life-threatening fluid and electrolyte losses requiring intensive intravenous fluid therapy are most likely to occur in a cat with:*

a. acute viral diarrhea
b. exocrine pancreatic insufficiency
c. chronic colitis
d. lymphocytic-plasmacytic enteritis
e. ascarid infection

570. *Narcotic analgesic opioids, such as lopermide and diphenoxylate, combat diarrhea by:*

a. enhancing intestinal peristalsis
b. inhibiting prostaglandins
c. decreasing rhythmic segmentation contractions of the gut
d. anticholinergic (parasympatholytic) activity
e. prolonging intestinal transit and inhibiting loss of fluid through the gut mucosa

571. *Dietary hypersensitivity has been associated with which feline enteropathy?*

a. lymphangiectasia
b. regional granulomatous enteritis
c. small intestinal bacterial overgrowth
d. lymphocytic-plasmacytic inflammatory bowel disease
e. lipofuscinosis

572. *Concerning lymphocytic-plasmacytic inflammatory bowel disease, which statement is most accurate?*

a. Only the small intestine is affected.
b. Dietary management does not play a role in treatment.
c. Endoscopy is not usually adequate for demonstrating lesions; full-thickness biopsies obtained at laparotomy are usually required.
d. The results of upper gastrointestinal barium radiography are usually unremarkable.
e. Costicosteroids should be avoided because of the risk of bacterial overgrowth.

Correct answers are on pages 140-171.

573. *In cats, oral lactulose is an effective treatment for:*

a. diarrhea
b. urinary tract infection
c. vomiting
d. anorexia
e. constipation

574. *Increased fecal mucus in cats is most likely to be associated with:*

a. gastric polyps
b. colitis
c. tapeworm infection
d. small intestinal bacterial overgrowth
e. pancreatitis

575. *In cats the most effective treatment for chronic recurrent obstipation associated with idiopathic megacolon is:*

a. intermittent phosphate enemas
b. low-fiber diet
c. mineral oil laxatives
d. cholinergic drugs
e. subtotal colectomy

576. *Which serum chemistry value is most likely to be* ***abnormal*** *in a cat with a congenital portosystemic shunt?*

a. alanine aminotransferase
b. albumin
c. bile acids
d. alkaline phosphatase
e. bilirubin

577. *Which liver disease is* ***not*** *a cause of jaundice in cats?*

a. hepatic lipidosis
b. cholangiohepatitis
c. hepatic lymphoma
d. pyogranulomatous hepatitis associated with feline infectious peritonitis
e. corticosteroid-induced hepatopathy

578. *Concerning serum alkaline phosphatase activity in cats, which statement is the* ***least*** *accurate?*

a. Elevated serum alkaline phosphatase activity indicates hepatic cholestasis.
b. Elevations of serum alkaline phosphatase activity in cats are generally of lesser magnitude than in dogs.
c. Serum alkaline phosphatase activity is frequently elevated in cats with idiopathic hepatic lipidosis syndrome.
d. Serum alkaline phosphatase activity is usually normal in cats with congenital portosystemic shunts.
e. Corticosteroid therapy causes elevated serum alkaline phosphatase activity in cats.

579. *Which anticonvulsant drug should* ***not*** *be used in cats?*

a. phenobarbital
b. phenytoin
c. diazepam
d. primidone
e. lorazepam

580. *Which electrolyte disturbance is most likely to be life threatening in a cat with urethral obstruction?*

a. hypocalcemia
b. hypokalemia
c. hyperkalemia
d. hyponatremia
e. hypernatremia

581. *What is the most common cause of dermatophytosis (ringworm) in kittens?*

a. *Microsporum canis*
b. *Microsporum gypseum*
c. *Microsporum audouinii*
d. *Trichophyton mentagrophytes*
e. *Trichophyton terrestre*

582. *Concerning acetaminophen toxicosis in cats, which statement is **least** accurate?*

a. Methemoglobinemia with cyanosis and acute respiratory distress may occur.
b. Heinz-body hemolytic anemia may occur.
c. An overdosage far exceeding the human dosage is required to produce toxicosis in cats.
d. Prolonged exposure to the drug may cause liver damage and jaundice.
e. *N*-acetylcysteine can be given for treatment of acute toxicosis.

583. *A cat with anorexia, depression, and vomiting has a blood urea nitrogen level of 98 mg/dl, serum phosphorus level of 11 mg/dl, serum calcium level of 7.3 mg/dl, total plasma protein level of 8.2 g/dl, and urine specific gravity of 1.066. The most likely mechanism underlying azotemia in this cat is:*

a. dehydration
b. acute primary renal failure
c. urinary tract obstruction
d. chronic renal failure
e. renal lymphoma

584. *Which of the following is **not** a manifestation of taurine deficiency in cats?*

a. dilative cardiomyopathy
b. central retinal degeneration
c. reproductive failure
d. cirrhosis
e. growth deformities in kittens

585. *Hypokalemia-induced "hanging head syndrome" is most likely to occur in a cat with:*

a. feline leukemia virus infection
b. hyperthyroidism
c. chronic renal failure
d. lower urinary tract disease ("feline urologic syndrome")
e. inflammatory bowel disease

586. *Hyperthyroidism in cats can be successfully controlled with:*

a. cyclophosphamide, vincristine, or thyroidectomy
b. prednisolone, iodine radioisotope, or thyroidectomy
c. methimazole, iodine radioisotope, or thyroidectomy
d. thyroxine, prednisone, or iodine radioisotope
e. somatostatin, cyclosporine, or cisplatin

587. *In cats what is the most common cardiac manifestation of hyperthyroidism?*

a. hypertrophic cardiomyopathy
b. mitral valve insufficiency caused by endocardiosis
c. pericardial effusion
d. dilative cardiomyopathy
e. sinus bradycardia

588. *Which of the following is **not** a typical manifestation of hyperthyroidism in cats?*

a. polydipsia and polyuria
b. diarrhea
c. weight loss
d. ravenous appetite
e. hepatic encephalopathy

589. *Which of the following is **not** a likely effect of corticosteroid treatment in cats?*

a. polyuria and polydipsia
b. increased appetite
c. elevated serum alkaline phosphatase activity
d. gluconeogenesis
e. suppression of inflammation

590. *Concerning diabetes mellitus in cats, which statement is most accurate?*

a. Diabetes mellitus is most prevalent in female cats.
b. Diabetic ketoacidosis does not occur in cats.
c. Diabetic cats always require daily insulin injections to maintain normoglycemia.
d. Insulin injections in cats typically have a longer duration of action than in dogs.
e. Cats do not develop diabetic cataracts.

Correct answers are on pages 140-171.

591. *In cats, diabetes mellitus may result from treatment with:*

a. tetracycline
b. azathioprine
c. aspirin
d. megestrol acetate
e. ketoconazole

592. *A diabetic cat is given insulin at 8 AM and fed at 8 AM and 6 PM. Blood glucose levels are 425 mg/dl at 8 AM, 225 mg/dl at 11 AM, 140 mg/dl at 2 PM, 260 mg/dl at 5 PM, and 355 mg/dl at 8 PM. What do these blood glucose values indicate?*

a. The cat is being fed at inappropriate times.
b. The cat is being fed excessive amounts.
c. The insulin dosage is too low.
d. The duration of action of this type of insulin is too short.
e. The cat has developed insulin resistance associated with hyperadrenocorticism.

593. *Which type of insulin has the longest duration of action?*

a. regular insulin
b. Ultralente insulin
c. Semilente insulin
d. NPH insulin
e. Lente insulin

594. *In cats, methimazole is used to treat:*

a. dilative cardiomyopathy
b. lymphoma
c. hyperthyroidism
d. renal secondary hyperparathyroidism
e. cholangiohepatitis

595. *As compared with dogs, cats have a prolonged half-life of elimination of:*

a. aspirin
b. insulin
c. prednisone
d. gentamicin
e. digitalis

596. *Heinz-body hemolytic anemia in cats is associated with:*

a. administration of aspirin
b. administration of chloramphenicol
c. warfarin poisoning
d. administration of acetaminophen
e. topical application of organophosphate insecticides

597. *In cats, hyperthyroidism is most often associated with:*

a. bilateral thyroid adenomas
b. unilateral thyroid adenoma
c. bilateral thyroid adenocarcinomas
d. unilateral thyroid adenocarcinoma
e. pituitary-dependent thyroid hypersecretion

598. *Which feline respiratory parasite causes thick-walled pulmonary cysts and passes yellow-brown single-operculated ova in the feces?*

a. *Capillaria*
b. *Paragonimus*
c. *Toxoplasma*
d. *Aelurostrongylus*
e. *Filaroides*

599. *Bilirubinuria is:*

a. an abnormal finding in both male and female cats
b. an abnormal finding in male cats only
c. an abnormal finding in female cats only
d. a normal finding in both male and female cats
e. only normal in cats younger than 4 months of age

600. *Which liver disease is **least** likely to cause jaundice in a cat?*

a. hepatic lipidosis
b. cholangiohepatitis
c. pyogranulomatous hepatitis associated with feline infectious peritonitis
d. congenital portosystemic shunt
e. hepatic lymphoma

DOGS AND CATS

D.W. Macy

Practice answer sheets are on pages 293-298.

601. *Concerning polydactylism in cats, which statement is most accurate:*
   a. Affected cats should have any extra toes removed.
   b. Owners should be advised that it is an inherited autosomal dominant disorder.
   c. It is a random congenital defect; no genetic information is available.
   d. It is seen most often in Siamese.
   e. It is seen most often in Rex cats.

602. *Passive immunity, derived from colostrum, can interfere with development of active immunity following vaccination for canine distemper. Until what age can this interference last in puppies born to immune bitches?*
   a. 4 to 6 weeks of age
   b. 8 to 10 weeks of age
   c. 14 to 16 weeks of age
   d. 18 to 20 weeks of age
   e. 22 to 24 weeks of age

603. *Concerning serum calcium, which statement is **least** accurate?*
   a. Approximately 50% is bound to albumin.
   b. Acidosis decreases ionized calcium levels.
   c. Alkalosis decreases ionized calcium levels.
   d. Approximately 5% of serum calcium is in the form of calcium salts.
   e. Lipemia may result in increased measured levels.

604. *Progestogens are used for controlling estrus in domestic animals. Which of the following is **not** a side effect of exogenous progestogens?*
   a. obesity
   b. behavior changes
   c. mammary gland dysplasia
   d. adrenal gland suppression in cats
   e. urinary incontinence

605. *Pain at the administration site, urticaria, and occasionally abscessation are most commonly associated with administration of:*
   a. bacterins
   b. killed-virus vaccines
   c. modified-live-virus vaccines
   d. genetically engineered vaccines
   e. intranasal vaccines

606. *When should the first panleukopenia-rhinotracheitis-calicivirus vaccination be given to a kitten?*
   a. 10 to 12 weeks
   b. 15 to 16 weeks
   c. 3 to 4 weeks
   d. 8 to 9 weeks
   e. 5 to 6 weeks

607. *Which breed of dog should **not** be given ivermectin at dosages above 200 μg/kg?*
   a. German shepherd
   b. collie
   c. dachshund
   d. poodle
   e. Labrador retriever

608. *All the following affect the immune response to vaccination **except:***
   a. nutritional status
   b. concurrent infections
   c. concurrent drug therapy
   d. diagnostic radiography
   e. route of vaccination

Correct answers are on pages 140-171.

609. *Which disease is **not** zoonotic?*

a. rabies
b. plague
c. leptospirosis
d. parvoviral enteritis
e. sporotrichosis

610. *With normal nursing behavior, what approximate percentage of a dog's circulating immunoglobulins is derived from absorption of colostrum in the neonatal period?*

a. 50%
b. 75%
c. 65%
d. 95%
e. 15%

611. *Which of the following is **not** a round-cell tumor?*

a. mast-cell tumor
b. lymphosarcoma
c. squamous-cell carcinoma
d. histiocytoma
e. transmissible venereal tumor

612. *In cats the tumor induced by exposure to ultraviolet radiation (sunlight) is the:*

a. melanoma
b. squamous-cell carcinoma
c. basal-cell carcinoma
d. histiocytoma
e. transmissible venereal tumor

613. *Based on the World Health Organization's TNM system of classifying tumors, which tumor has the **poorest** prognosis?*

a. T1, N2, MP
b. T2, N2, M0
c. T2, N0, M0
d. T1, N0, M0
e. T1, N3, M0

614. *Which of the following is the **least** commonly documented result of spaying in dogs?*

a. reduced incidence of mammary tumors if done before 2½ years of age
b. possible urinary incontinence
c. reduced incidence of pyometra
d. no attraction of male dogs
e. obesity

615. *Which anthelmintic is most effective against whipworms in dogs?*

a. fenbendazole
b. bunamidine
c. pyrantel pamoate
d. thenium closylate
e. praziquantel

616. *The daily caloric requirement for a 4-year-old German shepherd that is a house pet receiving a moderate amount of exercise is approximately:*

a. 35 to 40 kcal/lb
b. 20 to 30 kcal/lb
c. 10 to 15 kcal/lb
d. 40 to 45 kcal/lb
e. 40 to 55 kcal/lb

617. *What is the best fecal flotation solution to use if you suspect* Giardia *infection?*

a. Smith's sugar solution
b. zinc sulfate solution
c. magnesium sulfate solution
d. saturated sucrose solution
e. saturated sodium chloride solution

618. *Which hormones **decrease** sebaceous secretions in dogs?*

a. L-thyroxine and estrogens
b. growth hormone and L-thyroxine
c. androgens and estrogens
d. corticosteroids and estrogens
e. androgens and L-thyroxine

619. *Which fungal organism causes disease more commonly in cats than in dogs?*

a. *Cryptococcus neoformans*
b. *Coccidioides immitis*
c. *Blastomyces dermatitidis*
d. *Histoplasma capsulatum*
e. *Trichophyton simii*

620. *A 7-year-old intact male German shepherd has bilateral nonpruritic truncal alopecia. Skin scrapings and dermatophyte cultures are negative. Both testicles are descended and normal on palpation. The resting serum thyroxine (T_4) level is 3.5 μg/dl, and the resting triiodothyronine (T_3) level is 1.50 ng/ml. A skin biopsy reveals an "endocrine pattern." What is the **least** likely cause of this dog's dermatosis?*

a. Sertoli-cell tumor
b. pituitary-dependent hyperadrenocorticism
c. cortisol-secreting adrenal tumor
d. hypothyroidism
e. seminoma

621. *Currently, the most accurate test to determine if a dog has hyperadrenocorticism is the:*

a. ACTH stimulation test
b. low-dosage dexamethasone suppression test
c. TSH stimulation test
d. xylazine stimulation test
e. endogenous ACTH assay

622. *The test recommended for diagnosis of hypothyroidism in dogs is:*

a. baseline serum thyroxine (T_4) level
b. combination of baseline serum thyroxine (T_4) and triiodothyronine (T_3) levels
c. thyroid-stimulating hormone (TSH) response test
d. response to thyroid hormone supplementation
e. skin biopsy

623. *For pruritus to occur in a dog with hyperadrenocorticism, at least one of four clinical conditions must be present. Which of the following is **not** one of those conditions?*

a. pyoderma
b. seborrhea
c. thin skin
d. calcinosis cutis
e. demodicosis

624. *Which clinical sign is specific for Sertoli-cell tumor?*

a. seborrhea
b. hyperpigmentation
c. pruritus
d. truncal alopecia
e. linear preputial dermatosis

625. *Which of the following is **not** a potential complication of megestrol acetate therapy in cats?*

a. mammary hyperplasia and neoplasia
b. pyometra
c. diabetes mellitus
d. hypoadrenocorticism
e. diabetes insipidus

626. *Based on the causes of pruritic miliary dermatitides of cats in the United States, which of the following is the most rational and effective initial therapy for the problem?*

a. systemic corticosteroids
b. systemic antibiotics
c. topical and systemic antifungal therapy
d. flea control and systemic corticosteroids
e. hypoallergenic diet trial

Correct answers are on pages 140-171.

627. *Concerning feline-infectious peritonitis antibody titers, which statement is **least** accurate?*

a. A titer greater than 1:3200 is common in normal cats.
b. Titers do not always correlate with shedding of coronavirus.
c. The titer may be negative in terminally ill cats.
d. The titer is useful in helping detect carrier cats and eliminate coronavirus from catteries.
e. The titer may be positive in 20% to 40% of the cat population.

628. *Concerning diabetes mellitus in cats, which statement is **least** accurate?*

a. Diabetes mellitus generally develops in cats 6 years of age or older.
b. Stressed cats uncommonly develop blood glucose concentrations above 200 mg/dl.
c. Polyuria, polydipsia, polyphagia, and weight loss are common clinical signs in diabetic cats.
d. Hyperbilirubinemia is common in diabetic cats.
e. Protein zinc insulin is preferred for treatment of most diabetic cats.

629. *Concerning the cutaneous manifestations of food allergies in cats, which statement is **least** accurate?*

a. Pruritus may be quite refractory to systemic corticosteroids.
b. Food allergies may cause pruritic dermatitis restricted to the head and neck.
c. Food allergies may cause miliary dermatitis.
d. Food allergies are commonly associated with gastrointestinal signs (vomiting, diarrhea).
e. Diagnosis is supported by feeding a trial hypoallergenic diet (e.g., Gerber's lamb baby food) for 3 weeks.

630. *Concerning the skin of dogs and cats, which statement is **least** accurate?*

a. The supracaudal organ ("tail gland") area of dogs is restricted to the proximodorsal aspect of the tail, whereas in cats this tissue extends the entire length of the dorsum of the tail.
b. Feline acne and canine acne are similar in that both only affect young, prepubertal animals.
c. Stress exacerbates sebaceous-gland hyperplasia ("stud tail") in intact male cats.
d. Aluminum acetate solution is primarily used for its astringent properties in management of feline acne.
e. Feline acne is probably a manifestation of a focal, epidermal, keratinizing defect.

631. *Coronaviral vasculitis in cats is best treated with:*

a. azathoprine and corticosteroids
b. tylosin
c. methimazole
d. vitamin E
e. penicillin

632. *Concerning skin disease in cats, which statement is **least** accurate?*

a. Dermatophytosis may be intensely pruritic.
b. Superficial pyoderma is common in cats.
c. The Mackenzie toothbrush technique is used for dermatophyte culture in asymptomatic cats.
d. Intradermal testing can delineate sources of inhalant allergy.
e. The pruritus associated with inhalant allergy is usually responsive to systemic glucocorticoids.

633. *Which treatment is most likely to prevent permanent scarring in severe cases of juvenile cellulitis in dogs?*

a. systemic antibiotics
b. topical wet dressings/astringents
c. topical corticosteroids
d. systemic corticosteroids
e. topical antibiotics

634. *Which of the following is most commonly associated with griseofulvin toxicity in cats?*
   a. diabetes mellitus
   b. myelosuppression
   c. hypertrophic cardiomyopathy
   d. dilative cardiomyopathy
   e. uveitis

635. *Which of the following is **not** a recognized complication of mast-cell tumors?*
   a. shock
   b. hemorrhage
   c. erythema and edema
   d. delayed wound healing
   e. irregular heart rate

636. *Which tumor is **least** likely to spread to regional lymph nodes?*
   a. intracutaneous cornifying epithelioma
   b. anal sac adenocarcinoma
   c. mast-cell tumor
   d. hemangiopericytoma
   e. malignant melanoma

637. *Which tumor is **least** likely to yield cells on aspiration?*
   a. fibrosarcoma
   b. mast-cell tumor
   c. histiocytoma
   d. cutaneous lymphoma
   e. transmissible venereal tumor

638. *Concerning diabetes mellitus, which statement is **least** accurate?*
   a. Diabetes mellitus is a metabolic disorder characterized by disturbances of carbohydrate, lipid, and protein metabolism.
   b. Diabetes mellitus can result from an absolute or relative lack of insulin.
   c. Type-I diabetes mellitus in people is usually insulin dependent.
   d. In dog the age of onset is 4 to 14 years, and the disease is not usually insulin dependent.
   e. Hyperglucagonemia potentiates the effects of hypoinsulinism by increasing glucose production and by increasing fatty acid oxidation and ketogenesis.

639. *In cats, which of the following tumors is most common?*
   a. histiocytoma
   b. perianal-gland adenoma
   c. ceruminous-gland adenoma
   d. trichoepithelioma
   e. keratoacanthoma

640. *Excessive bleeding is frequently associated with mast-cell tumors and is thought to be caused by release of:*
   a. histamine
   b. proteolytic enzymes
   c. heparin
   d. Hageman factors
   e. ethylenediamine tetraacetic acid

641. *All the following are common features of both canine and feline fibrosarcomas **except:***
   a. recurrence following surgical removal
   b. caused by a retrovirus
   c. spindle-type cells
   d. required wide excision
   e. occur in many organs

642. *Which tumor is associated with hypercalcemia?*
   a. perianal-gland adenocarcinoma
   b. keratoacanthoma
   c. anal sac adenocarcinoma
   d. trichoepithelioma
   e. histiocytoma

643. *Which tumor is most likely to undergo spontaneous remission?*
   a. mast-cell tumor
   b. melanoma
   c. transmissible venereal tumor
   d. lymphosarcoma
   e. plasmacytoma

Correct answers are on pages 140-171.

644. *In dogs, which form of lymphosarcoma is most frequently associated with hypercalcemia?*

a. alimentary
b. mediastinal
c. generalized
d. osseous
e. ocular

645. *Which drug used in treatment of lymphosarcoma in dogs is limited by its cardiotoxicity?*

a. prednisolone
b. doxorubicin
c. vincristine
d. cyclophosphamide
e. L-asparaginase

646. *Which form of lymphosarcoma is most common in dogs?*

a. multicentric
b. alimentary
c. mediastinal
d. osseous
e. ocular

647. *Dogs with hypercalcemia commonly demonstrate:*

a. convulsions
b. hyperactivity
c. polyuria and polydipsia
d. ravenous appetite
e. twitching of facial muscles

648. *Which organ is most adversely affected by hypercalcemia?*

a. brain
b. heart
c. kidney
d. bladder
e. intestine

649. *Which breed of dog is most likely to lose its hair following therapy with doxorubicin?*

a. golden retriever
b. Labrador retriever
c. Doberman pinscher
d. Old English sheepdog
e. dalmatian

650. *Which feline virus is* ***least*** *contagious?*

a. feline leukemia virus
b. feline immunodeficiency virus (FIV)
c. feline rhinotracheitis virus
d. feline infectious peritonitis virus
e. feline calicivirus

651. *Which combination of drugs is used most commonly in treatment of lymphosarcoma in dogs and cats?*

a. cyclophosphamide, prednisone, vincristine
b. mitoxantrone, prednisone, methotrexate
c. doxorubicin, cyclophosphamide, vincristine
d. bleomycin, mitoxantrone, prednisone
e. bleomycin, mitoxantrone, prednisone

652. *In the United States the feline immunodeficiency virus infection rate is half that of feline leukemia virus. What percentage of the clinically healthy, low-risk cat population is infected with feline immunodeficiency virus?*

a. 2%
b. 5.5%
c. 10%
d. 11%
e. 17%

653. *Serologic tests for feline immunodeficiency virus infection detect:*

a. virus particles
b. antibody
c. antigen-antibody complexes
d. IgE
e. p27

654. *Which drug used in cancer therapy is termed* phase specific?

a. prednisolone
b. vincristine
c. cyclophosphamide
d. doxorubicin
e. prednisone

655. *Which tumor of dogs is curable with chemotherapy alone?*

a. lymphosarcoma
b. transmissible venereal tumor
c. fibrosarcoma
d. mast-cell tumor
e. mammary carcinoma

656. *Which clinical disease has **not** been associated with hypercalcemia?*

a. hypoadrenocorticism
b. lymphosarcoma
c. apocrine-gland tumors of the anal sac
d. parathyroid adenoma
e. histiocytoma

657. *Which fungal disease is most frequently seen in dogs in the southwestern United States?*

a. cryptococcosis
b. blastomycosis
c. coccidioidomycosis
d. histoplasmosis
e. sporotrichosis

658. *Throughout history, plague has killed large numbers of people. Which domestic animal is associated with 10% of the human cases of plague today?*

a. dog
b. cat
c. duck
d. cow
e. horse

659. *In dogs, skin biopsies are most useful in diagnosing:*

a. inhalant allergy
b. food allergy
c. pemphigus foliaceus
d. bacterial dermatitis
e. drug allergy

660. *Concerning eosinophilic ulcers (indolent ulcers, rodent ulcers) in cats, which statement is **least** accurate?*

a. They usually occur on the upper lip.
b. They may undergo malignant transformation to squamous-cell carcinoma.
c. They are typically associated with peripheral blood eosinophilia.
d. They have been associated with food allergies.
e. One recommended therapy is methylprednisolone acetate injection.

661. *Which pattern of alopecia suggests a sex hormone imbalance in a dog?*

a. hair loss beginning over the dorsum
b. hair loss beginning over the head and distal extremities
c. hair loss beginning in the perineum or flank
d. hair loss beginning with development of a "rat tail"
e. hair loss beginning in the axillae and ventral thorax

662. *The most consistent and diagnostically relevant laboratory abnormality in cats with feline infectious peritonitis is:*

a. high serum γ-globulin level
b. anemia
c. leukocytosis
d. *Hemobartonella* in red blood cells
e. feline leukemia virus positive

Correct answers are on pages 140-171.

663. *Which diagnostic procedure is recommended for diagnosis of pemphigus foliaceus in dogs?*
   a. direct immunofluorescence testing of formalin-fixed skin biopsies
   b. direct immunofluorescence testing of skin biopsies fixed in Bouin's solution
   c. indirect immunofluorescence testing of serum
   d. direct immunofluorescence testing of skin biopsies fixed in Michel's medium
   e. direct immunofluorescence testing of serum

664. *You are presented with a 3-year-old Labrador retriever with multiple lick granulomas on all its limbs. Treatment with oral prednisone stops the licking, and the lesions dramatically improve. Unfortunately, the lesions recur after discontinuation of corticosteroid therapy. The most likely underlying cause of the granulomas in this dog is:*
   a. a psychologic problem
   b. a systemic bacterial infection
   c. foreign bodies
   d. dermatophytosis
   e. an inhalant allergy

665. *Which tumor is frequently associated with fragmentation of red blood cells?*
   a. fibrosarcoma
   b. mast-cell tumor
   c. hemangiosarcoma
   d. melanoma
   e. histiocytoma

666. *Which tumor is frequently associated with excessive bleeding during excision?*
   a. fibrosarcoma
   b. mast-cell tumor
   c. squamous-cell carcinoma
   d. basal-cell carcinoma
   e. histiocytoma

667. *The antigen-presenting cell in the central nervous system (CNS) is the:*
   a. lymphocyte
   b. astrocyte
   c. microglial cell
   d. monocyte
   e. mast cell

668. *Blunt trauma to the central nervous system results in swelling that is:*
   a. primarily associated with edema
   b. almost completely associated with astrocyte swelling
   c. usually associated with a hematoma
   d. primarily associated with release of histamine from astrocytes
   e. primarily associated with degranulation of mast cells

669. *All the following can cause insulin resistance in dogs* ***except:***
   a. acromegaly
   b. hyperadrenocorticism
   c. bacterial bronchopneumonia
   d. uremia
   e. heartworm infection

670. *The most common primary site of hemangiosarcoma in dogs is the:*
   a. left atrium
   b. spleen
   c. lungs
   d. bladder
   e. liver

671. *Concerning insulin, which statement is* ***least*** *accurate?*
   a. Insulin is a two-chain polypeptide.
   b. Insulin is produced by the β-cells of the pancreas.
   c. Entry of glucose into red blood cells is an insulin receptor-dependent process.
   d. Insulin promotes nucleic acid formation into mononucleotides.
   e. Insulin inhibits gluconeogenesis.

672. *All the following tumors may be diagnosed through fine-needle aspiration of the spleen **except:***
   a. keratoacanthoma
   b. hemangiosarcoma
   c. mast-cell tumor
   d. lymphoma
   e. plasmacytoma

673. *In dogs, appropriate treatment for cholecalciferol rodenticide toxicity includes all the following **except:***
   a. saline
   b. furosemide
   c. calcitonin
   d. thiazide diuretic
   e. aluminum hydroxide

674. *Concerning hyperosmolar nonketotic syndrome in dogs, which statement is most accurate?*
   a. It is relatively common.
   b. Mild hyperglycemia and increased serum osmolality are usually present.
   c. Most affected dogs are ketotic.
   d. Development of cerebral edema during treatment is common.
   e. NPH insulin is the insulin of choice during the initial stages of management.

675. *Which agent is **not** appropriate for topical therapy of seborrhea in dogs?*
   a. sulfur
   b. salicylic acid
   c. tar
   d. captan
   e. benzoyl peroxide

676. *Which drug is **not** acceptable for long-term management of pruritus?*
   a. prednisolone
   b. methylprednisolone
   c. dexamethasone
   d. diphenhydramine
   e. essential fatty acid supplement

677. *Impetigo is another name for:*
   a. superficial pustular pyoderma
   b. juvenile pyoderma
   c. bacterial hypersensitivity
   d. skinfold pyoderma
   e. deep pyoderma

678. *The most common dermatophyte of cats is:*
   a. *Microsporum canis*
   b. *Microsporum felis*
   c. *Trichophyton mentagrophytes*
   d. *Trichophyton felis*
   e. *Microsporum gypseum*

679. *Copper toxicosis is seen in Bedlington terriers and other breeds. Copper toxicosis is appropriately treated with all the following **except:***
   a. dietary zinc supplementation
   b. dietary restriction of copper
   c. penicillamine
   d. tetramine
   e. dietary supplementation

680. *In treating infections of the liver, one should select an antimicrobial that is excreted in the bile. Which drug is **not** appropriate for treatment of liver infections because it is not excreted in bile?*
   a. ampicillin
   b. amoxicillin
   c. cephalexin
   d. cefadroxil
   e. gentamicin

681. *Which drug is **not** appropriate in treatment of bile duct infection in dogs with concurrent liver failure?*
   a. ampicillin
   b. chloramphenicol
   c. cephalexin
   d. cefadroxil
   e. amoxicillin

Correct answers are on pages 140-171.

682. *All the following drugs are potentially hepatotoxic in dogs or cats* ***except:***

a. halothane
b. griseofulvin
c. acetaminophen
d. primidone
e. cephalexin

683. *Which corticosteroid has the greatest glucocorticoid activity (is most potent)?*

a. hydrocortisone
b. prednisone
c. betamethasone
d. triamcinolone
e. prednisolone

684. *Which drug is* ***not*** *considered potentially toxic to the kidney?*

a. amphotericin B
b. gentamicin
c. thiacetarsamide
d. amoxicillin
e. cisplatin

685. *All the following drugs are used to stimulate appetite* ***except:***

a. diazepam
b. cyproheptadine
c. prednisolone
d. oxazepam
e. naloxone

686. *Toxoplasmosis is a zoonotic disease. Cats may play a role in transmission of the disease to people. At what age is a cat most likely to excrete oocysts in its feces?*

a. 3 to 5 years
b. 1 to 2 weeks
c. 2 to 12 months
d. 8 to 10 years
e. 5 to 7 years

687. *The recommended treatment for toxoplasmosis in cats is:*

a. ampicillin
b. amoxicillin
c. chloramphenicol
d. clindamycin
e. gentamicin

688. *Large-breed dogs are predisposed to appendicular osteosarcoma. Following amputation of the affected limb, what percentage of dogs survives at least 1 year with no other therapy?*

a. 30%
b. 50%
c. 10%
d. 70%
e. 90%

689. *Which antifungal agent is used primarily for treatment of cryptococcosis and is of limited use for other fungal infections?*

a. amphotericin B
b. ketoconazole
c. flucytosine
d. itraconazole
e. potassium iodide

690. *Left untreated, lymphosarcoma in dogs is typically fatal within 30 days. However, treatment with chemotherapeutic agents, such as doxorubicin, cyclophosphamide, vincristine, and prednisone, produces complete remission in approximately what percentage of treated dogs?*

a. 10%
b. 25%
c. 50%
d. 75%
e. 95%

691. *In dogs, chemotherapy for lymphosarcoma allows survival for an average of:*

a. 3 months
b. 10 months
c. 20 months
d. 30 months
e. 40 months

692. *What is the most common infectious cause of chronic nasal discharge in dogs?*
   a. cryptococcosis
   b. blastomycosis
   c. viral rhinotracheitis
   d. aspergillosis
   e. coccidioidomycosis

693. *Which common feline virus is most difficult to inactivate with disinfectants?*
   a. calicivirus
   b. coronavirus
   c. panleukopenia virus
   d. feline immunodeficiency virus
   e. feline leukemia virus

694. *Hypokalemic myopathy of cats is most similar in its clinical presentation to:*
   a. thiamin deficiency
   b. tetanus
   c. borreliosis
   d. cytauxzoonosis
   e. botulism

695. *Which drug is most effective in treatment of hyperthyroidism in cats?*
   a. cyclophosphamide
   b. doxorubicin
   c. cisplatin
   d. methimazole
   e. atropine

696. *A 12-year-old German shepherd has a chronic mucohemorrhagic discharge from its right naris. What is the most likely cause, but not necessarily the only possible cause, of this problem?*
   a. nasal tumor
   b. bacterial infection
   c. viral infection
   d. foreign body
   e. allergy

697. *You remove a hemangiosarcoma from the spleen of an 8-year-old German shepherd. The chance that the dog will survive at least 1 year after the surgery is:*
   a. less than 10%
   b. 30%
   c. 60%
   d. 80%
   e. greater than 90%

698. *Concerning management of uncomplicated diabetes mellitus in dogs, which statement is most accurate?*
   a. A glucose curve should be calculated the day diabetes mellitus is diagnosed.
   b. NPH insulin IV at 2.2 units/kg is a good starting dosage.
   c. Protein zinc insulin is the insulin of choice for initial use in dogs.
   d. Semimoist foods should be avoided because of their high sugar content.
   e. NPH insulin SC at 2.2 units/kg is a good starting dosage.

699. *Which of the following is **not** commonly associated with uncomplicated diabetes mellitus in dogs?*
   a. fasting hyperglycemia
   b. glycosuria
   c. hypercholesterolemia
   d. lipemia
   e. hypocalcemia

700. *Concerning insulin-producing islet-cell tumors in dogs, which statement is **least** accurate?*
   a. The amended serum insulin/glucose ratio is the most sensitive test for insulin-producing islet-cell tumors, but the diagnosis should not be based on this test alone.
   b. The glucagon tolerance test can be used to help confirm the diagnosis of insulin-producing islet-cell tumor.
   c. Insulin-producing islet-cell tumors are most common in older dogs.
   d. Insulin-producing islet-cell tumors can be solitary or multiple.
   e. Most insulin-producing islet-cell tumors are carcinomas, but metastasis is rare.

Correct answers are on pages 140-171.

F.W. Scott

701. *An adjuvant is a substance that:*

a. is used to adhere antibody to a plastic plate used in enzyme-linked immunosorbent assay
b. enhances antigenicity or antibody response when mixed with an antigen
c. enhances the activity of certain antiviral compounds
d. enhances the antigen response in natural viral infections
e. is used to adhere proteins to the nitrocellulose paper in the Western blot assay

702. *Which statement best characterizes an attenuated virus?*

a. The virulence of the virus has been reduced to an acceptable level for use as a vaccine.
b. The virus multiplies in the host animal but, by definition, cannot produce clinical signs.
c. The virus has been inactivated by chemical or physical means.
d. The virus has been altered by biotechnology.
e. The virus has been adapted to cell culture.

703. *Concerning capsomeres of the feline parvovirus virion, which statement is **least** accurate?*

a. Capsomeres are composed of the gp70 glycoprotein, which stimulates the primary immune response elicited by commercial vaccines against feline panleukopenia.
b. Capsomeres are morphologic units of the capsid of a virion.
c. Capsomeres are composed of polypeptides.
d. Capsomeres are composed of proteins.
e. Capsomeres contain the primary antigen responsible for stimulation of an immune response in the infected cat.

704. *Concerning the peplomer of the feline leukemia virus, which statement is **least** accurate?*

a. It is a glycoprotein unit that contains the antigen responsible for antigenicity and, hence, protective immunity.
b. It is the morphologic unit that protrudes from the surface of the viral envelope.
c. It is inserted into the altered cell membrane, which eventually becomes the envelope of the virus during viral replication.
d. It contains feline oncornavirus cell membrane antigen (FOCMA).
e. It contains the gp70 glycoprotein.

705. *After vaccination of a cat, humoral antibody to feline parvovirus generally appears in the serum after approximately:*

a. 1 day
b. 2 to 3 days
c. 6 to 7 days
d. 14 days
e. 28 days

706. *In kittens the half-life of passive maternal antibodies is approximately:*

a. 1 to 2 days
b. 3 to 4 days
c. 8 to 10 days
d. 14 to 16 days
e. 20 to 25 days

707. *A client's kitten has just died from feline panleukopenia (feline parvovirus), and she wants to replace it with an unvaccinated 14-week-old kitten from a neighbor. How long after vaccination of the kitten should she wait before taking it home?*

a. She can take the kitten home immediately.
b. 3 days
c. 1 week
d. 2 weeks
e. 1 year

708. *In most cases, to diagnose a disease in a cat by serum antibody titer determination, one must demonstrate a significant rise in titer in paired serum samples. What constitutes a "significant" rise in titer?*

a. a positive titer (>1:10) in both samples
b. two-fold increase
c. four-fold increase
d. ten-fold increase
e. 100-fold increase

709. *You collect paired serum samples 2 weeks apart from a group of five dogs with suspected canine distemper and submit the samples to the diagnostic laboratory. Which titers in the acute and convalescent samples, respectively, indicate acute canine distemper?*

a. 1:80 and 1:160
b. 1:320 and 1:320
c. 1:40 and 1:320
d. 1:320 and 1:40
e. 1:640 and 1:920

710. *"Blue eye" in dogs is caused by:*

a. canine adenovirus-1 vaccination
b. the immunosuppressive effect of canine parvovirus vaccination
c. parainfluenza virus vaccination
d. canine adenovirus-2 vaccination
e. canine distemper vaccination

711. *A new antiviral drug has specific action against DNA virus but no effect on RNA virus. Against which canine viruses is this drug likely to be effective?*

a. distemper virus, herpesvirus, parvovirus
b. infectious hepatitis virus, herpesvirus, parvovirus
c. distemper virus, infectious hepatitis virus, parainfluenza virus
d. parainfluenza virus, adenovirus-2, reovirus
e. distemper virus, reovirus, parvovirus

712. *A new antiviral drug is effective only against RNA viruses. Against which feline viruses is this drug likely to be effective?*

a. panleukopenia virus, calicivirus, rhinotracheitis virus
b. rhinotracheitis virus, calicivirus, infectious peritonitis virus
c. infectious peritonitis virus, leukemia virus, panleukopenia virus
d. calicivirus, infectious peritonitis virus, leukemia virus
e. immunodeficiency virus, leukemia virus, panleukopenia virus

713. *You suspect feline infectious peritonitis (FIP) in a 6-month-old Persian cat because of the severe clinical disease, including a persistent, nonresponsive fever, palpable lumps on the kidney, and progressive weight loss and anorexia. Despite heroic treatment, the cat develops progressive neurologic signs, and you and the owner reluctantly conclude that euthanasia is necessary. What single sample should be collected before euthanasia or at necropsy, and how should the sample be examined to confirm your diagnosis of FIP?*

a. blood smear examined for FIP virus by indirect fluorescent antibody test
b. serum examined for coronaviruses by indirect fluorescent antibody test
c. serum examined for FIP antibody titer by serum neutralization test
d. throat swab cultured for FIP virus
e. kidney tissue examined microscopically

714. *The commercial feline leukemia virus vaccine Leukocell (SmithKline) is a subunit vaccine containing two antigens, feline oncornavirus cell membrane and:*

a. p15E
b. p27
c. gp70
d. p70
e. gp27

715. *Which term best described a group of two or more feline calciviruses that contain the same major antigenic determinants and that are neutralized to a similar degree by antiserum to each of the separate viruses?*

a. subtype
b. serotype
c. isolate
d. strain
e. biotype

Correct answers are on pages 140-171.

716. *Feline infectious peritonitis (FIP) is a progressive, debilitating, highly fatal disease of cats caused by a:*

a. parvovirus
b. retrovirus
c. rhabdovirus
d. coronavirus
e. calicivirus

717. *The laboratory test used in most diagnostic laboratories as an aid to diagnosis of feline infectious peritonitis (FIP) is:*

a. direct fluorescent antibody testing of tissues to detect FIP virus
b. agar gel immunodiffusion of serum to detect coronavirus antigen (Coggins' test)
c. serum neutralization test to detect antibodies specific for FIP virus
d. indirect fluorescent antibody testing of serum to detect coronavirus antibodies
e. enzyme-linked immunosorbent assay (ELISA) of serum to detect coronavirus antibodies

718. *Cloudy, blue corneal edema in a dog 2 weeks after vaccination for infectious canine hepatitis is caused by:*

a. synergistic immunosuppressive effects of distemper virus and parvovirus in the vaccine
b. adenovirus-2 infection of the dog before vaccination
c. hypersensitivity to adenovirus-1
d. recrudescence of herpesviral infection because of the immunosuppressive effects of vaccination
e. formation of immune complexes in the cornea from interaction of *Bordetella* in the vaccine and anti-*Bordetella* antibodies

719. *Which antiviral drugs can be used as antiherpetic eye ointments for treatment of cats with ulcerative herpetic keratitis?*

a. ribavirin, adenine arabinoside
b. adenine arabinoside, idoxuridine
c. idoxuridine, ribavirin
d. amantadine, adenine arabinoside
e. amantadine, ribavirin

720. *The most common cause of vaccine failure in dogs and cats is:*

a. interference by maternally derived immunity with vaccine virus
b. loss of immunogenicity from improper handling of vaccines
c. low antigenic mass of vaccines
d. split dosages of vaccine to reduce cost of vaccination
e. inappropriate administration of vaccine (subcutaneous instead of intramuscular)

721. *A client's unvaccinated cat will soon be exposed to panleukopenia virus in a boarding establishment, and you must decide how to best protect the cat against infection. Ranking in order from most rapid to least rapid induction of immunity, what is the protective potential of available products?*

a. antiserum, killed-virus vaccine, modified-live-virus (MLV) vaccine
b. antiserum, modified-live-virus vaccine, killed-virus vaccine
c. killed-virus vaccine, modified-live-virus vaccine, antiserum
d. modified-live-virus vaccine, killed-virus vaccine, antiserum
e. modified-live-virus vaccine, antiserum, killed-virus vaccine

722. *Which of the following is an example of a heterotypic vaccine?*

a. canine parvovirus vaccine to protect against canine distemper
b. bovine virus diarrhea vaccine to protect against canine distemper
c. measles vaccine to protect against canine distemper
d. rinderpest vaccine to protect against bovine virus diarrhea
e. measles vaccine to protect against canine parvoviral infection

723. *Two caliciviruses are isolated at the state diagnostic laboratory from similar clinical disease outbreaks of upper respiratory disease in two breeding catteries. Vaccination of kittens at 8 to 10 weeks of age does not control the upper respiratory infections within these catteries because most kittens become infected before vaccination. You question whether a "new" virus has evolved, against which currently available vaccines are not effective. Characterization of these two viruses in the laboratory reveals that they both have the same major antigenic determinants. Which statement best characterizes the relationship between these two viruses?*

a. The viruses belong to the same virus serotype.
b. The viruses are subtypes of the same serotype.
c. The viruses are merely strains of the same virus.
d. The viruses are two new viral isolates.
e. The viruses are serotypes of the same subtype.

724. *In feline viral rhinotracheitis, herpesvirus-1 is spread from local lesions to sites of latent infection in the central nervous system by:*

a. macrophages
b. peripheral nerves
c. cell-free viremia
d. lymphatics
e. cell-associated viremia

725. *Concerning feline infectious peritonitis (FIP), which statement is **least** accurate?*

a. Clinical FIP is the result of Arthus-like interactions of antigen, antibody, and complement across vessel walls, accompanied by virus persistence within mononuclear phagocytes.
b. Coronaviral antibodies contribute to enhancement of the disease process by facilitating uptake of virus into mononuclear phagocytes.
c. A positive coronaviral antibody titer (as determined by immunofluorescence or enzyme-linked immunosorbent assay) in a clinically ill animal is diagnostic of FIP.
d. The mechanism responsible for immunity against FIP is not known but is suspected to be T-cell mediated.
e. The magnitude of the coronaviral antibody titer in a cat with FIP has little relationship to the chronicity of the disease process.

726. *Concerning feline leukemia virus (FeLV), which statement is **least** accurate?*

a. FeLV-associated diseases include lymphosarcoma, myeloproliferative disorders, nonregenerative anemia, and panleukopenia-like syndrome.
b. The reservoir of FeLV in nature is the chronically viremic carrier cat, which excretes infectious virus in respiratory secretions, feces, urine, and most importantly, saliva.
c. The persistent viremia in FeLV infection is frequently reversible.
d. A negative FeLV test, either by the slide test or enzyme-linked immunosorbent assay, in no way indicates past infection with integration of FeLV proviral DNA into host cells.
e. An effective FeLV control program begins with testing of all cats in the household and removal or permanent isolation of all persistently infected cats.

727. *Feline panleukopenia is caused by a:*

a. papovavirus
b. parvovirus
c. herpesvirus
d. calicivirus
e. lentivirus

728. *The longest time that feline panleukopenia virus may survive at room temperature in a contaminated environment is:*

a. 1 day
b. 1 week
c. 1 month
d. 6 months
e. more than 1 year

Correct answers are on pages 140-171.

729. *Chlorhexidine (Nolvasan) has virucidal activity against which feline viruses?*

a. panleukopenia virus, herpesvirus-1, and calicivirus
b. herpesvirus-1 but not calicivirus or panleukopenia virus
c. calicivirus but not herpesvirus-1 or panleukopenia virus
d. calicivirus and herpesvirus-1 but not panleukopenia virus
e. panleukopenia virus and calicivirus but not herpesvirus-1

730. *To be most effective by aerosol therapy for chronic respiratory tract infections in cats, an antimicrobial should be:*

a. rapidly absorbed from the respiratory mucosa, such as kanamycin or gentamicin
b. rapidly absorbed from the respiratory mucosa, such as penicillin or tetracycline
c. slowly absorbed from the respiratory mucosa, such as kanamycin or gentamicin
d. combined with an antiviral compound, such as idoxuridine
e. slowly absorbed from the respiratory mucosa, such as penicillin or tetracycline

731. *In treatment of tracheobronchitis in dogs, aerosol therapy with antibacterials:*

a. does not reduce numbers of bacteria in the trachea and does reduce clinical signs
b. reduces number of virus particles but not bacteria in the trachea and reduces clinical signs
c. reduces number of bacteria but not virus particles in the trachea and does not reduce clinical signs
d. reduces numbers of bacteria in the trachea and reduces clinical signs
e. has no local or clinical effect

732. *Feline parvovirus can replicate:*

a. only in mature enterocytes
b. only in cells undergoing mitosis
c. in both mature and mitotic cells
d. only in the cerebellum of newborn kittens
e. only if a helper virus is present, such as type-A feline leukemia virus

733. *Feline infectious peritonitis is caused by a:*

a. gammaherpesvirus
b. retrovirus
c. cell-associated renovirus
d. lentivirus
e. coronavirus

734. *In the environment, feline infectious peritonitis virus is:*

a. extremely resistant, surviving longer than 1 year at room temperature
b. moderately resistant, surviving several weeks at room temperature
c. moderately labile, surviving several days at room temperature
d. labile, surviving only 1 to 3 days at room temperature
e. very labile and is inactivated in less than 24 hours at room temperature

735. *Passive maternal immunity in kittens:*

a. persists as long as the kittens are nursing
b. is transferred to kittens via colostrum during the first 24 hours
c. is transferred to kittens only in utero
d. is transferred to kittens via colostrum during the first 4 weeks of life until they become immunocompetent
e. protects the kittens against in utero infection but has no protective benefits after birth

736. *Following initial vaccination of a cat against rhinotracheitis (herpesvirus-1), a secondary immune response can occur if a second dose of vaccine is given after:*

a. 1 day
b. 4 days
c. 7 days
d. 14 days
e. 21 days

737. *In cats, commercially available rhinotracheitis-calicivirus vaccines should be given:*

a. only intranasally
b. only intramuscularly
c. only subcutaneously
d. only by conjunctival inoculation
e. according to the manufacturer's recommendations

738. *In cats, corneal dendritic ulcers are usually caused by:*

a. feline parvovirus
b. feline herpesvirus-1
c. feline calicivirus
d. feline pneumonitis virus
e. feline immunodeficiency virus

739. *In cats, lingual ulcers are usually caused by:*

a. feline parvovirus
b. feline herpesvirus-1
c. feline calicivirus
d. feline pneumonitis virus
e. feline immunodeficiency virus

740. *In both the wet (effusive) and dry forms of feline infectious peritonitis, the most consistent finding is:*

a. hypergammaglobulinemia
b. chorioretinitis
c. nephritis
d. low specific gravity of any effusion
e. hepatitis

741. *In cats, Tyzzer's disease is caused by:*

a. the protozoan blood parasite *Eperythrozoon felis*
b. the bacterium *Bacillus piliformis*
c. an unclassified DNA virus
d. a systemic fungus, *Conidiobolus avis,* that is acquired from birds
e. the intestinal protozoan parasite *Giardia lamblia*

742. *In cats,* Salmonella typhimurium:

a. is nonpathogenic
b. causes mild, self-limiting gastroenteritis
c. can cause severe gastroenteritis in some cats, especially after stress, but often produces only subclinical infections
d. produces severe gastroenteritis in all infected cats, often with associated pyogranuloma formation throughout the abdominal organs
e. is a common cause of chronic upper respiratory infection, especially in cats with immunosuppression by feline immunodeficiency virus or feline leukemia virus

743. *Ranking in order from most effective to least effective, what is the efficacy of products to protect cats in animal shelters against feline panleukopenia?*

a. killed-virus vaccine, modified-live-virus vaccine, antiserum
b. killed-virus vaccine, antiserum, modified-live-virus vaccine
c. antiserum, modified-live-virus vaccine, killed-virus vaccine
d. modified-live-virus vaccine, killed-virus vaccine, antiserum
e. modified-live-virus vaccine, antiserum, killed-virus vaccine

744. *Concerning feline viral rhinotracheitis, which statement is most accurate?*

a. The serum neutralization titer is directly proportional to the degree of protection.
b. The minimum protective virus neutralizing antibody titer is 1:10.
c. The local antibody titer is the only significant protective titer.
d. Protection is determined by a combination of humoral antibody, local antibody, and cell-mediated immunity.
e. Protection is only provided by T-cell–mediated immunity.

Correct answers are on pages 140-171.

745. *Feline leprosy, a disease characterized by single or multiple skin nodules, some of which may ulcerate, is caused by:*

a. an acid-fast bacterium
b. feline leukemia virus
c. feline papovavirus
d. *Actinobacillus leprae*
e. *Leptospira felis*

746. *Under normal environmental conditions, feline rhinotracheitis virus (herpesvirus-1) contaminating a cage or ward is usually inactivated within:*

a. 1 hour
b. 1 day
c. 1 week
d. 1 month
e. 3 months

747. *In a cat with rabies, when is rabies virus excreted in the saliva?*

a. from 1 week before through 1 week after the onset of clinical signs
b. throughout the course of disease, beginning at the onset of clinical signs
c. for 1 week after the onset of clinical signs
d. from 1 days before through 3 days after the onset of clinical signs
e. from up to 6 months before the onset of clinical signs, throughout the course of disease

748. *"Chronic panleukopenia" or "panleukopenia-like syndrome" is caused by:*

a. *Salmonella typhimurium*
b. feline leukemia virus
c. *Bacillus piliformis*
d. feline panleukopenia virus
e. feline rotavirus

749. *For effective aerosol therapy of lower respiratory diseases in cats, a nebulizer should deliver an aerosol with a particle size of:*

a. less than 5 μm
b. 5 to 10 μm
c. 10 to 20 μm
d. 20 to 100 μm
e. more than 100 μm

750. *Concerning feline calicivirus vaccines, which statement is most accurate?*

a. They have limited value because of the multiple serotypes of calicivirus.
b. They protect cats against upper respiratory disease but not against pneumonia caused by calicivirus.
c. They protect cats against pneumonia but not against upper respiratory disease caused by calicivirus.
d. They protect cats against caliciviral enteritis but not against upper respiratory disease or pneumonia.
e. They protect against both upper respiratory infection and pneumonia caused by calicivirus.

751. *In viral respiratory infection of cats, virus may be shed from the pharyngeal area beginning 3 weeks after infection (so-called "carrier cat"), with virus shedding continuing for at least 1 year. Concerning patterns of virus shedding, which statement is most accurate?*

a. It occurs with rhinotracheitis virus but not with calicivirus.
b. It occurs with calicivirus but not with rhinotracheitis virus.
c. Both calicivirus and rhinotracheitis are shed continuously.
d. Rhinotracheitis virus is shed intermittently, whereas calicivirus is shed almost continuously.
e. Calicivirus is shed intermittently, whereas rhinotracheitis virus is shed continuously.

752. *The first feline infectious peritonitis vaccine was produced from a temperature-sensitive mutant virus. This vaccine virus grows at:*

a. 40° C but not at 37° C
b. 33° C better than at 37° C
c. 37° C but not at 40° C
d. 37° C but not at 33° C
e. 37° C but not at 35° C or 39° C

753. *In production of vaccines, viruses are frequently modified or attenuated in virulence. There are advantages and disadvantages to modified-live-virus (MLV) vaccines. When you, as a clinician, are faced with certain situations in practice, you must decide whether to use an inactivated (killed-virus) vaccine or an MLV vaccine. Concerning MLV feline vaccines, which statement is **least** accurate?*

a. MLV vaccines provide protection more quickly than inactivated vaccines.
b. MLV vaccines should not be used in a pregnant cat unless specifically approved for this use.
c. MLV vaccines are preferable for use in contaminated environments, such as animal shelters.
d. MLV vaccines can only be given as a monovalent vaccine because of viral interference if two or more viruses are combined into one vaccine.
e. MLV vaccines generally produce higher antibody titers than inactivated vaccines and therefore produce longer-lasting immunity in vaccinated cats.

754. *Concerning inactivated (killed-virus) feline panleukopenia vaccines, which statement is most accurate?*

a. Inactivated panleukopenia vaccines stimulate interferon production because the inactivation process releases nucleic acid, which is an interferon inducer.
b. Inactivated panleukopenia vaccines are usually preferable to modified-live-virus vaccines for vaccination of pregnant cats.
c. Inactivated vaccines are seldom used in veterinary medicine today because of the superior modified-live-virus vaccines.
d. Inactivated panleukopenia vaccines may be given effectively by the oral route.
e. Very effective inactivated vaccines have been developed using recombinant DNA technology, with insertion of the genome into *Escherichia coli.*

755. *In feline leukemia virus (FeLV) infection, a cat is described as persistently viremic if it has two or more positive FeLV tests during a period of at least:*

a. 1 week
b. 2 weeks
c. 3 weeks
d. 4 weeks
e. 12 weeks

756. *Concerning viruses you may encounter in your small animal hospital, and the ease with which these viruses can be inactivated by physical and chemical agents, which statement is most accurate?*

a. Rabies virus, canine distemper virus, and canine parvovirus are easily inactivated.
b. Feline herpesvirus, feline calicivirus, and feline parvovirus are easily inactivated.
c. Feline herpesvirus, canine distemper virus, and rabies virus are easily inactivated.
d. Canine distemper virus and feline parvovirus are easily inactivated, but not feline herpesvirus.
e. Feline leukemia virus, feline herpesvirus, and canine distemper virus are not easily inactivated.

757. *Following exposure to feline parvovirus (natural or vaccination), circulating antibodies are first detected in the serum of cats after approximately:*

a. 3 to 4 days
b. 6 to 7 days
c. 10 to 11 days
d. 14 to 15 days
e. 28 to 30 days

758. *The half-life of circulating antibodies in dogs and cats is approximately:*

a. 1 to 2 days
b. 3 to 4 days
c. 8 to 10 days
d. 20 to 25 days
e. 30 to 35 days

Correct answers are on pages 140-171.

759. *Concerning the serum neutralization test, which statement is **least** accurate?*

a. Results of this antibody assay are reported as a "titer."
b. The reaction in a positive serum neutralization test is not detectable, even with the aid of a microscope; therefore some indicator system, such as inoculation of susceptible cell cultures, embryonated eggs, or susceptible animals, must be used to indicate whether the infectious virus in an assay has been "neutralized."
c. The serum neutralization test is generally more expensive and more time consuming than enzyme-linked immunosorbent assay.
d. In many viral diseases, such as feline panleukopenia, there is an excellent correlation between positive serum neutralization titer and protection against infection with virus.
e. The serum neutralization test is highly specific but not very sensitive.

760. *Concerning use of electron microscopy in diagnosis of feline viral infections, which statement is most accurate?*

a. Electron microscopy can rapidly identify specific serotypes of viruses based on the morphology of the virion.
b. Electron microscopy is quite sensitive in diagnosing the cause of intestinal infections in that one can observe as few as one or two viral particles per gram of feces.
c. Electron microscopy can be used with specific antiserum to obtain an immune electron microscopy test by which one can identify serotypes of virus.
d. Electron microscopy is inexpensive and readily available.
e. The most common assay used with electron microscopy is the Western blot.

761. *Concerning enzyme-linked immunosorbent assay (ELISA), which statement is **least** accurate?*

a. An in-clinic ELISA kit is available for diagnosis of canine heartworm disease.
b. KELA is an ELISA that has been standardized and computerized to automatically calculate the titer of the antibody in the test serum.
c. ELISA can only be used to detect serum antibodies and cannot detect antigen.
d. ELISA is a very sensitive test.
e. An in-clinic ELISA kit is available for diagnosis of feline leukemia virus infection.

762. *Canine parvovirus produces severe enteritis in many susceptible dogs. Concerning canine parvovirus, which statement is **least** accurate?*

a. Canine parvovirus and feline parvovirus are antigenically very similar.
b. Canine parvovirus and minute virus of canines cannot be differentiated by electron microscopic examination of fecal samples.
c. Canine parvovirus is readily inactivated by most disinfectants and at normal room temperature within 30 days.
d. Mink enteritis virus cross reacts with canine parvovirus.
e. It is clear from retrospective studies on banks of canine serum samples that canine parvovirus did not exist in the canine population before it was recognized in 1978.

763. *The cause of "cat scratch disease" in people is:*

a. a gram-positive intracellular coccus, believed to be *Rhodococcus pyocyaneus*
b. *Cytauxzoon felis*
c. *Brugia pahangi*
d. feline leukemia virus
e. a gram-negative intracellular bacillus believed to be either *Afipia felis* or *Bartonella henselae*

764. *Concerning caliciviruses, which statement is **least** accurate?*

a. The name of the family (Caliciviridae) is derived from the morphology of the capsomeres of the virions, that is, they appear to be cup shaped when examined by electron microscopy.
b. Caliciviruses are enveloped DNA viruses that are almost never shed after infection and are easily inactivated by disinfectants and environmental conditions.
c. Caliciviral infection may cause ulcerative, respiratory, or enteric disease.
d. Caliciviruses contain single-stranded RNA.
e. Feline caliciviruses were originally called "feline picornaviruses."

765. *Concerning rabies, which statement is **least** accurate?*

a. Rabies virus can infect most warm-blooded animals, including people.
b. Rabies virus is classified as a Lyssavirus of the Rhabdoviridae family.
c. In cats, rabies is routinely diagnosed by identification of Negri bodies in sections of brain.
d. In cats, rabies may be manifested in the furious form or the paralytic (dumb) form.
e. Rabies virus travels to the central nervous system from the original site of infection via nerves.

766. *Parvoviruses of carnivores are similar in that antibodies stimulated against one virus protect against infection by a number of parvoviruses from other species. Concerning parvovirus, which statement is **least** accurate?*

a. The genomes of canine parvovirus-2 and feline parvovirus are similar, but there are slight variations between them.
b. The DNA of feline parvovirus, raccoon parvovirus, and mink enteritis is very similar.
c. Raccoon parvovirus is more closely related to feline parvovirus than to canine parvovirus.
d. Mink enteritis virus can be used as a vaccine for preventing feline parvoviral infection in cats.
e. Parvoviruses are extremely resistant to inactivation by chemical and physical agents because of their double-stranded DNA genomes.

767. *An IgG antibody titer against feline parvovirus in the serum of a 6-month-old, nonvaccinated cat indicates:*

a. chronic parvoviral infection
b. recent infection (within 2 weeks) with feline parvovirus or exposure to canine parvovirus-2
c. only that the animal was infected with this virus sometime in the past
d. persistent viremia
e. that the cat has passive immunity acquired from the queen

768. *Concerning enzyme-linked immunosorbent assay (ELISA), which statement is **least** accurate:*

a. ELISA can detect virus antigen if specific antibody is adhered to the test well or membrane.
b. ELISA can detect antibody if viral antigen is adhered to the test well or membrane.
c. ELISA can detect virus and antibody using the membrane technique.
d. ELISA can detect antibody titer if a kinetics test or KELA is used.
e. ELISA can detect antigen or antibody but not antibody titer.

769. *The indirect immunofluorescent assay for feline leukemia (Hardy test) detects antigen of the virus in:*

a. plasma
b. serum
c. peripheral blood leukocytes
d. erythrocytes
e. whole blood, but only after it is first processed in cell cultures

Correct answers are on pages 140-171.

770. *Concerning feline immunodeficiency virus infection, which statement is **least** accurate?*

a. The virus was first called feline T-lymphotropic virus.
b. The virus is not highly contagious within a group of socially stable cats.
c. The first commercial diagnostic test used to detect infected cats measure virus or viral antigen in the serum.
d. Most, if not all, infected cats remain persistently viremic for the remainder of their lives.
e. The primary method of transmission is via cat bites.

Questions 771 through 777

You receive a call from a fellow veterinarian concerning an outbreak of a fatal disease in cats within a local animal shelter. Your colleague wants to know if the state diagnostic laboratory can confirm the diagnosis of a certain disease by serologic tests. Further discussion reveals that kittens come into the shelter, are vaccinated, and then develop acute disease consisting of vomiting, diarrhea, dehydration, and death. A private home where orphan kittens were taken for rearing also is experiencing the same problems. Necropsy reveals dehydration, evidence of diarrhea, and edematous, hemorrhagic small intestines. Histopathologic changes reported by the local pathology laboratory are consistent with feline panleukopenia.

771. *Which of the following characterizes feline panleukopenia virus (feline parvovirus)?*

a. RNA virus, double-stranded genome, enveloped, labile
b. DNA virus, double-stranded genome, enveloped, labile
c. DNA virus, single-stranded genome, enveloped, labile
d. RNA virus, double-stranded genome, nonenveloped, resistant
e. DNA virus, single-stranded genome, nonenveloped, resistant

772. *What rapid diagnostic test could you perform in your office to be reasonably sure of your diagnosis before the results of gross and histopathologic examination are known?*

a. total plasma protein level
b. rectal temperature of infected kittens
c. total leukocyte count
d. total erythrocyte count
e. enzyme-linked immunosorbent assay for gp27 antigen

773. *Which virus is **not** antigenically related to feline parvovirus?*

a. bovine parvovirus
b. mink enteritis virus
c. raccoon parvovirus
d. canine parvovirus-2
e feline panleukopenia virus

774. *What disinfectant would you recommend to the director of the shelter for immediate use in contaminated cages, water/feed utensils, and on floors and other surfaces?*

a. chlorhexidine
b. povidone-iodine
c. sodium hypochlorite (household bleach)
d. ammonia
e. quaternary ammonium

775. *At what dilution should this disinfectant be used:*

a. undiluted from the container
b. diluted 1:10
c. diluted 1:32
d. diluted 1:128
e. diluted 1:640

776. *What type of panleukopenia vaccine should be used in this facility?*

a. inactivated (killed-virus) vaccine because it is safer
b. modified-live-virus vaccine because it evokes immunity more quickly
c. modified-live-virus vaccine for respiratory viruses, combined with an inactivated (killed-virus) vaccine for panleukopenia
d. intranasal inactivated (killed-virus) vaccine for local protection
e. an autogenous vaccine because it is specific for the bacteria as well as the viruses involved in this outbreak

777. *At what age should the kittens entering this facility be vaccinated?*

a. 4 weeks
b. 6 weeks
c. 8 weeks
d. 12 weeks
e. immediately on entry to the shelter

Questions 778 through 780

Feline immunodeficiency virus (FIV) infection is characterized by mild or subclinical infection initially. Clinical disease is associated with immunosuppression, resulting in a variety of secondary infections.

778. *The period from original infection with FIV until significant clinical disease develops in infected cats generally is:*

a. less than 1 week
b. between 1 and 2 weeks
c. 2 to 4 weeks
d. less than 1 year
e. 3 to 5 years

779. *Concerning the relationship between FIV and human immunodeficiency virus, which statement is most accurate?*

a. There is no similarity at all between these two viruses.
b. The two viruses belong to different families, but both infect T cells within the host.
c. Both viruses infect B cells within the host and impair humoral immune responses.
d. Both are lentiviruses, but there is no known cross infectivity between species (cats, people).
e. The two viruses are subtypes of the same virus and cross infectivity between species (cats, people) occurs.

780. *The primary means of transmission of FIV between infected and uninfected cats is by:*

a. sexual contact
b. direct contact of the queen with kittens
c. cat bites
d. contact with contaminated urine and feces in litter pans
e. aerosol transmission within a contaminated household

C.B. Waters

781. *An 8-year-old female Labrador retriever is presented because of polyuria and polydipsia. In obtaining the history, it is appropriate to ask the owner about all the following* ***except:***

a. appetite
b. general attitude and activity level
c. reproductive history
d. dental history
e. drugs given recently and currently

782. *A client complains that his dog has had diarrhea for 4 weeks. To determine if the diarrhea is of small-bowel or large-bowel origin, questions should include all the following* ***except:***

a. "Does the dog strain to defecate?"
b. "Does the stool appear bloody?"
c. "Does the dog eat with a hearty appetite?"
d. "Is there any mucus on the stools?"
e. "How many times per day does the dog defecate?"

Correct answers are on pages 140-171.

For Questions 783 through 787, select the correct answer from the five choices below:

a. ascites
b. melena
c. hematochezia
d. hematuria
e. icterus/jaundice

783. *Frank (red) blood in the stool*

784. *Dark, tarry stools containing occult (digested) blood*

785. *Accumulation of serous fluid in the abdominal cavity*

786. *Bloody urine*

787. *Yellow discoloration of the mucosae and sclerae*

Questions 788 and 789

A 6-year-old male Corgi is rushed to your clinic after the owner finds the dog prostrate at home. You quickly evaluate the dog and observe that the mucous membranes are pale and capillary refill time is 4 seconds. The dog is unable to stand, and the abdomen is markedly distended. The dog appears alert.

788. *Which of the following best describes this dog's condition?*

a. comatose and overhydrated
b. demented and cyanotic
c. weak and in shock
d. psychotic and polycythemic
e. semicomatose and dyspneic

789. *The dog has a rectal temperature of 37.2° C, a respiratory rate of 45 breaths per minute, a heart rate of 200 beats per minute, and 80 pulses palpated per minute. Which of the following best describes this dog's condition?*

a. hypothermic and eupneic, with pulse deficits
b. normothermic and eupneic, with pulse deficits
c. hypothermic and tachypneic, with appropriate pulses
d. hyperthermic and tachypneic, with pulse deficits
e. hypothermic and tachypneic, with pulse deficits

790. *A 13-year-old cat is presented because of lethargy and anorexia. You notice that the skin remains tented when you pinch it away from the body. The cat's mucous membranes feel very dry. In regard to hydration status, this cat is most likely:*

a. not dehydrated but not emaciated
b. 2% dehydrated
c. 4% dehydrated
d. 6% dehydrated
e. 8% or more dehydrated

791. *Damage to the spinal cord is **least** likely to cause:*

a. paresis
b. paralysis
c. loss of proprioception
d. head tilt
e. urinary or fecal incontinence

792. *Glaucoma is an ocular disease characterized by:*

a. inflammation of the conjunctiva
b. increased intraocular pressure
c. inflammation of the retina
d. corneal edema
e. corneal and conjunctival dryness

793. *Signs of proestrus in the bitch include all the following **except:***

a. vulvar swelling
b. bloody vulvar discharge
c. attraction of males
d. courtship play
e. standing to be mounted

794. *Normal puppies are characterized by all the following* ***except:***

a. crawl and right themselves at birth
b. open eyelids by 1 to 3 weeks of age
c. regulate their body temperature by 4 days of age
d. ear canals open by 13 to 17 days of age
e. suckle at birth

795. *Distichiasis is characterized by:*

a. ingrown eyelashes
b. a double row of eyelashes, one or both of which contact the eyeball
c. lack of eyelashes
d. increased intraocular pressure
e. opacification of the lens

796. *A client presents a 3-year-old basset hound with a 1-week history of a bloody nasal discharge. The clinical sign this dog is displaying is termed:*

a. hematemesis
b. hemoperitoneum
c. hemonasum
d. epistaxis
e. hemostaxis

797. *In dogs and cats, acceptable sites for venipuncture include all the following* ***except*** *the:*

a. jugular vein
b. cephalic vein
c. coccygeal (tail) vein
d. lateral saphenous vein (dog)
e. medial saphenous vein (cat)

798. *Serum values of which constituents are most likely to be increased in an azotemic dog?*

a. alanine aminotransferase and alkaline phosphatase
b. aspartate aminotransferase and creatine phosphokinase
c. urea nitrogen and creatinine
d. unconjugated bilirubin and cholesterol
e. γ-glutamyltransferase and glucose

799. *A 10-year-old dog with chronic renal failure has a blood urea nitrogen level of 90 mg/dl and a serum creatinine level of 4.0 mg/dl. The specific gravity of urine from this dog is most likely to be:*

a. between 1.020 and 1.040
b. between 1.006 and 1.025
c. less than 1.006
d. between 1.030 and 1.055
e. greater than 1.050

800. *The most sensitive laboratory test for detecting heartworm infection in dogs is:*

a. a direct blood smear
b. a modified Knott's test
c. a filter test
d. an antigen test
e. an antibody test

801. *After a dog is determined to be infected with heartworms, the most appropriate additional diagnostic tests before starting treatment include:*

a. thoracic radiographs and a serum biochemistry panel
b. abdominal radiographs and ultrasonographic examination
c. direct blood pressure measurements and blood gas analysis
d. pulmonary function tests and a liver biopsy
e. ophthalmologic examination and pelvic radiographs

802. *When performing cystocentesis, it is important to:*

a. direct the needle cranially before inserting it into the abdomen
b. aspirate as you withdraw the needle through the bladder and abdominal walls
c. insert the needle to the hub
d. stabilize the bladder before inserting the needle
e. use an 18-gauge, 1½ inch needle

Correct answers are on pages 140-171.

803. *The most common risk associated with bladder catheterization via the urethra is:*

a. damage to the urethra
b. damage to the bladder
c. bacterial infection
d. overinserting the catheter, causing the catheter to knot in the urinary bladder
e. damage to the ureters

804. *The earliest time in gestation that radiographs can be used to diagnose pregnancy in dogs and cats is:*

a. 20 days
b. 25 days
c. 35 days
d. 45 days
e. 55 days

Questions 805 and 806

805. *A cat is presented with pinpoint hemorrhages on the skin and mucous membranes. This condition is called:*

a. anemia
b. cyanosis
c. icterus
d. purpura
e. petechiation

806. *In this cat showing hemorrhages, what is the most likely hematologic abnormality?*

a. increased packed cell volume
b. decreased packed cell volume
c. increased platelet count
d. decreased platelet count
e. decreased bleeding time

807. *Concerning shock, which statement is* ***least*** *accurate?*

a. Shock is a maldistribution of blood flow, causing decreased delivery of oxygen to tissues.
b. Shock should be considered an emergency situation, warranting immediate treatment.
c. Shock causes a marked parasympathetic response.
d. Shock can be caused by hemorrhage, severe stress, infection, or anaphylaxis.
e. An animal in shock can develop tachypnea and tachycardia.

For Questions 808 through 812, select the correct answer from the five choices below.

a. calculus
b. stomatitis
c. enteritis
d. colitis
e. coprophagy

808. *Inflammation of the oral mucosa*

809. *An abnormal concretion, usually composed of mineral salts*

810. *Inflammation of the large intestine*

811. *Inflammation of the small intestine*

812. *Ingestion of feces*

For Questions 813 through 817, select the correct answer from the five choices below.

a. constipation
b. obstipation
c. anal sac impaction
d. perianal fistulae
e. rectal prolapse

813. *Eversion of the rectum out through the anus*

814. *Infected draining tracts around the anal region*

815. *Difficult evacuation of feces*

816. *Inability to pass a stool because of long-standing failure to evacuate feces*

817. *Common cause of "scooting" or rubbing the anal area along the ground*

818. *Regurgitation is:*
   a. commonly associated with hookworm infection
   b. preceded by retching
   c. the expulsion of undigested food
   d. a definitive sign of lead toxicity
   e. almost always seen in old dogs

819. *Pruritus is **least** likely to be seen in an animal with:*
   a. flea-allergy dermatitis
   b. demodicosis
   c. sarcoptic mange
   d. bacterial pyoderma
   e. endocrine alopecia

820. *Common signs of congestive heart failure include all the following **except:***
   a. ascites
   b. dyspnea
   c. exercise intolerance
   d. jugular distention
   e. muscle pain

821. *Common cutaneous and subcutaneous tumors of dogs include all the following **except:***
   a. lipoma
   b. mast-cell tumor
   c. malignant melanoma
   d. malignant fibrous histiocytoma
   e. histiocytoma

822. *Hip dysplasia:*
   a. most often affects small breeds of dogs
   b. is not hereditary
   c. resolves with age
   d. is diagnosed by ventrodorsal radiographs of the pelvis
   e. is common in cats

823. *Concerning osteomyelitis, which statement is **least** accurate?*
   a. Osteomyelitis is a bacterial or fungal infection of the bone.
   b. Osteomyelitis may require surgery and long-term medical therapy.
   c. Pain, fever, and lameness are frequently associated with osteomyelitis.
   d. The best way to determine which antibiotic is appropriate for treatment is usually with a gram-stained preparation.
   e. Radiographs can be helpful in making a definitive diagnosis.

824. *An 8-week-old collie puppy has had diarrhea for 3 days, and you suspect a parasite infection. Gastrointestinal parasites this puppy is most likely to have include all the following **except:***
   a. coccidia
   b. roundworms
   c. whipworms
   d. hookworms
   e. tapeworms

825. *You perform a fecal flotation on a dog's stool and observe whipworm eggs in the sample. The most appropriate anthelmintic for use in treating this dog is:*
   a. pyrantel pamoate (Nemex, Strongid-T)
   b. piperazine citrate
   c. praziquantel (Droncit)
   d. fenbendazole (Panacur)
   e. bunamidine hydrochloride (Scolaban)

826. *Enzyme-linked immunosorbent assay (ELISA) on serum from an apparently healthy cat is a positive for feline leukemia virus infection. The most appropriate course of action is to:*
   a. euthanize the cat immediately
   b. retest the cat by ELISA in 1 week
   c. retest the cat by ELISA or indirect fluorescent antibody test in 1 month or later
   d. permanently isolate the cat to prevent infection of other cats
   e. administer a broad-spectrum antibiotic at low levels for 6 months

Correct answers are on pages 140-171.

827. *A common yeast that often causes otitis in dogs is:*

a. *Candida albicans*
b. *Malassezia pachydermatis*
c. *Sporothrix schenckii*
d. *Blastomyces dermatitidis*
e. *Aspergillus flavus*

828. *The most common coccidial parasite of the gastrointestinal tract of dogs and cats is:*

a. *Eimeria*
b. *Isospora*
c. *Toxoplasma*
d. *Sarcocystis*
e. *Neospora*

829. *All the following are gastrointestinal parasites* ***except:***

a. *Ancylostoma caninum*
b. *Trichuris vulpis*
c. *Toxocara canis*
d. *Dipylidium caninum*
e. *Paragonimus kellicotti*

830. *All the following are caused solely by a virus* ***except:***

a. feline infectious peritonitis
b. canine distemper
c. kennel cough
d. rabies
e. feline panleukopenia

831. *Of the following agents, which is the only one that can destroy parvovirus?*

a. phenol
b. detergents
c. formaldehyde
d. chlorine bleach
e. alcohol

832. *Of the following sets of diseases, which set consists only of zoonotic diseases?*

a. leptospirosis, ringworm, salmonellosis, toxoplasmosis
b. leptospirosis, Rocky Mountain spotted fever, feline immunodeficiency virus infection, sarcoptic mange
c. leptospirosis, canine parvovirus infection, salmonellosis, giardiasis
d. rabies, brucellosis, canine adenovirus infection, cryptosporidiosis
e. rabies, salmonellosis, toxoplasmosis, feline immunodeficiency virus infection

833. *Concerning demodectic mange in dogs, which statement is* ***least*** *accurate?*

a. It is caused by the mite *Demodex canis.*
b. Occasional mites may be seen on skin scrapings of normal dogs.
c. The dam transmits the mite to her puppies by direct contact.
d. This is primarily a disease of mixed-breed dogs.
e. Generalized demodicosis can be a sign of immunodeficiency.

834. *Dermatophytosis (ringworm) in dogs and cats can be caused by* Microsporum *and* Trichophyton. *Concerning dermatophytosis, which statement is* ***least*** *accurate?*

a. Approximately 50% of *Microsporum* species cause fluorescence of lesions on exposure to a Wood's lamp.
b. Lesions caused by *Trichophyton* species do not fluoresce on exposure to a Wood's lamp.
c. *Microsporum canis* is the most common genus in dogs and cats.
d. *Microsporum canis* is more common in dogs than in cats.
e. Systemic treatment may be necessary with generalized dermatophytosis.

835. *If a puppy is infected with heartworm* (Dirofilaria immitis) *microfilariae on the second day of life, what is the earliest time at which the animal will test positive for microfilariae?*
   a. 2 months of age
   b. 3 months of age
   c. 6 months of age
   d. 8 months of age
   e. 9 months of age

836. *Heartworm infection can be prevented by use of any of the following* ***except:***
   a. ivermectin
   b. milbemycin
   c. fenbendazole
   d. diethylcarbamazine
   e. diethylcarbamazine with oxibendazole

Questions 837 and 838

837. *A drug given to dogs by careful intravenous injection to kill adult heartworms is:*
   a. thiobenzamine
   b. thiacetarsamide
   c. ivermectin
   d. diethylcarbamazine
   e. levamisole

838. *Major side effects of this drug are:*
   a. hepatic and renal toxicity
   b. cardiac and otic toxicity
   c. anaphylaxis and shock
   d. hematuria and melena
   e. lymphadenopathy and uveitis

839. *In cats, all the following diseases may* ***directly*** *cause upper respiratory disease* ***except:***
   a. rhinotracheitis
   b. calicivirus infection
   c. chlamydial infection
   d. feline leukemia virus infection
   e. bacterial rhinitis

840. *A 3-year-old golden retriever is receiving 1 grain of phenobarbital every 12 hours for epilepsy. One grain is equivalent to:*
   a. 100 mg
   b. 65 mg
   c. 10 mg
   d. 1000 mg
   e. 50 mg

841. *A 28-lb cocker spaniel has congestive heart failure and requires furosemide per os at 2 mg/kg of body weight BID. At this dosage, this dog should be given:*
   a. 50 mg every 4 hours
   b. 25 mg every 12 hours
   c. 12.5 mg every 24 hours
   d. 100 mg every 12 hours
   e. 10 mg every 8 hours

842. *A 55-lb dog develops acute pulmonary edema. The veterinarian orders treatment with 5% furosemide intravenously at 2 mg/kg of body weight. What quantity of furosemide should you give?*
   a. 1 ml
   b. 0.5 ml
   c. 1.5 ml
   d. 5 ml
   e. 10 ml

843. *A 28-lb mongrel has been vomiting for 3 days and is estimated to be 8% dehydrated. What approximate fluid volume should you give to rehydrate this dog?*
   a. 500 ml
   b. 1000 ml
   c. 2000 ml
   d. 2240 ml
   e. 1500 ml

Correct answers are on pages 140-171.

844. *When administering intravenous fluids to a cat or dog, care must be taken to monitor for overhydration. The best initial indicator of overhydration is:*

a. edematous skin
b. pulmonary edema
c. polyuria
d. continued weight gain after the animal has been rehydrated appropriately
e. tachypnea

845. *You are using a microdrip to administer intravenous fluids to a cat. The cat must receive 360 ml of fluid during a 24-hour period. At what rate should the fluid be infused:*

a. 15 drops/min
b. 15 drops/sec
c. 150 drops/hr
d. 15 ml/min
e. 36 ml/hr

846. *You are attempting to infuse intravenous fluids in a cat, but the fluid is not flowing well. What is the* ***least*** *likely cause of this problem?*

a. The infusion line is kinked.
b. The vein is obstructed.
c. The bottle is held above the level of the vein.
d. The needle or catheter has become dislodged from the vein.
e. The air vent is obstructed.

847. *An example of an isotonic fluid is:*

a. 50% dextrose
b. distilled water
c. 0.9% saline
d. 10% calcium gluconate
e. lactated Ringer's solution with 2.5% dextrose

848. *Concerning total parental nutrition (intravenous feeding), which statement is most accurate?*

a. The solution usually contains equal volumes of B vitamins and dextrose.
b. If a dextrose solution in a concentration of 10% or higher is used, the fluid should be infused into the jugular vein.
c. The catheter should be flushed thoroughly with saline before administering any intravenous medications.
d. Laboratory tests are seldom necessary as long as asepsis is strictly observed.
e. Solutions can be mixed in a bowl that has been sterilized in a dishwasher.

849. *The preferred enema solution for cats and dogs is:*

a. sodium phosphate
b. soapy water
c. warm tap water
d. mineral oil
e. vegetable oil

850. *Complications of enema administration may include all the following* ***except:***

a. hypothermia
b. vomiting
c. anemia
d. constipation
e. diarrhea

J.P. Thompson

851. *Which disorder is* ***least*** *likely to be associated with splenomegaly?*

a. bone marrow erythroid hypoplasia
b. myasthenia gravis
c. immune-mediated hemolytic anemia
d. hemobartonellosis
e. lymphoma

852. *An excess of which element has been associated with hemolytic anemia in dogs?*

a. copper
b. silver
c. sodium
d. zinc
e. carbon

853. *Which assessment would be **least** helpful in differentiating possible causes of anemia in a dog?*

a. fecal examination
b. splenic palpation
c. mucous membrane evaluation
d. conscious proprioception evaluation
e. urinalysis

854. *Which dog breed has naturally occurring erythrocyte macrocytosis?*

a. poodle
b. cocker spaniel
c. golden retriever
d. Scottish terrier
e. coon hound

855. *A dog has a hematocrit (packed cell volume) [PCV] of 18%, marked erythrocyte polychromasia, and 18% reticulocytes. The equation to calculate the reticulocyte index (RI) in the presence of polychromasia is RI = [(Patient's PCV ÷ 45) × Reticulocyte percentage] ÷ 2. A reticulocyte index above 2.5 is considered evidence of regenerative anemia. What is this patient's reticulocyte index?*

a. 3.6
b. 1.8
c. 7.2
d. 4.0
e. 2.0

856. *Which disorder is **least** likely to be associated with nonregenerative anemia?*

a. chronic renal failure
b. immune-mediated hemolytic anemia
c. iron-deficiency anemia
d. acute blood loss (within the first 48 to 96 hours)
e. hypothyroidism

857. *Which of the following is **least** likely to be associated with neutropenia?*

a. myelophthisis
b. chemotherapy for neoplasia
c. parvovirus infection
d. endotoxic shock
e. bacterial infection

858. *Which neoplasm is most likely to be associated with disseminated intravascular coagulation?*

a. hemangiosarcoma
b. perianal-gland adenoma
c. oral squamous-cell carcinoma
d. ocular melanoma
e. osteosarcoma

859. *Which disorder has been associated with monoclonal gammopathy?*

a. feline infectious peritonitis
b. ehrlichiosis
c. pyometra
d. leishmaniasis
e. systemic mycosis

860. *Which disorder has **not** been associated with retrovirus infections in cats?*

a. lymphoma
b. multicentric fibrosarcoma
c. immunodeficiency
d. bone marrow aplasia
e. hyperthyroidism

861. *Which sample should be submitted to the clinical pathology laboratory to perform a direct Coombs' test?*

a. serum
b. blood
c. plasma
d. urine
e. joint fluid

862. *A positive antinuclear antibody test result is considered one of the necessary laboratory criteria in diagnosis of:*

a. systemic lupus erythematosus
b. immune-mediated hemolytic anemia
c. immune-mediated thrombocytopenia
d. pemphigus vulgaris
e. rheumatoid arthritis

Correct answers are on pages 140-171.

863. *Which antineoplastic drug is **not** contraindicated in the presence of significant thrombocytopenia (platelet count below 10,000/μl)?*

a. azathioprine
b. doxorubicin
c. vincristine
d. cyclophosphamide
e. methotrexate

864. *Which antineoplastic drug has been associated with transitional-cell carcinoma of the bladder or sterile hemorrhagic cystitis?*

a. cyclophosphamide
b. azathioprine
c. doxorubicin
d. vincristine
e. methotrexate

865. *All the following diagnostic tests should be strongly considered in evaluating a patient with a fever of unknown origin **except:***

a. thoracic and abdominal radiographs
b. serial blood cultures
c. antinuclear antibody test
d. urinalysis
e. cardiac catheterization

866. *Which component of the immune system is considered nonspecific in its functions?*

a. B cells
b. T cells
c. immunoglobulin G (IgG)
d. complement
e. immunoglobulin M (IgM)

867. *Which clinical sign is most consistent with left-sided congestive heart failure?*

a. pulmonary congestion and edema, leading to coughing, tachypnea, and dyspnea
b. venous congestion, leading to high central venous pressure
c. hepatic and splenic congestion
d. pleural effusion
e. ascites

868. *Which of the following is **least** likely to cause syncope or intermittent weakness?*

a. hypoglycemia
b. hypoadrenocorticism
c. tachyarrhythmia (paroxysmal ventricular tachycardia)
d. stress-associated hyperglycemia
e. anemia

869. *Any of the following conditions may be associated with cyanotic mucous membranes **except:***

a. right-to-left shunting congenital cardiac defect
b. sepsis
c. methemoglobinemia
d. hypoventilation
e. shock

870. *Which disorder is most likely to be associated with sinus bradycardia?*

a. hyperthermia
b. hypoxia
c. hypothyroidism
d. hypotension
e. chocolate intoxication

871. *Right atrial enlargement is commonly associated with:*

a. mitral insufficiency
b. patent ductus arteriosus
c. ventricular septal defect
d. pulmonic stenosis
e. subaortic stenosis

872. *Which of the following is **least** likely to be associated with acute thromboembolic disease in a cat?*

a. acute caudal paresis
b. cool distal limbs
c. pale foot pads
d. cyanotic nail beds
e. hypoglycemia

873. *Which abnormality is **least** likely to be associated with thromboembolic disease in a cat?*

a. azotemia
b. increased serum lactate dehydrogenase activity
c. lymphopenia
d. neutropenia
e. disseminated intravascular coagulation

874. *Which of the following is **least** likely to be a sequela of infectious endocarditis?*

a. heart murmur
b. infarction
c. septic or immune-mediated arthritis
d. fever
e. pulmonary thromboembolism

875. *Which radiographic finding is most likely to be observed in a patient with congenital patent ductus arteriosus?*

a. right atrial enlargement
b. left ventricular enlargement
c. reduced blood flow through pulmonary vessels
d. normal blood flow through pulmonary vessels
e. caudal vena cava dilation

876. *Concerning thiacetarsamide therapy for heartworm disease in dogs, which statement is **least** accurate?*

a. Thiacetarsamide toxicity may occur during or within 1 week after therapy.
b. Thiacetarsamide may cause hepatotoxicity or nephrotoxicity.
c. Laboratory abnormalities associated with thiacetarsamide toxicity may include azotemia, tubular casts in the urine sediment, and bilirubinemia.
d. Icterus and persisting vomiting are indications to discontinue thiacetarsamide treatment immediately.
e. Thiacetarsamide therapy should be discontinued on documentation of elevated serum liver enzymes.

877. *Concerning pure transudates, which statement is most accurate?*

a. Pure transudates are slightly cloudy and generally have a pinkish tinge.
b. Pure transudates have a cellularity of 15,000 to 30,000 cells/μl.
c. Pure transudates have a low protein content (less than 2.5 to 3.0 g/ml).
d. Pure transudates have a specific gravity above 1.030.
e. Pure transudates are commonly associated with the "wet" (effusive) form of feline infectious peritonitis.

878. *What is the most common complication of pericardiocentesis?*

a. cardiac arrhythmia secondary to cardiac injury or puncture
b. coronary artery laceration
c. myocardial infarction
d. lung laceration, leading to pneumothorax
e. lung laceration, leading to hemothorax

879. *A mucopurulent nasal discharge is **least** likely to be observed in a patient with:*

a. nasal *Aspergillus* infection
b. nasal bacterial infection
c. acute nasal trauma
d. nasal neoplasia
e. allergic rhinitis

880. *Cryptococcus neoformans:*

a. is a parasite that infects dogs and, less commonly, cats
b. is found in the soil and can remain viable for months to years in pigeon droppings
c. enters the body though the gastrointestinal tract following ingestion
d. rarely infects the nasal cavity or central nervous system
e. most commonly infects the proximal jejunum

881. *Causes of inspiratory distress include all of the following* ***except:***

a. laryngeal paralysis
b. tracheal hypoplasia
c. nasopharyngeal polyps
d. intrathoracic tracheal collapse
e. elongated soft palate

882. *What is the most common cause of laryngeal paralysis?*

a. hypothyroidism
b. hypocalcemia
c. neoplasia affecting the recurrent laryngeal nerve
d. trauma
e. idiopathic factors

883. *Causes of pulmonary vascular enlargement observed on thoracic radiographs include all of the following* ***except:***

a. heartworm disease
b. pulmonary hypertension
c. hypoadrenocorticism
d. thromboembolic disease
e. left heart failure

884. *Which disorder is most frequently associated with an alveolar pattern on thoracic radiographs?*

a. allergic bronchitis
b. pulmonary edema
c. bronchiectasis
d. pulmonary parasitism
e. bacterial bronchitis

885. *Concerning* Blastomyces dermatitidis, *which statement is* ***least*** *accurate?*

a. It is commonly found in soil.
b. At room temperature it usually exists as a mold.
c. At body temperature it usually exists as a yeast.
d. It is most often transmitted directly from animal to animal.
e. In the United States it is distributed primarily along the Ohio, Missouri, and Mississippi River valleys.

886. *Pulmonary thromboembolization has been reported with each of the following disorders* ***except:***

a. hyperadrenocorticism
b. tetanus
c. immune-mediated hemolytic anemia
d. nephrotic syndrome
e. dirofilariasis

887. *Which of the following is* ***least*** *likely to be associated with ptyalism?*

a. nausea
b. hepatic encephalopathy in a cat
c. seizures
d. xerostomia
e. organophosphate intoxication

888. *Which virus has as its genetic material a single strand of DNA?*

a. poxvirus
b. parvovirus
c. adenovirus
d. herpesvirus
e. coronavirus

889. *Which disorder is* ***least*** *likely to be associated with protein-losing enteropathy?*

a. intestinal lymphangiectasis
b. alimentary histoplasmosis
c. alimentary lymphoma
d. lymphocytic-plasmacytic enteritis
e. rectal adenocarcinoma

890. *Which disorder is* ***least*** *likely to be associated with tenesmus and/or dyschezia?*

a. rectal neoplasia
b. perineal hernia
c. proctitis
d. prostatomegaly
e. intestinal lymphangiectasia

*891. Which disorder is **least** likely to be associated with renomegaly?*

a. lymphoma
b. hydronephrosis
c. polycystic renal disease
d. renal amyloidosis
e. chronic renal insufficiency

*892. All the following oral tumors are considered potentially malignant **except:***

a. squamous-cell carcinoma
b. melanoma
c. fibrosarcoma
d. fibromatous epulis
e. lymphoma

*893. Which coagulation factor is **not** dependent on vitamin K?*

a. factor II
b. factor VII
c. factor IX
d. factor X
e. factor XII

*894. Which enzyme is **not** secreted by or found in the exocrine pancreas?*

a. trypsinogen
b. chymotrypsinogen
c. gastrin
d. lipase
e. procarboxypeptidase A

*895. Polyuria is commonly associated with any of the following disorders **except:***

a. chronic renal failure
b. hepatic insufficiency
c. normoglycemic glucosuria
d. cystitis
e. hyperadrenocorticism

896. Which bacterium is most commonly isolated from the urine of dogs with urinary tract infections?

a. *Pseudomonas aeruginosa*
b. *Klebsiella pneumoniae*
c. *Escherichia coli*
d. *Enterobacter aerogenes*
e. *Proteus vulgaris*

*897. All the following are common clinicopathologic abnormalities associated with hyperadrenocorticism **except:***

a. hypocholesterolemia
b. stress leukogram
c. elevated serum alkaline phosphatase activity
d. hyposthenuria or isosthenuria
e. urinary tract infection

*898. Hypocalcemia may be observed with any of the following **except:***

a. puerperal tetany
b. chronic renal failure
c. phosphate enema administration
d. primary hyperparathyroidism
e. acute pancreatitis

*899. Electrocardiographic findings associated with hyperkalemia include all the following **except:***

a. absent or flattened P waves
b. shortened P-R interval
c. widened QRS complex
d. bradycardia
e. sinoatrial or ventricular arrhythmias

900. Which antineoplastic drug has been implicated in inducing acute pancreatitis?

a. cyclophosphamide
b. chlorambucil
c. azathioprine
d. cisplatin
e. methotrexate

Correct answers are on pages 140-171.

Answers

1. **c** Chronic renal disease does not produce the same degree of cardiovascular, neuromuscular, or metabolic insult as the other four choices.
2. **b** Left-sided, not right-sided, heart failure usually produces coughing.
3. **e** All the other answers are seen with left-sided heart disease (answers a, b,and c) or pulmonic stenosis and right-to-left shunting (answer d). Answer e is the only one pertaining to right-sided cardiac enlargement, as seen in heartworm disease.
4. **c** Other than aspergillosis, the other fungal diseases listed rarely affect the nasal cavity in dogs.
5. **a** Adenocarcinoma is the most common nasal tumor of dogs. Fibrosarcoma is also common but is not given as an answer.
6. **c** Radiation therapy is much more effective than other therapies or no therapy at all.
7. **e** Viral infections, such as canine distemper, are less likely causes of epistaxis than the other answers listed.
8. **e** Bronchitis is the only lower airway disease listed. Upper airway diseases are most likely to result in inspiratory distress.
9. **d** In dogs, pythiosis is a disease of the gastrointestinal system or the skin.
10. **b** The right middle bronchus arises from the floor of the right main-stem bronchus. This is part of the reason the right middle lung lobe is so commonly affected in dogs with aspiration pneumonia.
11. **d** Hyperventilation would be a response to acidemia, producing alkalemia.
12. **b** Terbutaline is a β_2-agonist. Aminophylline and oxtriphylline are methylxanthine derivatives. Atropine is a parasympatholytic. Atenolol is not a bronchodilator and is a β-blocker.
13. **a** The lungs are the portal of entry, and the skin and eyes are the two most commonly affected organ systems.
14. **b** The lungs are the portal of entry, and the gastrointestinal tract is the most common organ system affected. The gastrointestinal tract may serve as a second portal of entry. Bones are also commonly affected.
15. **e** Hypothyroidism can cause nonregenerative anemia.
16. **d** All the answers can cause thrombosis, but aortic valve vegetative endocarditis produces systemic thromboses, whereas the other conditions listed result primarily in pulmonary thromboembolism.
17. **a** Dogs with nephrotic syndrome have glomerular protein loss and hypoalbuminemia, which can then result in transudative effusions. The other answers produce modified transudates, hemorrhagic effusions, or exudates.
18. **c** Trimethoprim-potentiated sulfonamide can cause keratoconjunctivitis sicca as a side effect.
19. **d** Answers a, b, c, and e are all seen with vomiting but not regurgitation. The time relative to eating is variable in both vomiting and regurgitation.
20. **e** Hyperadrenocorticism typically does not produce megaesophagus.
21. **a** Alkaline phosphatase is not a liver-specific enzyme; each of the other answers depends on liver function.
22. **d** The age, breed, clinical signs, and microcytosis all point toward a portosystemic vascular anomaly.
23. **e** Diazepam may worsen the signs of hepatoencephalopathy.
24. **d** Each of the other breeds has been affected by familial liver disease involving copper. The liver disease of cocker spaniels does not involve copper.
25. **d** Methionine is contraindicated in dogs with hepatoencephalopathy. Each of the other treatments would be indicated in a dog with hepatic failure and coma, given the information available.
26. **a** Although the BUN level is often increased with pancreatitis, it is a nonspecific finding and would more likely indicate renal disease or prerenal azotemia from other causes, such as dehydration.
27. **b** Sulfasalazine is an enteric sulfonamide used in treatment of colitis; it has no antacid effect. Aluminum hydroxide is a locally active antacid. Famotidine and cimetidine are H_2-receptor antagonists. Omeprazole is a proton pump inhibitor.
28. **e** Fenbendazole is not effective against coccidian organisms.

29. **d** Hemoconcentration with a normal total plasma protein level in a dog with acute onset of the signs described suggests hemorrhagic gastroenteritis.
30. **a** Nonsteroidal antiinflammatory drugs are very ulcerogenic in dogs.
31. **a** Trypsinlike immunoreactivity is a sensitive and specific test for exocrine pancreatic insufficiency and is decreased in affected dogs.
32. **c** Any of these disorders may respond to therapy, but eosinophilic gastroenteritis has a good prognosis and is usually very responsive to corticosteroids. In cats, eosinophilic gastroenteritis is very difficult to treat and has a guarded prognosis.
33. **e** Lymphangiectasia is a cause of protein-losing enteropathy, which results in loss of albumin and globulins. Rocky Mountain spotted fever, liver disease, and glomerular disease may result in hypoalbuminemia, but serum globulin levels remain normal or are increased. Blood loss can result in decreased albumin and total plasma protein levels, but in chronic blood loss the PCV would be decreased and the protein level would likely be normal.
34. **e** This combination of anticholinergics (Darbazine) has some efficacy in treatment of small intestinal diarrhea but is not effective in idiopathic colitis. Of the therapies listed, dietary therapy is most useful, followed by sulfasalazine, prednisone, and metronidazole.
35. **d** Female Dobermans are more commonly affected than males. This disease rarely is seen in young or very old dogs.
36. **b** Histoplasmosis commonly affects the gastrointestinal tract, causing significant granulomatous infiltration.
37. **d** Coccidioidomycosis occurs in hot, dry, dusty climates, from west Texas to the San Joaquin Valley of California. Blastomycosis and histoplasmosis occur in the central and southeastern United States, especially along the Mississippi and Ohio River valleys. Aspergillosis and sporotrichosis occur sporadically throughout the United States.
38. **e** Aspergillosis most commonly causes nasal disease. Systemic infection, fungal pneumonia, renal disease, and diskospondylitis are less commonly seen with aspergillosis.
39. **a** Blastomycosis is a budding yeast at body temperature. The skin and eyes are most likely to yield organisms for diagnosis.
40. **c** Sporotrichosis is a cutaneous fungal infection that rarely becomes systemic.
41. **a** Hemophilia A is caused by factor VIII deficiency, which affects only the intrinsic coagulation pathway. PTT tests the intrinsic and common pathways and thus would be prolonged in a dog with hemophilia A. PT tests the extrinsic and common pathways. Warfarin toxicity, hepatic failure, and disseminated intravascular coagulation result in decreased factors in all three pathways (intrinsic, extrinsic, common), so PT and PTT would be prolonged. Ehrlichiosis results in thrombocytopenia but does not affect PT or PTT.
42. **c** Sound would travel unimpeded through the fluid-filled cyst, resulting in a hypoechoic appearance.
43. **a** Glomerulonephritis, renal amyloidosis, hyperadrenocorticism, and systemic lupus erythematosus all may result in glomerular protein loss that can be quantified by the urinary protein/creatinine ratio (UPCR). Urinary tract infection may result in inflammation that increases the UPCR, so the UPCR would not be useful in monitoring urinary glomerular protein loss. UPCR should not be used in dogs with urinary tract infections.
44. **d** Cardiomyopathy typically causes decreased cardiac output, with normal blood pressure or systemic hypotension.
45. **e** Primidone is potentially hepatotoxic. The other drugs listed can cause significant nephrotoxicity.
46. **b** Infusion rates above 0.5 mEq/kg/hr may result in cardiotoxicity.
47. **a** Pancreatitis can lead to hypocalcemia and calcification of the peripancreatic fat. The other choices are potential causes of hypercalcemia.
48. **d** *E. coli* is involved in approximately 40% of canine urinary tract infections.
49. **d** Cephalexin is concentrated in the urine. Bacteria showing in vitro sensitivity to this antibiotic by the Kirby-Bauer technique would also show sensitivity using a mean inhibitory concentration.
50. **a** Medical dissolution is not generally effective for oxalate urolithiasis. Prevention measures would include urinary alkalinization and feeding a low-protein diet. Potassium citrate is often recommended for alkalinization.

51. **e** Chronic pancreatitis is a predisposing factor, along with genetic predisposition, infection, insulin antagonistic diseases and drugs, and immune-mediated ileitis.
52. **c** Functional pancreatic β-cell tumors produce high concentrations of insulin, resulting in hypoglycemia.
53. **b** Dexamethasone has no mineralocorticoid effects and no effect on potassium. Deoxycorticosterone pivalate and fludrocortisone have significant mineralocorticoid effects. Insulin, dextrose, and sodium bicarbonate shift extracellular potassium to the intracellular space.
54. **e** Potassium bromide, in conjunction with phenobarbital, is very useful in management of refractory epilepsy. The half-life of diazepam is too short to be of benefit in long-term management. Increasing the dose of phenobarbital would not be indicated if the concentration is well within the therapeutic range.
55. **e** The head tilt and falling to the right, together with horizontal nystagmus with the fast phase to the left, suggest a right-sided vestibular lesion. The right-sided miotic pupil, ptosis, and enophthalmos indicate Horner's syndrome on the right. These findings in a dog with no other neurologic abnormalities indicate a lesion of the right inner and middle ear.
56. **a** These signs indicate left-sided facial nerve (cranial nerve VII) paralysis. The most common causes of facial nerve paralysis are middle ear disease on the affected side or idiopathic disease. Of the other answers, only hypothyroidism might cause cranial nerve disease; it is not a common cause.
57. **d** Neurologic deficits are uncommon in dogs with corticosteroid-responsive meningitis. Cervical pain, vertebral pain, and fever are typical.
58. **b** A fourfold rise in IgG titers over 3 weeks, a single positive IgM titer, and biopsy demonstrating organisms are all supportive of toxoplasmosis.
59. **d** Bilateral trigeminal nerve paralysis results in difficulty with prehension of food, a mouth that hangs open, and atrophy of masticatory muscles. Affected dogs can swallow normally. Other findings of physical examination are usually normal. Dogs with masticatory myositis may have atrophy of the muscles of mastication but more typically have difficulty opening the mouth.
60. **c** Doxorubicin causes acute cardiotoxicity, characterized by arrhythmias. Chronic doxorubicin cardiotoxicity is characterized by dilative cardiomyopathy.
61. **e** Cough typically occurs with disease of the airways from the trachea distally (caudally).
62. **a** Spherocytosis indicates an extravascular hemolytic process. Autoimmune hemolytic anemia is more common than babesiosis.
63. **c** The high triglyceride and low cholesterol levels are diagnostic of a chylous effusion.
64. **c** Human recombinant epoetin alfa is a recombinant erythropoietin. The drug quickly increases the red blood cell mass if the dog does not also have iron deficiency or anemia from some chronic disease.
65. **d** Renal adenocarcinoma and chronic pulmonary disease are secondary causes of polycythemia; polycythemia vera is a primary cause. Hemorrhagic gastroenteritis and dehydration cause relative polycythemia, but a dehydrated animal would also have an increased total plasma protein level, whereas a dog with hemorrhagic gastroenteritis would not.
66. **a** Parvovirus infection typically causes vomiting, bloody diarrhea, and leukopenia. The other answers listed may cause vomiting and bloody diarrhea but not leukopenia.
67. **b** Corticosteroids are contraindicated. Immunostimulants are not helpful and do not take the place of antibiotics. Mitaban, Ivomec, and Interceptor are effective. Continued estrous cycling could cause recrudescence.
68. **e** Dogs with hypothyroidism tend to gain weight, but this is caused by a decreased metabolic rate, not an increased appetite.
69. **a** The other answers are rare causes of hypothyroidism in dogs.
70. **a** Many medications and illnesses can alter the baseline T_4 level. T_3 is intracellular and cannot be measured accurately in the serum. Blood levels of thyroid hormone are much lower in dogs than in people. Borderline results should be evaluated with more definitive tests.
71. **a** Abnormalities commonly seen with hyperadrenocorticism are polyuria, polydipsia, polyphagia (not anorexia), eosinopenia, neutrophilia (not neutropenia), hepatomegaly (not splenomegaly), and increased serum alkaline phosphatase activity.

72. **b** The ACTH stimulation test is the only test that detects inability of the adrenal glands to produce cortisol on stimulation.
73. **b** Ketoconazole, mitotane, and deprenyl are effective in treating hyperadrenocorticism.
74. **a** High-dosage dexamethasone suppression and endogenous ACTH levels are used to differentiate the types of hyperadrenocorticism. They are used after the disease is diagnosed with a screening test, such as the ACTH stimulation test or low-dosage dexamethasone suppression.
75. **b** Dexamethasone has no mineralocorticoid effects.
76. **c** Calcium deposition in tissue is not seen in hypothyroidism but is seen in hyperadrenocorticism.
77. **c** An osmotic gradient is created by the increased glucose in the urine, causing polyuria with compensatory polydipsia.
78. **c** Normal daily water consumption averages 20 to 40 ml/lb.
79. **c** Insulinoma is characterized by excessive insulin production.
80. **a** The hallmark of the uveodermatologic syndrome is bilateral anterior uveitis, with cutaneous depigmentation. Ocular disease usually precedes noticeable cutaneous changes.
81. **d** The primary inflammatory reaction is apparently attributable to a cellular response to melanocyte cell-surface receptors and melanin, which induces a granulomatous lymphocytic reaction.
82. **a** Pituitary tumor is the most common cause of hyperadrenocorticism, with resultant hyperplastic adrenal cortices and excessive production of cortisol.
83. **c** With a large adrenal tumor, excessive cortisol production decreases release of ACTH by the pituitary. Decreased ACTH causes atrophy to the nontumorous adrenal gland.
84. **a** Dogs with hyperadrenocorticism have increased fat deposition over the thorax, muscle wasting, and weakness of respiratory muscles. Pressure on the diaphragm is increased by fat accumulation in the abdomen and hepatomegaly. Affected dogs also have an increased incidence of thromboembolism.
85. **b** Pyelonephritis (from untreated urinary tract infection), pulmonary thromboembolism, congestive heart failure (from volume overload), and diabetes mellitus (glucocorticoids cause insulin antagonism) are all associated with hyperadrenocorticism.
86. **b** The insulin requirement decreases with time because the insulin antagonism of glucocorticoids is lessened by reduced production of glucocorticoids.
87. **c** Hyperglycemia (not hypoglycemia) is a cause of hypercholesterolemia/hyperlipidemia in dogs.
88. **e** Hypercalcemia (not hypocalcemia) is a cause of polyuria and polydipsia.
89. **e** The urine cortisol/creatinine ratio is a good screening test for hyperadrenocorticism. A normal ratio rules out hyperadrenocorticism, but a high ratio warrants further testing.
90. **c** Bacteria and many white blood cells in the urine indicate a urinary tract infection.
91. **e** A high urine protein/creatinine ratio indicates glomerular protein loss unless there is evidence of inflammation on the urinalysis. With the inflammation present in this dog, the protein/creatinine ratio is not indicative of any specific disease process.
92. **c** Alkalinization from sodium bicarbonate administration shifts ionized calcium to the bound (non-ionized) form of calcium. The total serum calcium level is not affected, but the level of ionized calcium is reduced.
93. **d** The high chloride content of saline (NaCl) solution reduces resorption of Cl, Na, and Ca from the ascending limb of the loop of Henle.
94. **a** Bilirubinuria can be a nonspecific finding in dogs. The normal canine kidney can conjugate and excrete bilirubin.
95. **a** Bile acid levels are used as a test of liver function.
96. **b** Trypsinlike reactivity (TLI) is a measure of free and bound trypsin and trypsinogen in the serum. Decreased TLI indicates exocrine pancreatic insufficiency.
97. **b** Corticosteroid administration would likely result in lymphopenia.
98. **d** Thrombocytopenia may be seen but not thrombocytosis. Babesiosis causes hemolytic anemia in dogs.
99. **d** Because the dog had been vaccinated before being bitten and has not bitten any people since the incident, quarantine is not necessary. As a safety precaution, the dog should be revaccinated against rabies immediately to boost the immune response.

100. **c** *Ehrlichia canis* is a rickettsial organism sensitive to tetracyclines.

101. **b** Amphotericin is extremely nephrotoxic and must be administered carefully with saline loading and by slow intravenous infusion.

102. **e** The compression bandage is almost useless. Intravenous infusion of physiologic saline solution will simply dilute the remaining red blood cells in the intravascular compartment. Immediate surgery will almost certainly kill the dog. Infusion of 1 unit of packed red blood cells is helpful but not nearly enough in a 57-kg dog. Fresh whole blood would be preferred. Vitamin K_3 will not help if there is rodenticide intoxication; vitamin K_1 would be indicated. Autotransfusion is the best chance of keeping the client alive until the bleeding slows and either adequate whole blood transfusion plus vitamin K_1 therapy or exploratory surgery is possible.

103. **a** The agar gel immunodiffusion test for blastomycosis is one of the few serologic tests for fungal infections with high sensitivity (>90%) and high specificity (>90%).

104. **a** The other items listed are used to treat encephalopathy (lactulose, neomycin, low-protein diet) or help control ascites (low-salt diet). Dexamethasone may exacerbate bacterial cholangitis or may further diminish hepatic function by causing steroid hepatopathy.

105. **d** Barium enemas are rarely indicated because they are relatively insensitive and are technically difficult.

106. **c** The description of the wound suggests an anaerobic infection. Metronidazole has excellent antianaerobic activity.

107. **a** Preincubation with food does not have a significant impact on the efficacy of powdered pancreatic enzyme supplements.

108. **c** Coagulopathy is a rare cause of hematemesis. *Helicobacter pylori* is thought to play a role in ulcer formation in people but not in dogs. The two parasites listed do not cause gastrointestinal bleeding.

109. **c** The description of the wound (discoloration, crepitus, odor) suggests an infection with anaerobic bacteria as the predominant type, as opposed to aerobic bacteria as the predominant type. *Bacteroides* and *Clostridium* are common anaerobic bacteria.

110. **e** Prostatomegaly, a common cause of tenesmus, would be difficult to diagnose on physical examination of such a large dog. It would be difficult to reach the prostate via the rectum and difficult to isolate it on abdominal palpation. Perineal hernia, perianal fistulae, anal sac carcinoma, and anal sacculitis should be easy to diagnose on physical examination.

111. **a** Cefazolin is a first-generation bactericidal cephalosporin with a relative broad antibacterial spectrum. It is relatively safe (nontoxic). Gentamicin is nephrotoxic and must be given by injection. Lincomycin has a narrow antibacterial spectrum. Tetracycline would be effective against *Ehrlichia,* but there is no reason to suspect ehrlichiosis in this dog. Also, tetracycline is bacteriostatic. Trimethoprim should not be used alone, but rather in conjunction with a sulfa drug.

112. **e** Polyuria and polydipsia are often seen in dogs with chronic hepatic insufficiency, especially when the blood urea nitrogen level is decreased. This sign is rarely present in dogs with acute, fulminating hepatic failure. All other signs may be seen in animals with acute or chronic hepatic insufficiency.

113. **d** Nocardiosis can cause pleural effusion. The age and occupation of this dog suggest nocardiosis, as does the inflammatory nature of the exudate.

114. **a** The effusion is a pure (low-protein) transudate, typically seen in hypoproteinemic animals. Renal disease can result in severe hypoalbuminemia if the glomeruli are affected. The other four diseases usually cause modified transudates (also called high-protein transudates) or exudates.

115. **e** The "grains" are tapeworm segments. Praziquantel is effective for eliminating cestodes.

116. **e** The dog has a modified transudate (high-protein transudate), which is usually caused by hepatic disease (especially cirrhosis), right-heart failure, or abdominal neoplasia. Serum bile acid concentrations would help determine if hepatic disease (especially cirrhosis) is present. Abdominal radiographs would probably be useless because of the fluid in the abdomen. Intestinal biopsy and a urine protein/creatinine ratio can detect causes of hypoalbuminemia. Culture would detect infection, a cause of an exudate.

117. **b** All dogs with blastomycosis should be treated. Although amphotericin B is toxic, it is effective. Ketoconazole can be used if there is substantial kidney disease (i.e., amphotericin B is contraindicated). Current data suggest that itraconazole may be the preferred therapy.

118. **d** The fluid is an exudate. Bile acid determinations are used to diagnose hepatic disease, which is not a serious consideration in this case. Empiric antibiotic therapy is reasonable while attempting to determine if the exudate is septic. Culture might detect an infection (septic peritonitis). Ultrasonography may reveal a tumor. A complete blood count and serum chemistry profile are needed to ascertain electrolyte balance, renal function, and coagulation, which may be seriously disturbed in a dog with septic peritonitis.
119. **a** Corticosteroids and anticonvulsants are common causes of iatrogenic hepatic disease. Arsenicals may also produce this problem (primarily seen in dogs treated for adult heartworms).
120. **b** The fluid is a pure (low-protein) transudate, almost certainly caused by hypoalbuminemia. Thoracic radiographs would be useful in evaluating the heart, but heart failure is not expected in this patient. Urine protein:creatinine ratio, endoscopic biopsy, and serum bile acid concentrations would help determine why the albumin level is decreased. Ultrasonography would help evaluate the liver.
121. **c** Although corticosteroids (e.g., triamcinolone) may cause some gastric disease, nonsteroidal antiinflammatory drugs (e.g., ibuprofen) are the most consistent cause of severe ulceration.
122. **c** The fluid is exudate. The nondegenerate neutrophils suggest nonseptic peritonitis. Creatinine determinations can detect uroabdomen, a cause of nonseptic exudates. The dog is not icteric, so biliary tract rupture is very unlikely. If there were intestinal leakage, you would expect to see bacteria, food particles, and/or degenerate neutrophils on abdominocentesis. You should not perform surgery until you know whether uroabdomen is present. If uroabdomen is present, you should perform a contrast radiographic examination first to determine the location of the leakage.
123. **e** Cirrhosis may result in reduced liver size. Determining the cause of the cirrhosis may allow you to arrest or reverse the process that initiated the disease and thereby help maintain the animal in remission.
124. **e** The presence of blood clots shows that the hemorrhage is almost certainly iatrogenic. The other choices listed would not cause clots in the abdominal fluid. Abdominal distention does not necessarily mean that an effusion is present. Inability to ballotte a fluid wave makes copious abdominal effusion less likely.
125. **d** Bordetellosis is a likely cause of this dog's disease. A complete blood count would not diagnose tracheal infection. Theophylline is a mild antitussive, but it would not help resolve the infection. Prednisolone without antibiotics would probably allow the infection to persist. Terbutaline is used to treat asthma.
126. **b** Many dogs with acute Rocky Mountain spotted fever do not have circulating antibodies when signs of disease are first seen. Ampicillin and gentamicin would not be useful in treatment of the two common tick-borne diseases, ehrlichiosis or Rocky Mountain spotted fever. A positive *Borrelia* titer does not indicate clinical borreliosis. Most dogs with acute ehrlichiosis do not have hyperglobulinemia.
127. **a** The fluid is an exudate and probably septic, based on the apparent septic shock (hypothermia and injected mucous membranes). The very high white blood cell count is also suggestive of septic peritonitis. Alimentary tract leakage is a common cause of septic peritonitis. Cirrhosis causes a modified transudate. Pancreatitis rarely causes peritoneal effusion and then usually in meager amounts. Hemangiosarcoma would probably cause hemoabdomen. Hemangiosarcoma and carcinomatosis rarely cause intestinal perforation, septic peritonitis, or septic shock.
128. **c** Chronic aspergillosis often mimics nasal neoplasia in signs and turbinate osteolysis. Occasional fungal hyphae can be found in nasal samples from unaffected dogs. The preferred treatment is flushing the nasal cavity with clotrimazole.
129. **e** The dog has signs of small intestinal diarrhea. Colonic adenocarcinoma would produce large bowel signs.
130. **a** Pancreatic insufficiency is the only one of these diseases that would be very unlikely to cause such severe hypoalbuminemia.
131. **e** Examination of capillary blood smears is the most common diagnostic test for babesiosis, which often causes Coombs'-positive, regenerative anemia. (Indirect fluorescent antibody testing is also useful for diagnosis of babesiosis). Doxycycline is useful for treatment of rickettsial infection but not babesiosis. There is no appreciable human health risk.

132. **b** The dog is regurgitating and should have its esophagus evaluated. Acute regurgitation of solids but not liquids may suggest an esophageal foreign body. Therefore plain films are indicated first. There is no reason to think the dog is dehydrated at this time.
133. **e** This dog obviously has hepatic insufficiency. Doberman pinschers often develop chronic hepatitis. Steroid hepatopathy and lipidosis are almost never symptomatic in dogs and rarely, if ever, cause cirrhosis. Pancreatitis does not cause hepatic insufficiency. Lymphosarcoma is possible, but it typically causes hepatomegaly from infiltrative disease.
134. **d** Any organ can be affected. The other four systems are commonly affected in dogs with blastomycosis.
135. **e** *Bordetella bronchiseptica* is the most common bacterial cause of infectious tracheobronchitis in dogs. Herpesvirus is a rare cause.
136. **c** The dog appears to be regurgitating because of esophageal disease. Aspiration pneumonia is a major cause of death in these dogs.
137. **c** Vitamin K_1 would not prevent bleeding from an ulcer or erosion. Abdominal compression bandages are not effective. You cannot autotransfuse when the blood is entering the stomach. Cimetidine and sucralfate often do not work quickly enough in animals that appear to be exsanguinating. In this animal you must eliminate the source of the hemorrhage by resecting the ulcer.
138. **d** Dogs do not develop the skin lesions typically observed in affected people. Dogs may have high titers but not have clinical disease. It is uncertain if kidney disease is caused by borreliosis. Thrombocytopenia is found in rickettsial infection (borreliosis is a bacterial infection).
139. **b** Salmon poisoning requires therapy with tetracycline. Metronidazole is useful for anaerobic infections and intestinal protozoal infections and as an immunomodulator in inflammatory bowel disease.
140. **c** The feces can be assayed for the causative toxin, but rarely are the causative bacteria isolated. Once the toxin has bound to the nerves, antitoxin will not affect it. Flaccid paralysis and normal pain perceptions are classic findings.
141. **a** Chronic tenesmus and dyschezia suggest inflammation or obstruction of the rectum. The easiest and most sensitive way to detect obstruction (likely in an old German shepherd) is by digital rectal examination. Urecholine should never be given if obstruction is a possibility.
142. **b** Congenital shunts rarely cause hepatocellular membrane damage; therefore serum alanine aminotransferase activity is rarely increased.
143. **a** The rapid slide test is not specific (there are many false-positive reactions). Human infections are usually mild. Infected male dogs may shed the bacteria for weeks after infection. Minocycline with an aminoglycoside is the treatment of choice. The asymptomatic nature of many infections is one reason why the disease can be spread so easily.
144. **c** Campylobacteriosis is an acute enteritis of dogs that is transmissible to people. Salmonellosis is possible but unlikely. Giardiasis would probably not cause bloody diarrhea. Yersiniosis is very rare in dogs.
145. **b** This dog has chronic hemoabdomen. Compression bandages are almost useless. Autotransfusion is used in emergencies, but this is a chronic problem. One unit of fresh, whole blood might help in rodenticide intoxication, but this is too chronic for that. Surgery may be useful, but it would be better to perform ultrasonography, looking for areas suggestive of hemangiosarcoma (common in older German shepherd dogs and often manifested as described). If such a tumor were present and if it were found throughout the abdomen, you might avoid unnecessary surgery.
146. **d** The disease is principally found in and around Texas. There is no effective therapy for most symptomatic dogs. Diagnosis is usually made at necropsy, after the dog dies suddenly from acute heart failure.
147. **b** The dog is not dehydrated and is unlikely to become so; therefore fluid therapy is not warranted. Most acute diarrhea is caused by diet, parasites, and/or infections. Except for clostridial colitis (best treated with amoxicillin or tylosin), antibiotics are seldom indicated in young animals with mild diarrhea.
148. **d** Osseous coccidioidomycosis has an extremely poor long-term prognosis and often does not have any other obvious disease preceding it. This is in contrast to acute coccidioidomycosis, which is often respiratory in nature and self-limiting. Osseous coccidioidomycosis can resemble osteosarcoma on radiographs.

149. **e** Ascites is common in dogs with severe cirrhosis and does not cause decompensation.
150. **c** Hypertonic enemas should never be administered to cats or small dogs, especially if the animal is obstipated. These can kill the animal by fluid and electrolyte shifts.
151. **d** The other diseases listed do not cause fever, emaciation, and lymphadenopathy and tend not to be chronic. Cryptococcosis does not usually affect the lungs in dogs.
152. **d** Trientine is used to reduce the body copper concentration, a common problem in Bedlingtons.
153. **b** Lactated Ringer's solution can increase the body pH and exacerbate hepatic encephalopathy. Phenobarbital would deepen the coma. "Lipotropic agents" are contraindicated.
154. **c** Chronically inflamed anal sacs can produce such blood on otherwise normal stools. The normal stool consistency suggests that there is not colonic disease; hence dietary fiber and pelvic radiographs are not needed. Coagulopathy is very unlikely to cause chronic bleeding from the anal region.
155. **e** Schnauzers are at increased risk for idiopathic hyperlipidemia. Fasting hyperlipidemia seems to be a risk factor for acute pancreatitis in dogs.
156. **d** The most commonly affected breeds are Boston terriers, boxers, collies, Pekingese, and Welsh corgies.
157. **d** Cytologic examination is not useful. Mortality is rare unless the patient is septicemic. Fecal shedding can be protracted, especially if inappropriate antibiotic therapy has been administered (e.g., gentamicin).
158. **d** These media produce poor contrast because they draw water from the body into the intestines. Thus they may further decrease extracellular fluid volume and should not be used in dehydrated animals.
159. **a** Diet, infection, and parasites are the most common causes of diarrhea in young animals. Parasympatholytics are inferior for treatment of diarrhea. Fiber is used for chronic large bowel disease, not for acute diarrhea in a young animal. Barium contrast radiographs are seldom needed in diarrheic animals. Bacterial infection is seldom identified as a cause of such diarrhea except for colitis, which cause different signs. Antibiotics are rarely indicated in these patients. Clostridial colitis is treated with amoxicillin.
160. **d** Histoplasmosis rarely affects bone. *Helicobacter* affects the stomach. *Yersinia pestis* causes plague. *Norcardia* usually causes pyothorax or chronic draining tracts. Borreliosis best fits the signs described.
161. **d** Polyps principally occur in the rectum. They may have a very broad head, and the stalk may be short and difficult to see. Polyps can also be multiple. They rarely cause constipation.
162. **c** Dietary therapy (a trial elimination diet or a fiber-enriched diet) is often successful in so-called "mild" lymphocytic-plasmacytic colitis. Prednisolone and azathioprine are rarely needed in such cases. Long-term prednisolone therapy may cause significant side effects in dogs. Diarrhea and/or fecal mucus are the most common signs. There is no known association between colonic inflammatory bowel disease and lymphosarcoma in dogs.
163. **b** Enamel hypoplasia suggests prior distemper infection. Inclusion bodies are rarely seen on the complete blood count. Lymphopenia is nonspecific. Central nervous system signs may occur now, later, much later, or never.
164. **a** Lymphangiectasia causes hypoalbuminemia. Salmonellosis is a rare cause of chronic diarrhea. Granulomatous enteritis is very rare. It is doubtful the animal would have lived this long or would be this healthy if it had lymphosarcoma.
165. **e** Respiratory infection is commonly seen in acute coccidioidomycosis. The most common radiographic sign is hilar lymphadenopathy. The organism is often hard to find cytologically, and culture is almost never recommended. Central nervous system involvement is very difficult to treat. Disseminated disease often involves bones and is difficult or impossible to cure.
166. **b** Although tubular forms of regurgitated food suggest esophageal disease, they are rarely seen. Bile indicates that duodenal fluid is present; hence the animal is vomiting. Animals may vomit or regurgitate anytime after eating. Retching is part of the centrally mediated reflex associated with vomiting, as opposed to regurgitation. Cervical dilation is not commonly seen.
167. **c** Many dogs with lymphangiectasia can be treated for substantial periods. Dogs with protein loss caused by inflammatory bowel disease can often be treated if treatment is begun early enough.

168. **b** Vomiting dogs may be significantly alkalotic; therefore bicarbonate supplementation is inappropriate unless you have strong reason to suspect severe acidosis. Mild acidosis is best treated by volume replacement.
169. **c** This diet would prevent further engorgement of lacteals and subsequent protein loss. Medium-chain triglycerides would allow the animal to assimilate calorie-rich fats.
170. **b** The obvious pain in the perineal area would best be explained by inflammation or a foreign object. Severe inflammation is often caused by perianal fistulae, which are common in German shepherds. Polyps are an unlikely cause of constipation.The other causes listed would not be likely to cause such intense pain.
171. **d** This is the characteristic appearance of diffuse infiltrative intestinal disease on positive-contrast radiographs.
172. **d** Epistaxis is seen in 50% of affected animals. At least 14 days of treatment are needed to effect a cure with tetracycline. Ticks are the major reservoir, and doxycycline is not nephrotoxic.
173. **b.** The most common sites of esophageal foreign bodies are the thoracic inlet, base of the heart, and the lower esophageal sphincter.
174. **c** Biopsy of the band should be done because it may be caused by neoplasia, histoplasmosis, pythiosis, or scar tissue. Surgery would probably make the dog incontinent and would not help the dog if it had a malignancy.
175. **a** The esophagus is a muscular tube; therefore diseases that affect muscular tone may affect the esophagus. Causes of lower motor neuron disease are important causes of acquired esophageal dysfunction. These dogs very rarely recover from this disease spontaneously. Cimetidine and prophylactic antibiotics are not useful in this disease.
176. **b** Acute bloody diarrhea and vomiting in a mature small-breed dog with severe hemoconcentration are almost diagnostic for hemorrhagic gastroenteritis. Parvoviral enteritis does not usually cause such hemoconcentration. Ulceration causes anemia. Arsenic intoxication is very rare in dogs and does not typically cause hemoconcentration.
177. **a** The virus is not particularly resistant to the environment. Serologic examination would be of dubious value. Both distemper and ehrlichiosis may cause thrombocytopenia. Distemper is thought to be a relatively common cause of seizures in young dogs.
178. **c** Finding *Isospora* oocysts does not warrant therapy, because there are no clinical signs. The nematode infections should be treated to prevent infection of other dogs and people. Only fenbendazole will eliminate both*Toxocara* and *Ancylostoma.*
179. **a** Intestinal and kidney silhouettes do not help diagnose microhepatia.
180. **b** Radiographs made with the animal in left lateral recumbency sometimes do not allow the clinician to discern the "shelf" of tissue in the dilated stomach that indicates torsion. A stomach tube can often be passed when an animal has gastric torsion. Animals with chronic gastric torsion may bloat intermittently.
181. **c** Thrombocytopenia is the most common clinicopathologic change in dogs with acute ehrlichiosis. Morulae are rarely, if ever, seen. Any titer (including those <1:128) is significant. You cannot repeat the serologic examination to see if the dog is cured; the titer stays high for some time after successful therapy. Plasma cells are found in the bone marrow, but they do not cause myelophthisis.
182. **c** Many cases recur after surgery.
183. **a** The dog is regurgitating; therefore it has esophageal disease as opposed to gastrointestinal dysfunction. A vascular ring anomaly is most likely, because it is the only cause of esophageal disease.
184. **a** Although metoclopramide is not the ideal antiemetic, it is the only central-acting drug listed among the answer choices and, as such, is much more effective than the drugs listed. Methscopolamine is a parasympatholytic. Bismuth subsalicylate is a local-acting drug. Misoprostol is used for ulceration. Diphenhydramine (Benadryl) is an antihistamine that rarely helps stop vomiting in dogs.
185. **b** The small intestine functions to absorb food. Loss of weight strongly suggests small intestinal involvement. The low frequency of diarrhea plus the absence of blood, mucus, and tenesmus (often seen in large intestinal diarrhea) further suggests small intestinal diarrhea, as opposed to large intestinal diarrhea.
186. **e** Management of hypovolemic shock is the first concern. Flunixin is used for septic shock. Flunixin plus dexamethasone are likely to cause severe gastric ulceration. Lidocaine is used after arrhythmias occur, not before. This is far too much potassium to add to fluids being infused in large volumes to treat shock.

187. **c** Triamcinolone is a commonly used corticosteroid. Corticosteroids commonly increase serum alkaline phosphatase activity, with less effect on serum alanine aminotransferase activity.
188. **a** Free gas strongly suggests a ruptured viscus, which would produce septic peritonitis. Peritonitis is consistent with depression, vomiting, and abdominal pain. The abdomen must be lavaged and the ruptured viscus repaired to prevent further contamination. This should be done as soon as the animal can withstand anesthesia.
189. **c** Dogs with acute disease often die before they become icteric. Corneal edema is a chronic manifestation. Thrombocytopenia occurs because of disseminated intravascular coagulation associated with acute hepatic failure.
190. **c** Septic shock causes acidosis, disseminated intravascular coagulation, and azotemia. Regurgitation is caused by esophageal disease, which is unlikely in this case.
191. **c** Retroflexion of the urinary bladder into the perineal hernia is the reason why perineal hernia can become an emergency.
192. **d** This tends to be a chronic disease that is diagnosed by finding the organism in circulating white blood cells or in muscle biopsies. Thrombocytopenia is found in many rickettsial infections and some viral infections but uncommonly in hepatozoonosis. Periosteal changes are not consistent, especially in the early stages.
193. **c** Ascites is commonly found in cirrhotic dogs with acquired portosystemic shunting. Although ascites may be found in dogs with congenital portosystemic shunt (caused by hypoalbuminemia), it is rare in these dogs.
194. **d** Mucosal hypertrophy rarely causes ulceration. Gastric malignancy can easily cause upper gastrointestinal bleeding. Metoclopramide, intravenous fluids, and antibiotics are inadequate therapy for gastrointestinal ulceration, although fluids may reasonably be incorporated into a therapeutic regimen with H_2 blockers and/or sucralfate.
195. **e** The most common necropsy finding is petechiation in the kidneys and liver. You cannot find the virus in white blood cells. Antibiotics are ineffective.
196. **c** Acepromazine is a central-acting antiemetic and is the most effective antiemetic of the drugs listed as answers. Misoprostol and cimetidine are used for gastric ulceration but are not antiemetics. Kaopectate is a poor antiemetic. Atropine is a parasympatholytic with only mediocre antiemetic efficacy.
197. **d** Serologic tests are not very sensitive for histoplasmosis. Osseous lesions are rare in this disease. *Cryptococcus* organisms have a capsule, whereas *Histoplasma* organisms do not. Most dogs with disseminated disease are presented because of weight loss and/or large bowel diarrhea.
198. **d** Inflammatory and neoplastic infiltrates usually produce a thickened gastric mucosa that is often, but not always, ulcerated; plus, infiltration of the underlying wall is common. Mucosal hypertrophy is usually found in older, small-breed dogs and only affects the mucosa. *Physaloptera* is a grossly visible nematode parasite.
199. **e** The prostate gland is ventral to the colon in the pelvic canal. If it is enlarged, it displaces the colon dorsally. Prostatomegaly is a common cause of constipation in dogs.
200. **b** Blastomycosis often affects the eyes. Histoplasmosis and coccidioidomycosis may affect the eyes but are uncommon. Sporotrichosis almost never affects the eyes. Coccidioidomycosis and cryptococcosis rarely cause marked peripheral lymphadenopathy.
201. **a** Chlorpromazine is an effective antiemetic but is not effective in treating ulceration.
202. **e** The acute fever, lymphadenopathy, and especially the pitting edema are very suggestive of Rocky Mountain spotted fever, which is characterized by vasculitis. This is especially likely in an outdoor dog in summer. Borreliosis usually causes pain, not edema or lymphadenopathy.
203. **b** Hematochezia originates from infarcted gut mucosa, whereas vomiting is caused by obstruction and pain. Hypoproteinemia and profuse diarrhea are sometimes seen in animals with chronic intussusception. Abdominal distention is very rare in this condition, as is prolapse of the intussusception from the anus.

204. **a** Microhepatia is characteristic of hepatic atrophy (seen with portosystemic shunts). Decreased serum albumin and urea nitrogen levels also suggest hepatic insufficiency. Changes in serum alanine aminotransferase and alkaline phosphatase activities and/or bilirubin levels are possible but uncommon in these animals. Decreases in serum γ-glutamyltransferase and alanine aminotransferase activities and bilirubin levels are meaningless.

205. **b** Although it is relatively uncommon, reversible hepatic disease may occur and cause anorexia, vomiting, and/or icterus.

206. **a** Contrast radiographs are notoriously insensitive for detecting gastric ulcers. Many affected animals can be treated successfully. Peripheral white blood cell counts are usually normal to modestly increased, unless perforation has occurred. Serum iron levels are low if intestinal bleeding has been chronic. Ulcers sometimes can be detected by ultrasonography, but it is not known how sensitive ultrasonography is for this purpose.

207. **d** A large amount of intraabdominal fat would cause abdominal distention and provide excellent serosal detail on radiographs. Fat causes the intestines (which have a water density) to have excellent contrast. Effusion would obscure serosal contrast in the abdomen. Lymphadenopathy would probably decrease serosal contrast. Hepatic failure would cause weight loss and/or ascites, both of which would decrease contrast.

208. **e** Renal failure is more often seen in subacute and chronic leptospirosis. Renal biopsy may reveal the organisms in chronically affected kidneys. It is difficult to culture the organism, and special media are needed if the attempt is to be made. Most leptospiral infections in dogs are probably chronic or subclinical.

209. **a** The described topical therapy is usually effective in animals with an initial episode of acute anal sacculitis.

210. **b** Keratoconjunctivitis sicca may occur after use of any sulfa drug. Azulfidine is salicylazosulfapyridine and has caused keratoconjunctivitis sicca in dogs. The salicylate moiety is thought to be the effective portion of the drug. The drug's main indication is for chronic or nonresolving large-bowel diarrhea. Although it may cause salicylate toxicity in cats, it can be used, albeit carefully.

211. **d** H_2 blockers are not totally effective in protecting against ulceration induced by nonsteroidal antiinflammatories. Sucralfate is an effective treatment for existing ulcers. Affected animals are not helped by kaolin-pectin or bland diets. Metoclopramide does not significantly increase gastric blood flow.

212. **a** The history suggests a portosystemic shunt. Serum bile acid concentrations would be most useful in identifying this disorder.

213. **d** Flunixin meglumine is a nonsteroidal antiinflammatory drug that can readily produce gastrointestinal ulceration. Aminopentamide does not facilitate ulcer healing but may lessen vomiting secondary to an ulcer.

214. **d** Of the diseases listed, leptospirosis is the most likely to cause icterus and fever. Blastomycosis could cause both, but this is unlikely.

215. **c** This dog probably has extrahepatic biliary tract obstruction associated with acute pancreatitis. The history of vomiting and abdominal pain is consistent with pancreatitis. Schnauzers seem particularly prone to pancreatitis.

216. **e** The dog has an anal sac abscess, which should be lanced once it develops a discernible "head" or soft spot. Systemic antibiotics are indicated in animals with abscesses, as opposed to those with uncomplicated anal sacculitis.

217. **e** This is a progressive central nervous system disease that is usually fatal. Diagnosis requires histopathologic or serologic examination.

218. **a** Correction of the vascular ring does not ensure that the regurgitation will resolve. Some treated animals continue to vomit. Other congenital cardiac abnormalities, although possible, are not widely recognized. Likewise, congenital esophageal weakness is not recognized as a common problem in these animals. German shepherds appear to have a predisposition for this disease.

219. **a** Prostatic disease has not been reported, but all the other conditions listed have been associated with use of trimethoprim-sulfa combinations.

220. **a** Loss of gastric acid depletes body acid (hence metabolic alkalosis) and chloride stores (hence hypochloremia). Vomiting for almost any reason may produce hypokalemia.

221. **c** *Nocardia* grows aerobically and may require long incubation before growth is evident. Sulfonamides are the drugs of choice. These animals are not human health risks.

222. **d** Of the organs listed, the urinary bladder is the most caudal organ in the abdominal cavity and can become greatly distended if the animal cannot urinate.
223. **d** This dog probably has acute pancreatitis, not pancreatic insufficiency. The latter is not commonly associated with acute pancreatitis. Ultrasonography (to rule out other diseases and confirm pancreatitis), nothing per os, and intravenous fluids are indicated in dogs with suspected pancreatitis.
224. **c** Standard fecal flotation is often diagnostic. Fenbendazole or praziquantel is the treatment of choice. The life cycle requires an intermediate host. Coughing is the most common presenting complaint.
225. **b** Aspiration pneumonia is probably the most common cause of death, aside from euthanasia. Esophagitis is an uncommon cause of symptomatic esophageal disease in dogs. Surgery is usually contraindicated. H_2 blockers are used to diminish gastric acid production and are only useful in animals with esophagitis.
226. **d** Corticosteroids are useful for reducing the hepatic inflammatory response in dogs with chronic hepatitis. Lactulose, neomycin, and low-protein diet are used for hepatic encephalopathy. Trientine is used for copper storage disorder.
227. **e** Despite the fact that many recognized cases of parvoviral enteritis are very severe, it is believed that most infections are relatively mild. The severity of the disease depends on the size and virulence of the inoculum, presence or absence of other intestinal disease (e.g., parasites), and the pup's maternal immunity. Fecal enzyme-linked immunosorbent assay for parvoviral antigen is usually negative at 2 to 3 weeks after the onset of signs.
228. **c** There appears to be an association between hepatic failure and gastrointestinal ulceration. Cirrhotic dogs that suddenly become worse may have a bleeding duodenal ulcer, which in turn causes hepatic encephalopathy from the large amount of protein passing into the intestines.
229. **c** Metronidazole, amoxicillin, and clindamycin are the only drugs listed with good anaerobic efficacy. Metronidazole only kills anaerobic bacteria. Clindamycin is not very effective against gram-negative bacteria, which would be expected in peritonitis caused by intestinal leakage. Ampicillin plus amikacin has excellent aerobic efficacy. Combinations of β-lactam antibiotics (e.g., cephalothin with amoxicillin) are rarely useful.
230. **d** There is no currently recognized effective medical therapy. Serologic testing is currently useless. The gastrointestinal tract is commonly affected. Distal appendicular lesions are principally found in horses.
231. **d** Cardiac arrhythmias and gastric motility disturbances are common. Disseminated intravascular coagulation occurs in animals with severe, advanced gastric dilation/volvulus. Ulcers may develop because of poor mucosal perfusion.
232. **a** Loperamide is an opiate that increases segmental contraction and decreases intestinal secretion. Parasympatholytics are much less effective. Kaopectate is of dubious value.
233. **a** Although rare and controversial, there are reports of dogs living relatively long periods (weeks or months) despite rabies. Purulent or suppurative meningoencephalitis does not occur in rabies. Phenolic disinfectants are not needed to cleanse wounds.
234. **e** Copper storage disease is a very common cause of hepatic disease in Bedlington terriers.
235. **e** Both Rocky Mountain spotted fever and ehrlichiosis can cause thrombocytopenia. Chloramphenicol is very effective in treatment of Rocky Mountain spotted fever. Many animals with acute Rocky Mountain spotted fever have a negative titer. *Rhipicephalus sanguineus* is the principal vector in the United States for ehrlichiosis, not Rocky Mountain spotted fever.
236. **c** Lipemia in a vomiting miniature schnauzer strongly suggests acute pancreatitis. The laboratory results are consistent with this diagnosis. Serum lipase activity is an inaccurate indicator of pancreatitis, and affected dogs may have normal values.
237. **e** Oral antacids must be given frequently (4 to 6 times/day) to maintain a high gastric pH. Even then they may be vomited. H_2 blockers and proton pump inhibitors (omeprazole) are more effective and for longer periods.
238. **b** Most affected dogs die if they are not treated. Diagnosis is principally by finding the organism in fine-needle aspirates of swollen lymph nodes. Finding fluke ova in the feces is suggestive but not diagnostic.

239. **e** The description of the feces is suggestive of whipworms. The parasites are often missed by fecal examination because they shed eggs periodically and the eggs are relatively heavy (they sink if the flotation solution is not made properly). Salmonellosis and protothecosis are rare.

240. **c** Ultrasonographic examination is the most sensitive and specific means of diagnosing an intussusception.

241. **c** Serologic testing has not been well evaluated in dogs. Dogs often have very few organisms in cutaneous lesions (as opposed to cats, which often have numerous organisms). The recommended therapy is with potassium iodide or possibly itraconazole.

242. **b** The dog obviously has chronic small intestinal diarrhea, meaning that it has malabsorption or maldigestion. Maldigestion is particularly common in German shepherds. Serum trypsinlike immunoreactivity is the best test for maldigestion in dogs. Abdominal radiographs are rarely useful in dogs with either malabsorption or maldigestion. Because five fecal examinations have been negative, it is doubtful that another would be useful. Biopsy should be postponed until maldigestion has been ruled out.

243. **a** Dogs are relative resistant to tetanus. Antitoxin is not effective once the toxin has bound to nerves. Phenobarbital and acepromazine are sometimes very helpful in management of these clients.

244. **a** This dog appears to be regurgitating because of esophageal disease, not gastrointestinal disease. Thoracic radiographs are needed to evaluate the esophagus.

245. **a** Cats usually are infected by *Mycobacterium bovis* and show gastrointestinal signs. Dogs usually are infected by *Mycobacterium tuberculosis* and show respiratory signs. Histopathologic and cytologic examinations are better means of diagnosis. Affected dogs should probably be euthanized because of the human health risk.

246. **e** Nonsteroidal antiinflammatory drugs (NSAIDs) are a major cause of gastrointestinal ulceration in dogs. Corticosteroids have comparatively low ulcerogenic potential compared with NSAIDs.

247. **d** The latex agglutination test for cryptococcosis detects circulating antigen. It is one of the few sensitive, specific serologic tests for fungal infection. Aspergillosis is more common than cryptococcosis in the nose of dogs. *Cryptococcus* has a capsule, which makes cytologic diagnosis relatively easy. Ketoconazole is generally ineffective against central nervous system cryptococcosis, but fluconazole is effective.

248. **e** Endoscopy is not as good as fluoroscopy in demonstrating esophageal dysfunction. Metoclopramide does not improve esophageal function. Although some affected animals can be managed well with dietary therapy, the prognosis is guarded, since many die from aspiration pneumonia. Cisapride appears to be of benefit in rare cases, possibly in dogs with gastroesophageal reflux.

249. **a** Hypocalcemia is occasionally associated with pancreatitis. Hypercalcemia is not caused by pancreatitis, although it theoretically could cause pancreatitis. However, this is not thought to be clinically significant in dogs and cats.

250. **d** Chlorpromazine is a very effective central-acting antiemetic. Cimetidine is not an antiemetic. Atropine and aminopentamide are parasympatholytics and are not nearly as effective as chlorpromazine.

251. **a** Abdominal palpation may fail to detect an intestinal obstruction. Oral iodine contrast agents result in poor-quality gastrointestinal radiographs. Endoscopy is not useful if the foreign object is farther into the intestines than the endoscope can reach. Contrast radiographs are only needed if plain radiographs are not diagnostic. Dilated air- or fluid-filled intestinal loops are the most common finding on plain radiographs.

252. **c** The description of these protozoa suggests giardiasis. Fenbendazole is an accepted therapy for these parasites.

253. **a** The dog is regurgitating and has aspiration pneumonia. Therefore abdominal radiographs and sonograms would be of dubious value. The dog's old age means that this is an acquired esophageal disease. Neuromuscular disease causes acquired esophageal weakness in dogs.

254. **d** Immunoproliferative enteropathy is a common cause of protein-losing enteropathy in basenjis. These dogs often have increased serum globulin levels despite intestinal protein loss.

255. **a** *Coccidioides immitis* is a large organism containing small internal structures. An encapsulated yeast is likely *Cryptococcus.* Pleomorphic cigar-shaped organisms are likely *Sporothrix.* Nonseptate hyphae may be those of various other fungi.
256. **c** Boston terriers are suspected to be at increased risk.
257. **b** Prednisolone may kill the dog if it has histoplasmosis (a reasonable differential diagnosis in this dog). Pyrantel would not kill whipworms, the parasite most likely to cause large bowel diarrhea. Sulfasalazine (Azulfidine) can cause side effects. Dietary intolerance and fiber-responsive disease are common causes of diarrhea and are safe to administer.
258. **e** The oocysts indicate coccidiosis. These protozoa are occasionally problematic in young dogs but rarely in older animals. This infection need not be treated. Also, none of the drugs listed is effective for coccidiosis.
259. **d** Corticosteroids commonly produce vacuolar hepatopathy, which characteristically increases serum alkaline phosphatase activity, but they have few other effects on the liver. The lymphopenia also suggests a corticosteroid effect. Portosystemic shunts often do not affect serum alanine aminotransferase or alkaline phosphatase activities. When cirrhosis or copper storage disease increases hepatic enzyme activities, alanine aminotransferase activity is typically increased.
260. **c** Portosystemic shunts are sometimes first considered in animals that do not recover from anesthesia as expected (because of hepatic insufficiency and slowed drug metabolism). Yorkshire terriers seem predisposed to portosystemic shunts.
261. **b** In right lateral recumbency the pylorus is the most dependent part of the stomach; thus barium is most likely to pool there.
262. **b** Bismuth subsalicylate is an effective antisecretory agent (because of the salicylate moiety). Sucralfate and cimetidine are used for gastrointestinal ulceration. Atropine is a parasympatholytic and is much less effective than an opiate.
263. **b** Acute nosocomial diarrhea caused by *Clostridium* has been reported in dogs, especially those hospitalized in veterinary clinics.
264. **a** Many dogs with ulcers do not vomit blood. Ulcers would be a reason the barium is retained in two discrete areas of the stomach. Metoclopramide and chlorpromazine, although good antiemetic agents, are not useful for healing ulcers. Pancreatitis and foreign bodies are uncommon causes of gastric ulcers.
265. **b** Approximately 70% of affected dogs have bacterial overgrowth in the small intestine. Fecal film digestion tests are worthless. Many animals do not respond to supplementation of pancreatic enzymes because the product used is inferior or is used with a high-fat diet. Hypoproteinemia is rare in affected animals. The most common cause is pancreatic atrophy.
266. **a** Xylazine is a satisfactory emetic in cats but not in dogs. Syrup of ipecac and salt water are very unreliable antiemetics. Apomorphine is the most consistently effective emetic in dogs.
267. **a** These puppies almost certainly became infected with hookworms from the dam. Pyrantel pamoate is safe and effective for such an infection.
268. **c** The mucus, absence of weight loss, and softness of the lst portion of the fecal mass strongly suggest large-bowel disease.
269. **e** Affected animals are often clinically normal. It is rare to find inclusions in platelets because of the periodicity of their appearance and the diminished number of platelets present at these times. Pancytopenia is not expected in this infection. Ticks carry both rickettsiae, and concurrent infections are probably common.
270. **d** Bones are common foreign bodies and are usually seen with plain radiographs. Even if the foreign object is radiolucent, there is often gas around it, which makes it visible radiographically. Barium in only contraindicated if a perforation is suspected. Contrast esophagograms may not reveal an esophageal perforation that is present.
271. **e** This description is classic for a congenital hepatic portosystemic shunt causing hepatic encephalopathy with polyuria and polydipsia.
272. **c** This is a common history for acute parvoviral enteritis. Coronaviral enteritis is usually relatively mild. Salmonellosis is uncommon. The dog's age makes garbage ingestion unlikely. Foreign bodies usually do not produce severe diarrhea.

273. **d** Marked hemoconcentration is the hallmark of hemorrhagic gastroenteritis.
274. **e** Gastric dilation/volvulus is a major cause of unproductive retching and abdominal pain in giant-breed dogs. Plain abdominal radiographs are usually diagnostic if physical examination is not.
275. **e** Histiocytic ulcerative colitis is almost only found in young to middle-aged boxers. Some clinicians refer to the disease as "boxer colitis."
276. **b** Ascites is possible but very unlikely in a dog with a congenital portosystemic shunt, unless very severe hypoalbuminemia is present.
277. **e** *Dipylidium caninum* is the most common tapeworm of dogs and cats. Its intermediate hosts are the flea and louse. Most affected animals do not show clinical evidence of infection.
278. **b** Parvovirus does not destroy villi directly, but destruction of crypts leads to subsequent loss of villi.
279. **d** The black, tarry stools suggest upper gastrointestinal bleeding, such as from an ulcer. Pancreatitis rarely causes gastric or duodenal ulceration.
280. **a** Xylazine paralyzes esophageal musculature and allows the organ to dilate with air. Thus the patient appears to have megaesophagus on esophagograms.
281. **c** Liquid barium reaches the area of the ileocolic valve within 2 hours.
282. **c** You must determine if the protruding mucosa is associated with rectal prolapse (the most common cause) or an ileocolic intussusception that is so long that it protrudes from the rectum. A rectal prolapse forms a cul-de-sac near the rectum, but an ileocolic intussusception does not. Repelling the end of an ileocolic intussusception back into the descending colon would not benefit the client.
283. **a** Bacterial metabolism of malabsorbed carbohydrates is probably the most common cause of flatulence. For example, beans often cause flatulence in people because raffinose in the beans is not absorbed and colonic bacteria metabolize it, producing gas.
284. **e** Hypoadrenocorticism commonly causes vomiting but not hyperadrenocorticism.
285. **d** This is a likely cause of parvoviral enteritis. Many affected clients do not show leukopenia if tested only once, early in the course of the disease. The severity, fever, and acute onset suggest viral enteritis. Parasitism and bacterial enteritis rarely cause fever like that seen in this puppy.
286. **d** Although tetracycline or doxycycline usually used for ehrlichiosis, chloramphenicol is also effective. The diagnostic tests listed would probably not aid in diagnosis or change your therapy.
287. **a** Ascites is a very rare finding with acute pancreatitis.
288. **e** Sudden gagging up of food or mucus, without prodromal nausea or retching, suggests regurgitation caused by esophageal disease.
289. **c** Icterus is often not seen in significant hepatic disease in dogs. Pancreatitis (not exocrine pancreatic insufficiency) may cause icterus. Gallstones are rarely symptomatic in dogs. Steroid hepatopathy generally does not cause clinical problems in dogs.
290. **a** This correctly describes the position of the duodenum on ventrodorsal radiographs.
291. **d** Serum γ-glutamyltransferase activity is not as sensitive as serum alkaline phosphatase activity in detecting liver disease.
292. **c** The history is classic for congenital portosystemic shunt. This therapy is appropriate to symptomatically treat hepatic encephalopathy. High-protein meals and anticonvulsants are contraindicated because of the likely diagnosis.
293. **c** Only intravenous fluids and preventing oral intake have been agreed on as important in treating pancreatitis. Antibiotics are of uncertain value, because septic pancreatitis is very rare in dogs and cats. No food must be offered during the acute phase.
294. **c** This accurately describes the normal position of the cecum on ventrodorsal radiographs.
295. **d** Acute febrile gastroenteritis in a young dog is suggestive of parvoviral infection. Intussusception, gastrointestinal parasitism, and dietary intolerance typically do not cause fever. Gastric ulceration is very unlikely in a 5-month-old dog.

296. **d** A hepatoma arising from the right side of the liver would displace the pylorus caudomedially as described. Lymphosarcoma is a possibility, but it is often multicentric and unlikely to cause a solitary large mass in the cranial right abdominal quadrant. Hemangiosarcoma is possible, but it is more likely to affect the spleen on the other side of the abdomen. A linear foreign body may displace the intestines, but it is doubtful that it would displace the pylorus as described.
297. **e** The dog probably has acute gastritis or perhaps a foreign body. Endoscopy (which requires anesthesia) is not indicated unless the dog's condition worsens or radiographs suggest a foreign body. Also, you would not perform endoscopy without first ascertaining if the client was a good anesthetic risk.
298. **a** Liquid barium normally passes into the duodenum from the stomach within 30 minutes.
299. **d** There may be some inflammatory effusion immediately surrounding the pancreas, which is why the cranial right quadrant is hazy on a ventrodorsal abdominal radiograph. Profuse ascites is rare.
300. **e** Most congenital hepatic portosystemic shunts are single vessels that anastomose with the azygos vein or the caudal vena cava.
301. **c** The clinical signs are referrable to neuromuscular weakness and muscular pain.
302. **f** Serum creatine phosphokinase activity increases as a result of leakage of the enzyme from damaged muscle.
303. **b** β-Blockers cause bronchoconstriction and, as such, are contraindicated for use in asthmatic cats.
304. **a** Abyssinians are predisposed to renal amyloidosis.
305. **c** In cats, amyloid is deposited in the renal medulla, versus the glomeruli in dogs.
306. **e** Lymphosarcoma is the most common renal tumor of cats and is typically associated with a negative FeLV status. Renomegaly may be unilateral or bilateral.
307. **a** Hyperglobulinemia frequently occurs secondary to FIP and is usually classified as a polyclonal gammopathy.
308. **d** Although cats demonstrate hypersensitivity reactions, IgE has not yet been identified in this species.
309. **e** In comparison, the blood volume of dogs is about 7% to 8% of body weight.
310. **b** Historically, thiamin deficiency was always considered the first differential diagnosis for cervical ventroflexion in cats. Potassium deficiency should now also be given strong consideration.
311. **d** Affected cats have a better prognosis for long-term survival than do dogs.
312. **a** Bile acid concentrations are very useful for detecting liver disease in cats.
313. **b** Meningioma is the most common primary brain tumor of cats.
314. **c** Aortic thromboembolism is a frequent complication of hypertrophic cardiomyopathy.
315. **c** Horner's syndrome results from loss of sympathetic innervation.
316. **a** Diaphragmatic hernia muffles the heart and lung sounds.
317. **b** Hyperkalemic myocardiotoxicity and metabolic acidosis are classic findings with prolonged lower urinary tract obstruction.
318. **e** Deficiency of factor XII is commonly recognized in cats.
319. **b** Respiration may cease with an incompatible transfusion; vomiting may occur when the rate of blood administration is excessively rapid.
320. **d** Arginine is an essential amino acid for cats. It is needed to "drive" the urea cycle, because it transforms ammonia to urea. Therefore a deficiency of arginine may potentiate hepatic encephalopathy.
321. **c** Digoxin is contraindicated because it is a positive inotrope.
322. **b** The recognized blood groups of cats are A, B, and AB. Severe transfusion reactions occur most frequently in type-B cats receiving type-A blood; type-B cats carry alloantibodies to type A. Of interest is the apparently higher incidence of type-B blood in purebred cats.
323. **e** None of the life cycle of *Giardia* takes place in the large intestine.
324. **a** *Mycobacterium lepraemurium* causes feline leprosy.
325. **d** Visceral mast-cell tumors are much more common in cats than in dogs. They should always be included in the differential diagnoses for splenomegaly. Cutaneous mast-cell tumors are less aggressive in cats than in dogs.

326. **c** Growth hormone is a powerful insulin antagonist and therefore exerts a diabetogenic effect.
327. **b** Cryptococcosis is distributed on a worldwide basis and is therefore most common; however, some geographic areas have another predominant mycosis, such as histoplasmosis.
328. **d** Latent infection is virtually impossible to demonstrate in everyday clinical practice. Bone marrow cultures must be submitted to special laboratories.
329. **c** The normal heart rate in cats is approximately 160 to 240 beat/min.
330. **b** Methemoglobinemia reduces the oxygen-carrying capacity of blood.
331. **d** Acetylcysteine helps replenish hepatocellular supplies of glutathione.
332. **d** All the aminoglycosides may cause neuromuscular blockade. This danger is potentiated with anesthesia.
333. **b** *Microsporum canis* is the most common cause of ringworm in cats.
324. **d** Amitraz is inappropriate for treatment of dermatophytosis. It is used to treat demodicosis in dogs.
325. **d** In cats, acromegaly is caused by pituitary tumors. In dogs, it is usually related to progestagens, either endogenous (intact bitch) or exogenous. Progestagens stimulate release of growth hormone. Insulin resistance occurs because of the antagonism of growth hormone to insulin.
336. **e** Cats have a a higher renal threshold for glucose than dogs. Dogs have a threshold of about 180 mg/dl. Interestingly, diabetic cats appear to have a lower threshold (about 200 mg/dl) for glucose spillage than nondiabetic cats.
337. **d** "Walking dandruff" is *Cheyletiella* infestation.
338. **c** Cerebellar hypoplasia may be caused by panleukopenia virus, a parvovirus of cats.
339. **c** This is a classic presentation for food allergy in cats.
340. **b** It is important to change to a truly hypoallergenic diet and not just another commercial brand of diet. The diet should be tried for a minimum of 3 weeks.
341. **a** Some argue that cats are not infected by whipworms, yet the literature (and most current text) indicate that it occurs sporadically.
342. **d** Digitoxin has a half-life of over 100 hours in cats. It undergoes extensive hepatic metabolism. It should not be used in cats.
343. **e** Phosphate-containing enemas are extremely dangerous in cats and small dogs. They can cause severe electrolyte disturbances, such as hypocalcemia and hypernatremia. Their use frequently results in death of the animal.
344. **e** Cats with hepatic lipidosis are notorious for their refusal to eat.
345. **c** This is a classic presentation for squamous-cell carcinoma on the head.
346. **d** This presentation is more representative of autoimmune skin disease.
347. **e** Basophilic stippling is not diagnostic of any particular disease. In cats, however, it can be supportive evidence of regenerative anemia.
348. **d** The kidneys, liver, spleen, and mesenteric lymph nodes often provide diagnostic samples. The noneffusive form of FIP, usually more difficult to diagnose than the effusive form, shows pyogranulomas and vasculitis on tissue sections.
349. **a** Benzyl alcohol is a preservative frequently added to intravenous fluid products and sterile water (for drug reconstitution) intended for human use. The neurologic disturbance may ultimately be fatal, dictating that the veterinarian should use caution when purchasing fluids for use in cats.
350. **e** FIP produces a high-protein exudate that is nonseptic and contains relatively few cells. The relative cellularity may vary with the stage of the disease, however.
351. **b** Feline leukemia virus is readily transmitted by contact with the saliva of an infected cat.
352. **c** Electrical alternans is an occasional electrocardiographic finding in cats with pericardial effusion.
353. **a** The mitral valve is usually the most commonly affected valve. The aortic valve is probably the second most commonly affected valve.
354. **c** In dogs, pleural effusion is generally recognized on radiographs after accumulation of about 100 ml of fluid in the pleural space.
355. **a** Chemotherapy is typically disappointing with this tumor.
356. **a** Canine insulin is identical to porcine insulin. Feline insulin, although not identical, is most similar to bovine insulin.

357. **c** Because many cats have occult infections, microfilariae are seldom identified. The occult test may be negative because fewer adults develop in cats than in dogs, and thus less antigen is present. The occult (antigen) test is becoming more reliable, however, as the sensitivity of this test increases. The antibody test is unreliable.

358. **d** Lymphoma is the most common gastrointestinal tumor of cats.

359. **e** Hemorrhage, thrombosis, petechiae, and large number of parasites characterize cytauxzoonosis.

360. **e** *Mycobacterium lepraemurium* does not cause conjunctivitis.

361. **a** Propylthiouracil is not commonly used because it can induce immune-mediated hemolytic anemia in treated cats.

362. **d** Lymphoid hyperplasia, or reactive hyperplasia, is the most common cause of lymphadenomegaly in cats.

363. **e** Hyperglycemia and/or glucosuria are relatively common in stressed cats. One should never institute insulin therapy based on a single finding of either. If in doubt about diabetes mellitus, hospitalize the cat (allow time to acclimate) and continue to recheck glucose levels. A stressed cat can have a serum glucose level of 300 mg/dl.

364. **b** This antigen stimulates the immune system but does not elicit a virus-neutralizing response.

365. **b** Older cats are more likely to be infected with FIV than are younger cats.

366. **e** The upper third premolar is the carnassial tooth.

367. **a** This test must be done by a diagnostic laboratory. Several stool samples are submitted.

368. **d** Aminoglycosides are relatively ototoxic in cats.

369. **d** Depletion of vitamin K–dependent factors prolongs prothrombin time and partial thromboplastin time.

370. **a** Anticoagulant rodenticide intoxication depletes the body of vitamin K–dependent factors.

371. **d** Latex agglutination is particularly useful because it is an antigen test. It can be helpful in monitoring therapy.

372. **d** A positive FIP titer may be generated in response to coronaviruses other than FIP virus. A positive titer is only evidence of exposure to a coronavirus, not specifically FIP virus.

373. **a** The adult cat has 30 teeth.

374. **b** An animal in diastolic failure should not receive intravenous fluids.

375. **d** Multicentric (generalized) lymphadenopathy is an uncommon presentation for feline lymphoma.

376. **a** Metronidazole is used most commonly.

377. **c** Vomiting during blood transfusion frequently indicates an excessive rate of administration.

378. **a** Acute onset of blindness with ocular hemorrhage in a geriatric cat should initiate an investigation into renal disease and its attendant hypertension.

379. **d** Sinus tachycardia is a common finding in stressed cats. It is also the most common arrhythmia in dogs. Ventricular tachycardia is the second most common arrhythmia of cats and dogs.

380. **d** Excessive chordae tendinae/papillary muscle cardiomyopathy is not a recognized form of cardiomyopathy in cats or dogs.

381. **d** Cats with persistent FeLV viremia often die of secondary bacterial infections related to immunosuppression.

382. **c** This is a frequent finding in orange cats, and owners commonly ask the significance of the pigmentation. It is a benign lesion.

383. **e** Culture of the effusion of pyothorax typically yields a mixed population of gram-negative anaerobic bacteria.

384. **e** Once the fluid is drained, antibiotics given intravenously reach adequate levels in the pleural space. Infusing antibiotic solutions into the chest exacerbates pleuritis.

385. **a** Metronidazole has good activity against most anaerobes, particularly *Bacteroides.* Penicillins may also be good choices. The cephalosporins have variable activity against anaerobes and may not be effective against *Bacteroides.* Aminoglycosides do not work in anaerobic environments. Base treatment on culture and sensitivity results.

386. **d** Brain tumors are among the more common causes of forebrain dysfunction. Meningioma is the most common primary brain tumor of cats.

387. **d** T_3 suppression is a relatively new test for diagnosing hyperthyroidism in cats with normal basal T_4 values.

388. **b** *Ctenocephalides felis* most commonly infests cats.

389. **e** Electric heating pads may cause thermal burns. These are particularly dangerous for the unconscious or immobile patient. These have no place in clinical practice, and their use only invites a lawsuit.
390. **c** Nonenveloped (hydrophilic) viruses, such as calicivirus and parvovirus, are difficult to kill with routine disinfection. Household bleach (sodium hypochlorite, Clorox) at 1:32 dilution is probably best.
391. **b** Cats often become infected by ingesting infected prey animals, such as mice.
392. **b** The serum IgM titer is used to diagnose toxoplasmosis.
393. **c** Clindamycin has been used more commonly recently.
394. **b** Oocysts do not sporulate for at least 24 hours after excretion. Ideally, someone other than the pregnant woman should clean the litter box. The pregnant women may be at greater risk for contracting toxoplasmosis from eating undercooked meat than from contact with cats.
395. **c** Portosystemic shunts in cats are typically single and extrahepatic; they often occur as congenital defects.
396. **d** Aromatic amino acids worsen the signs of hepatic encephalopathy; branched-chain amino acids do not.
397. **c** Dilative cardiomyopathy has become increasingly rare because of taurine supplementation in most cat foods.
398. **a** Tetracycline can induce fever in cats.
399. **c** Cats with ischemic encephalopathy are unlikely to show a crossed-extensor reflex.
400. **b** FIV is a lentivirus.
401. **d** Chloramphenicol is not used today as much as it has been in the past because of the concern for bone marrow suppression, both in the cat and the person administering the drug. The client should always be told to wear latex gloves when handling the drug. It may cause aplastic anemia in people.
402. **b** The same maximal rate of administration of 0.5 mEq/kg/hr should be used for dogs.
403. **d** Pulmonic stenosis is not a common congenital defect in cats.
404. **d** The feline liver fluke is primarily found in Puerto Rico and Florida.
405. **c** Praziquantel is used to treat liver fluke infection in cats.
406. **c** Hypothyroidism is unrelated to insulin resistance in diabetic cats.
407. **e** The normal flora in a cat's mouth is a "mixed bag" of bacterial types.
408. **a** Amoxicillin or perhaps amoxicillin–clavulanic acid would be a good first choice to treat a bite abscess. A cephalosporin may not be indicated unless the less expensive β-lactams are ineffective. Drainage of the abscess is as important as the antibiotic used.
409. **d** Lymphoma is the most common hepatic tumor in cats. It is usually metastatic from a distant site.
410. **a** Persian and Himalayan breeds are particularly sensitive to the effects of griseofulvin.
411. **d** This is a classic cause of nonobstructive feline urologic syndrome. The more currently accepted terminology is *feline lower urinary tract disorder.*
412. **e** Both the obstructive and nonobstructive lower urinary tract syndromes are invariably associated with sterile urine.
413. **a** Stomatitis and gingivitis are "markers" for immunosuppression.They are frequently found in cats with retroviral immunosuppression.
414. **a** These are classic signs of dysautonomia.
415. **d** Steatitis is an inflammatory condition of adipose tissue. Diets high in polyunsaturated fats, such as fish and fish oils, require large amounts of vitamin E to prevent oxidation of fat. Vitamin E, the body's main defense against lipid peroxidation, is scant in many types of fish.
416. **b** Steatitis is treated with vitamin E supplementation.
417. **d** Cats typically shed all of their temporary teeth by 6 months of age.
418. **c** Propranolol may be used for hypertrophic cardiomyopathy but is not recommended if the cat has embolism.
419. **d** Cats with intestinal lymphoma do not demonstrate eosinophilia.
420. **b** Thyroid tumors are typically benign adenomas in cats. They are usually malignant in dogs.
421. **e** Tyzzer's disease is caused by *Bacillus pisiformis.*
422. **d** Mast cells produce histamine, an agonist for parietal cells.

423. **c** Dextrose-containing solutions should be avoided because of deranged glucose metabolism. Saline at 7% is hypertonic. Saline at 0.45% is hypotonic. Saline at 0.9% is the fluid of choice.
424. **b** Ptyalism is a prominent sign of hepatic encephalopathy in cats.
425. **e** 5-Fluorouracil is a potent neurotoxin in cats, and its use is likely to result in death of the client.
426. **a** Deficiency of glucuronyl transferase limits the cat's ability to conjugate compounds to glucuronic acid and increase the water solubility of a compound.
427. **b** Cats do not have a glucocorticoid-induced isoenzyme of alkaline phosphatase.
428. **a** Phenobarbital is useful for long-term control of seizures.
429. **e** Bile acids are conjugated with taurine in cats.
430. **b** Eosinophilic linear granuloma is a common cause of lower lip swelling.
431. **e** Hemangiomas are uncommon in cats.
432. **e** *Felicola subrostrata* is the feline louse.
433. **d** Microscopic examination of conjunctival scrapings often reveals the cause of conjunctivitis.
434. **c** The higher osmolality is less favorable for bacterial growth.
435. **b** Thiacetarsamide has been recommended in the older literature. However, recent research suggests that it may be less effective than once thought and, in higher dosages such as those used to treat heartworms, it may be toxic. Arsenical compounds have an affinity for capillary beds.
436. **c** Cyanosis occurs as a result of life-threatening methemoglobinemia.
437. **b** *Hemobartonella felis* may be seen on feline red blood cells after splenectomy.
438. **b** Hyperthyroidism has not been reported as a sequel to use of megestrol acetate. This is a progestational agent.
439. **d** Cardiomyopathy caused by hyperthyroidism is sometimes called "thyrotoxic" heart disease.
440. **b** Although the clinical signs of heart failure vary with the form of cardiomyopathy, ascites is a rarely recognized sign of heart failure in cats.
441. **b** About half of infected cats have nasal cavity involvement.
442. **c** The indirect fluorescent antibody test detects p27 antigen.
443. **c** Notoedric mange is intensely pruritic.
444. **d** Stress and anorexia predispose to hepatic lipidosis in obese cats.
445. **e** Mycosis fungoides is not characterized by miliary dermatitis.
446. **a** FeLV is an oncornavirus.
447. **d** Five-percent dextrose in water is an unacceptable choice. The dextrose is metabolized to free water and leaves the vascular compartment for the intracellular and interstitial tissues. Any of the others would be reasonable choices, depending on the electrolytes they contain.
448. **a** In reality, any of the signs listed may be seen. It is interesting, however, that vomiting is the most common clinical sign.
449. **c** These lesions can be treated with various applications or the affected tooth can be extracted, because the lesions are painful.
450. **b** Cats have a very high threshold for bilirubin elimination by the kidney (approximately 9 times higher than that of dogs). It is always an abnormal finding. The stressed cat may occasionally spill glucose into the urine because of stress hyperglycemia.
451. **c** Cisplatin causes fulminant pulmonary edema in cats.
452. **b** Hypocalcemia will occur if the parathyroid glands cannot be preserved. In some cats, calcium homeostasis is transiently disrupted postoperatively, even if the parathyroids are preserved.
453. **c** Atropine is used to treat carbamate toxicity.
454. **c** Organ meats have a high vitamin A content.
455. **b** Steatitis is associated with vitamin E deficiency.
456. **b** Infected cats tend to become depressed, whereas infected dogs exhibit excitement.
457. **a** Rabid cats have a pronounced "furious" stage. "Dumb" rabies is less common in cats.
458. **a** Such autoagglutination is diagnostic of one type of autoimmune hemolytic anemia (AIHA).
459. **b** Failure of autoagglutinated cells to disperse on addition of a drop of saline is diagnostic of AIHA.
460. **e** Treatment consists of immunosuppressive doses of corticosteroids. Tetracycline may be added to the protocol. *Hemobartonella felis* organisms are present but not identified.
461. **c** Chronic illness typically causes normocytic normochromic anemia.

462. **d** Although serum iron levels are decreased, bone marrow iron stores are increased; hence the anemia is normochromic.
463. **e** A brain tumor would be less likely because of the cat's age.
464. **d** Cranial mediastinal lymphoma commonly produces an effusion containing neoplastic cells.
465. **b** These are classic signs of cerebellar hypoplasia.
466. **b** Cats have four pairs of mammary glands.
467. **d** There appears to be little relation between hormones and mammary tumor development in cats. This is not the case in dogs.
468. **c** Normal cats suppress serum T_4 levels with the T_3 suppression test.
469. **c** Dietary taurine deficiency causes central retinal degeneration in cats.
470. **b** Methimazole is associated with severe bone marrow suppression in some cats. Monitor the complete blood count (CBC) closely.
471. **d** Bethanechol is used to enhance bladder tone after urethral obstruction is relieved.
472. **e** The uvea is most likely to exhibit changes associated with FIP.
473. **c** Heartworms live about 5 years in dogs.
474. **a** Cats not living with other cats commonly exhibit play aggression toward their owners.
475. **c** Viral upper respiratory infection predisposes kittens to secondary bacterial infection.
476. **a** The gingival sulcus is normally up to 1 mm deep.
477. **d** Many domestic cats are overfed and become obese.
478. **d** The response to prednisone is poor; these cats have a guarded prognosis.
479. **e** Thoracic organs and vessels are often damaged in falls from heights.
480. **c** The lateral saphenous vein is frequently used in dogs. The medial saphenous vein is used in cats.
481. **c** Griseofulvin is extremely teratogenic.
482. **d** These seven diseases are responsible for most cases of uveitis in cats.
483. **a** *Hemobartonella* is a rickettsial blood parasite.
484. **b.** Caution is warranted when administering most drugs to cats with liver disease.
485. **b** *Ollulanus* is the stomach worm of cats.
486. **e** A urine specific gravity above 1.035 should be attainable in cats with normal renal function.
487. **d** The plantigrade stance associated with diabetes mellitus is probably the major metabolic neuropathy of cats.
488. **c** These lesions are likely the breathing hole of *Cuterebra* larvae.
489. **a** Toxoplasmosis is unlikely to cause jaundice.
490. **d** Thymic atrophy and subsequent immunodeficiency are thought to cause this syndrome.
491. **a** Large doses of trimethoprim-sulfa are a good first choice to treat nocardiosis.
492. **c** The feline red blood cell is too small to detect spherocytosis. If immune-mediated hemolytic anemia is suspected, the erythrocyte fragility test may be useful.
493. **c** The dog tapeworm, *Dipylidium caninum,* is also common in cats.
494. **a** Feline rhinotracheitis virus is a herpesvirus.
495. **a** *Escherichia coli* is commonly involved in feline pyometra.
496. **a** Squamous-cell carcinoma is the most common oral tumor of cats.
497. **c** This oily accumulation is known as stud tail.
498. **d** Calcium ions oppose the cardiotoxic effects of hyperkalemia but do not lower serum potassium levels.
499. **b** This is a classic description of Chédiak-Higashi syndrome.
500. **d** Cats with Chédiak-Higashi syndrome have a defect in neutrophil function, which renders them more susceptible to recurrent infections.
501. **c** Cytoplasmic inclusions are characteristic of chlamydial conjunctivitis. The other agents listed do not produce inclusions.
502. **a** Feline herpesvirus has a predilection for corneal epithelium. Keratitis is a common manifestation of feline herpesviral infection.
503. **c** Feline calicivirus has a predilection for oral epithelium. Vesicles that develop into ulcers are common on the tongue of infected cats.
504. **d** Calicivirus has a predilection for the lower respiratory tract. Virulent strains cause pulmonary lesions in young kittens.
505. **c** These signs are typical of upper respiratory infections caused by herpesvirus.
506. **d** Once infected, cats remain latent carriers of herpesvirus for life. Stress can cause recrudescence of the infection.
507. **d** Tetracycline is the drug of choice for treatment of *Chlamydia* infection.

508. **a** Idoxuridine is the only drug listed with efficacy against herpesvirus.
509. **a** Generalized peripheral lymph node lymphoma is the most common form in dogs, but is relatively rare compared with other forms in cats.
510. **e** Latent FeLV is nonreplicating by definition and therefore is undetectable by ELISA or the IFA test.
511. **d** Typically, erthrocytes in FeLV-infected cats are macrocytic, not microcytic.
512. **e** FeLV ELISAs are accurate if performed properly, but they often yield false-positive results because of technical error. Answers b and d improve accuracy.
513. **c** FeLV is excreted in massive amounts in saliva. Normal feline grooming behavior promotes transmission of the virus.
514. **b** More than 50% of cats with alimentary lymphoma are FeLV negative.
515. **a** Saliva testing is subject to a greater rate of false-positive and false-negative results. The other answers listed enhance test accuracy.
516. **d** Latent FeLV infection is not detected by conventional testing, only by in vitro isolation from cultured bone marrow cells.
517. **b** ELISAs are more sensitive, detect earlier stages of infection, and are more prone to yield false-positive results.
518. **e** The result of ELISA becomes positive earlier than the result of the IFA test.
519. **b** Intestinal lymphoma occurs in aged cats; the other forms occur in young cats.
520. **c** FIV is commonly transmitted via cat bites.
521. **d** FIV antibody indicates exposure and infection. FIV infection is for life.
522. **b** Although the other listed signs occur, oral cavity lesions are present in well over 50% of cats with clinical disease related to FIV.
523. **d** Pyogranulomatous exudate is typical of effusive FIP.
524. **a** Immune-complex vasculitis is the key event in FIP coronavirus infection.
525. **b** Exudative anterior uveitis caused by vasculitis is a common manifestation of FIP.
526. **d** This is a very nonspecific test and not a confirmatory diagnostic test of FIP.
527. **a** Feline enteric coronavirus is very prevalent in cats. It elicits antibodies indistinguishable from antibodies directed against FIP coronavirus.
528. **a** Cats ingest *Toxoplasma* cysts in muscles (raw meat) of rodents and meat-producing animals.
529. **e** An IgG antibody titer can indicate previous infection from years earlier; an IgM titer indicates recent or active infection.
530. **d** Of the drugs listed, only tetracycline is effective against hemobartonellosis.
531. **a** The capsule is characteristic of *Cryptococcus.*
532. **d** *Chlamydia* causes conjunctivitis but no internal ocular involvement.
533. **a** Panleukopenia virus can interfere with cerebellar development in the fetus.
534. **c** Serologic testing cannot distinguish between FIP and enteric coronaviral antibodies.
535. **e** Ketoconazole is the oral drug of choice for treatment of histoplasmosis.
536. **e** Hyperglobulinemia is a common finding in FIP but not in the other listed infections.
537. **a** Injection pain and systemic side effects are caused by vaccine adjuvants.
538. **c** In groups of cats, viruses are most likely to be transmitted by contact or aerosol.
539. **b** Asthma causes prominence of bronchial structures on radiographs. Air bronchograms indicate an alveolar fluid density, as occurs in pneumonia or edema
540. **b** Terbutaline is an oral β_2-adrenergic agent used as a bronchodilator.
541. **a** A bronchodilator is indicated; the only one listed is aminophylline.
542. **c** Nasopharyngeal polyps are common in cats.
543. **d** This lesion is typical of chronic lipidoid aspiration pneumonia.
544. **a** Eosinophils are typical in airway aspirates from asthmatic cats.
545. **e** Anaerobes are the most common type of bacteria found in pyothorax of cats.
546. **d** The twisted lung lobe and its air spaces become engorged with blood, producing a radiopaque lobe.
547. **d** Drainage and lavage of the pleural space are used in treatment of pyothorax.
548. **d** The fibrosing, walling-off process in pyothorax may encapsulate fluid into one hemithorax.
549. **d** A space-occupying cranial mediastinal mass, such as lymphoma, reduces compliance of the feline thorax.
550. **e** Air in the pleural space (pneumothorax) is resonant and tympanic on percussion.

551. **c** This is the definition of orthopnea.
552. **b** Aspiration pneumonia is a frequent complication of esophageal regurgitation.
553. **b** Fluid therapy promotes fluidity and enhances expectoration of respiratory secretions.
554. **d** *Cryptococcus* has a predilection for the nasal cavity of cats.
555. **d** Failure of the laryngeal orifice to open and close properly during respiration indicates laryngeal neuromuscular dysfunction.
556. **b** This treatment is for the pulmonary edema that results from electrocution.
557. **a** In asthma, bronchoconstriction is a major contributor to the signs of airway obstruction.
558. **c** With extensive thoracic wall injury, the flail or floating segment of the chest wall collapses (rather than expands) on inspiration (negative intrapleural pressure).
559. **d** Stridor is a high-pitched inspiratory sound associated with upper airway (laryngeal) obstruction.
560. **a** Mediastinal and subcutaneous free air originates from an airway leak.
561. **d** Foreign bodies abruptly cause unilateral signs. The other answers are chronic or bilateral.
562. **b** *Campylobacter* infects many animal species and is of public health concern because of the potential for animal-to-human transmission.
563. **b** Metronidazole is not effective against *Salmonella.*
564. **d** Sulfasalazine is specifically indicated for treatment of colonic inflammation.
565. **b** Melena indicates upper gastrointestinal tract bleeding.
566. **a** Histamine from neoplastic mast cells stimulates gastric acid hypersecretion.
567. **c** Inflammatory bowel disease is usually lymphocytic or lymphocytic-plasmacytic.
568. **a** Intestinal adenocarcinomas often appear as circumferential stenosing intramural masses in older cats.
569. **a** Hypovolemia and shock are serious complications of viral gastroenteritis.
570. **e** These drugs enhance rhythmic segmentation contractions, delay transit, and reduce mucosal fluid loss in diarrhea.
571. **d** Some cats respond to dietary management, such as hypoallergenic diets.
572. **d** This disease is characterized by a mucosal inflammatory process detected by histopathologic examination but not be radiography.
573. **e** Lactulose is a poorly absorbed disaccharide that induces osmotic catharsis.
574. **b** Mucus is secreted from the abundant goblet cells in the colon in response to local irritation or inflammation.
575. **e** Medical therapy is not effective, and the nonfunctional colon must be removed.
576. **c** Serum bile acid determinations are the most sensitive screening test for shunts. The results of other tests of liver function (such as enzymes) are often normal.
577. **e** Cats are inherently resistant to corticosteroid hepatopathy, and it is unlikely to cause jaundice.
578. **e** Cats do not develop a corticosteroid-induced isoenzyme of alkaline phosphatase.
579. **b** Phenytoin is dangerous to cats. Phenobarbital is the preferred anticonvulsant.
580. **c** Acidosis and progressive hyperkalemia are typical of urethral obstruction.
581. **a** *Microsporum canis* is common in cats. The other organisms listed are rare.
582. **c** Even standard human dosages of acetaminophen can be fatally toxic in cats.
583. **a** Azotemia with concentrated urine suggests prerenal azotemia caused by dehydration.
584. **d** Cirrhosis is not an effect of taurine deficiency, but the other signs listed do occur.
585. **c** There are many causes, but chronic renal failure is the most common clinical setting for chronic hypokalemia.
586. **c** Each of these three is effective in restoring euthyroidism.
587. **a** Excessive thyroxine causes secondary cardiac hypertrophy and cardiomyopathy.
588. **e** Encephalopathy is not a manifestation of hyperthyroidism, whereas the other signs listed are very typical.
589. **c** A corticosteroid-induced isoenzyme of alkaline phosphatase does not occur in cats.
590. **e** Unlike dogs, cats do not develop diabetic cataracts because of a difference in their lens metabolic pathway.
591. **d** Megestrol is a progestational drug used for dermatologic and behavior therapy. It can cause diabetes mellitus in some cats.

592. **d** In this cat the peak insulin effect (glucose nadir) occurs early and then wanes, as indicated by the afternoon and evening rise in glucose levels. This indicates a short duration of action of the insulin and the need for a longer-acting insulin or twice-daily insulin administration.
593. **b** Ultralente is the longest-acting insulin available.
594. **c** Methimazole can be used to maintain euthyroidism in hyperthyroid cats.
595. **a** Salicylates are very slowly metabolized in the feline species.
596. **d** Acetaminophen toxicity in cats causes methemoglobinemia and Heinz-body anemia.
597. **a** More than 70% of hyperthyroid cats have bilateral adenomas of the thyroid glands.
598. **b** These findings describe lungworm infection.
599. **a** Bilirubinuria is abnormal in any cat and is an important indicator of liver disease.
600. **d** Portosystemic shunts typically have minimal effect on serum bilirubin levels or enzyme activities.
601. **b** Polydactylism is inherited as an autosomal dominant trait in cats.
602. **c** Interference of colostral antibodies with the response to vaccination can persist until 4 months of age.
603. **b** Ionized calcium predominates in acidemic animals.
604. **e** Urinary incontinence is not a side effect of progestogens.
605. **a** Bacterins elicit this type of reaction more commonly than do vaccines.
606. **d** Kittens should be first vaccinated at 8 or 9 weeks of age.
607. **b** Some collies have an adverse reaction to large doses of ivermectin.
608. **d** Routine radiographic procedures have no effect on immune function.
609. **d** Parvovirus does not infect people.
610. **d** Approximately 95% of a nursing puppy's immunoglobulins are derived from colostrum.
611. **c** Squamous-cell carcinoma is not a round-cell tumor.
612. **b** Light-skinned cats can develop squamous-cell carcinoma from chronic exposure to sunlight.
613. **a** Tumors in this classification have the poorest prognosis.
614. **e** Although spayed dogs may become obese, it stems from overfeeding rather than from the surgery.
615. **a** Fenbendazole is effective in treating whipworm infection.
616. **b** A daily intake of 20 to 30 kcal/lb should be sufficient for this dog.
617. **b** *Giardia* is best detected in feces using zinc sulfate flotation solution.
618. **d** Corticosteroids and estrogens cause sebaceous gland atrophy.
619. **a** Cryptococcosis is more common in cats than in dogs.
620. **d** These findings are consistent with hypothyroidism.
621. **b** Hyperadrenocorticism is diagnosed with low-dosage dexamethasone suppression.
622. **c** Hypothyroidism is diagnosed with the TSH response test.
623. **c** Although affected dogs may have thin skin, this is unrelated to pruritus.
624. **e** Linear preputial dermatosis is a cardinal sign of Sertoli-cell tumor.
625. **e** Megestrol therapy is unlikely to cause diabetes insipidus.
626. **d** Flea infestation is the most common cause of miliary dermatitis in cats.
627. **a** Normal cats would not have a high titer.
628. **b** Hyperglycemia induced by stress is relatively common and must be differentiated from that associated with diabetes mellitus.
629. **d** In cats, food allergy tends to be manifested as pruritus, rather than as gastrointestinal signs.
630. **b** Acne tends to occur in young dogs but can occur in cats of any age.
631. **a** Azathioprine and corticosteroids are most effective for this disorder.
632. **b** Superficial pyoderma is relatively uncommon in cats.
633. **d** Systemic corticosteroids are most effective in preventing scarring associated with juvenile cellulitis.
634. **b** Myelosuppression is an adverse effect of griseofulvin use in cats.
635. **e** Mast-cell tumors are unlikely to produce arrhythmias.
636. **a** Cornifying epitheliomas tend to remain localized.
637. **a** It can be difficult to obtain cells for cytologic examination by aspiration of fibrosarcomas.

638. **d** Nearly all diabetic dogs require exogenous insulin (insulin dependent).
639. **c** Of those listed, ceruminous-gland tumors are most common in cats.
640. **c** Release of heparin from mastocytomas predisposes to bleeding.
641. **b** Sarcoma virus, a retrovirus, causes fibrosarcoma in cats but is not the cause of fibrosarcoma in dogs.
642. **c** Up to 90% of female dogs with anal sac adenocarcinoma have hypercalcemia.
643. **c** Transmissible venereal tumors may regress spontaneously.
644. **b** Mediastinal lymphosarcoma is most commonly associated with hypercalcemia.
645. **b** Doxorubicin can be cardiotoxic.
646. **a** Lymphosarcoma is usually multicentric in dogs.
647. **c** Polyuria and polydipsia are commonly associated with hypercalcemia.
648. **c** Hypercalcemia can lead to dystrophic calcification and renal dysfunction.
649. **d** Long-haired breeds, such as Old English sheepdogs, often lose their hair after doxorubicin therapy.
650. **b** Cats are most commonly infected by FIV through bite wounds rather than by casual contact.
651. **a** This combination of drugs is most effective in treating lymphosarcoma.
652. **a** It is estimated that only 2% of healthy cats are infected with FIV.
653. **b** FIV infection is detected using enzyme-linked immunosorbent assay for FIV antibodies.
654. **b** Vincristine is a phase-specific chemotherapeutic agent.
655. **b** Transmissible venereal tumors need not be surgically reduced or totally resected before chemotherapy.
656. **e** Histiocytomas have not been associated with hypercalcemia.
657. **c** Coccidioidomycosis is most common in dogs living in the southwestern United States.
658. **b** Cats are involved in 10% of human cases of plague.
659. **c** Pemphigus foliaceus is diagnosed by histologic examination and indirect immunofluorescence testing of skin biopsies.
660. **c** Circulating eosinophilia is rare in affected cats.
661. **c** Alopecia related to a hormonal imbalance typically begins in the perineal or flank region.
662. **a** Infected cats may develop polyclonal gammopathy, with elevated α-, β-, and γ-globulin levels.
663. **d** See answer 659.
664. **e** These findings are consistent with inhalant allergy.
665. **c** Red blood cell fragmentation is a common finding in animals with hemangiosarcoma.
666. **b** Of the tumors listed, mastocytomas tend to bleed most profusely during excision because of their tendency to produce heparin.
667. **b** Astrocytes serve as antigen-presenting cells in the CNS.
668. **b** Astrocytes respond to trauma by swelling.
669. **e** Heartworm infection is unlikely to be associated with insulin resistance.
670. **b** In dogs the spleen is most commonly affected by hemangiosarcoma.
671. **c** Hypoglycemia is associated with insulin excess, rather than with a deficiency of insulin.
672. **a** Keratoacanthoma (intracutaneous cornifying epithelioma) occurs in the skin and does not affect the spleen.
673. **d** Diuresis is induced with saline infusion and use of furosemide.
674. **d** These clients are often severely dehydrated, and fluids must be formulated and infused carefully to avoid cerebral edema, based on serum electrolyte levels.
675. **d** Captan is an antifungal and is not used in treating seborrhea.
676. **c** Prolonged use of dexamethasone, a relatively long-acting glucocorticoid, may reduce Cushingoid signs.
677. **a** Impetigo is more accurately termed *superficial pustular pyoderma.*
678. **a** *Microsporum canis* is the most common cause of ringworm in cats.
679. **e** Supplementation with copper tends to worsen the toxicity.
680. **e** Gentamicin is excreted through the kidneys.
681. **b** Chloramphenicol is metabolized in the liver by glucuronide conjugation and should not be used in animals with liver disease.
682. **e** Cephalosporins are more likely to be nephrotoxic than hepatotoxic.

683. **c** Of those listed, betamethasone is the most potent glucocorticoid.
684. **d** Penicillins are very unlikely to cause nephrotoxicity.
685. **e** Naloxone is an opioid antagonist and is not used as an appetite stimulant.
686. **c** Cats contract toxoplasmosis by eating infected mice. Cats usually begin to hunt at 2 to 12 months of age. Once infected, cats only shed oocysts for 1 to 2 weeks. Even if reinfected, they do not again shed oocysts.
687. **d** Clindamycin is used to treat toxoplasmosis in cats.
688. **c** Only approximately 10% of affected dogs survive for 1 year after limb amputation.
689. **c** Flucytosine is most effective against cryptococcosis.
690. **d** Approximately 75% of dogs treated with this regimen achieve complete remission.
691. **b** Chemotherapy prolongs survival for an average of 10 months.
692. **d** Aspergillosis is the most common cause of a chronic nasal discharge in dogs.
693. **c** Panleukopenia virus is very resistant to common disinfectants but can be inactivated with 6% sodium hypochlorite solution.
694. **a** Clinical signs resemble those of thiamin deficiency.
695. **d** Methimazole is most effective in treating hyperthyroidism in cats.
696. **a** The dog's age and the chronic clinical course strongly suggest a nasal tumor.
697. **a** Less than 10% of affected dogs survive 1 year after surgery.
698. **d** None of the other answers is accurate.
699. **e** Dogs with uncomplicated diabetes mellitus are not hypocalcemic.
700. **e** About half of islet-cell tumors metastasize to the liver and regional lymph nodes.
701. **b** Adjuvants are included in vaccines to enhance the antibody response.
702. **a** The key is reduction in virulence while still maintaining viability.
703. **a** gP70 is present in feline leukemia virus, not parvovirus. Parvoviruses have no glycoprotein because they are non-enveloped.
704. **d** FOCMA is a cell membrane antigen and not a viral antigen.
705. **c** Antibodies generally appear 6 or 7 days after vaccination.
706. **c** The half-life of maternal antibodies is approximately 8 to 10 days in nursing kittens.
707. **d** The general recommendation is to wait 2 weeks after vaccination, even though immunity may be generated before this time.
708. **c** A four-fold increase in titer is the general standard for a rising titer.
709. **c** This is the only choice showing a four-fold increase in titer between samples.
710. **a** CAV-1 (infectious canine hepatitis) vaccines may induce an antigen-antibody reaction in the cornea, producing the "blue eye" reaction.
711. **b** ICH, CHV, and CPV are all DNA viruses.
712. **d** FCV, FIP, and FeLV are all RNA viruses.
713. **e** Histopathologic examination is the only test that is diagnostic for FIP. Lesions are in the kidney.
714. **c** gp70 glycoprotein of the peplomer or spike of the virus is the key immunogen to stimulate neutralizing antibodies against FeLV.
715. **b** All viruses within one serotype are antigenically very similar and thus stimulate similar antibody titers.
716. **d** FIP is caused by a coronavirus.
717. **e** ELISA is the most common test for antibodies to FIP virus.
718. **c** Such hypersensitivity reactions are first apparent about 1 week after vaccination and usually persist for up to 1 month.
719. **b** Both drugs are commercially available as eye ointments for antiherpes therapy.
720. **a** This is the reason animals are not vaccinated early in life.
721. **b** Antiserum can provide rapid but temporary protection, whereas MLV vaccines stimulate protection faster than inactivated.
722. **c** Both measles virus and canine distemper virus are morbilliviruses that stimulate cross-reactive protection.
723. **a** Viruses with the same antigenic determinants are of the same serotype.
724. **b** Like herpes simplex of people, local infection results in transport of virus via peripheral nerves to the nerve ganglia, where latent infection is established.
725. **c** FIP antibody titers are not diagnostic but only indicate previous infection with a coronavirus, possibly FIP virus.
726. **c** Persistent viremia is only rarely reversible (less than 5% of infected cats).

727. **b** Panleukopenia is caused by a parvovirus.
728. **e** Panleukopenia virus may persist for years without a decrease in infectivity.
729. **b** Chlorhexidine is effective against herpes viruses, such as feline herpesvirus, but has no effect on nonenveloped viruses, such as feline calicivirus and parvovirus.
730. **c** Gentamicin and kanamycin remain on the mucosa of the respiratory system much longer than penicillins and other antibiotics and hence are more effective in aerosols.
731. **d** Aerosol therapy can greatly reduce the number of bacteria and reduce clinical signs.
732. **b** Feline parvovirus requires an actively dividing cell for replication; hence, the clinical signs produced in panleukopenia are related to lysis of replicating cells.
733. **e** Feline infectious peritonitis is caused by a coronavirus.
734. **b** Although FIP virus was once though to be labile, studies have shown that the virus can persist up to 7 weeks at room temperature.
735. **b** Transfer only occurs within the first few hours after nursing, until the gut "closes" to antibody uptake.
736. **e** An anamnestic response to rhinotracheitis virus occurs at 21 days but not if the vaccine is given earlier. Hence, one should not give two rhinotracheitis vaccines sooner than 3 weeks apart.
737. **e** They may be given by various routes, depending on the specific vaccine.
738. **b** Feline herpesvirus-1 is the most common cause of ulcers on the cornea of cats.
739. **c** Some strains of calicivirus commonly cause tongue ulcers.
740. **a** Hypergammaglobulinemia is common to both forms of FIP.
741. **b** *Bacillus pisiformis* causes Tyzzer's disease.
742. **c** *Salmonella* may cause subclinical infections but also may produce fatal infections.
743. **c** Because cats are frequently exposed to panleukopenia virus almost immediately on entering some shelters, the efficacy of vaccines and antiserum (although rarely used now) is directly related to the speed of antibody induction.
744. **d** All three types of immunity provide protection against infection.
745. **a** Feline leprosy is caused by *Mycobacterium lepraemurium.*
746. **c** Feline herpesvirus is quite labile and rapidly inactivated, but it may take a few days to completely inactivate the virus.
747. **d** Rabies virus excretion in infected cats and dogs begins shortly before clinical signs appear.
748. **b** FeLV infection of the crypt cells of the small intestine produces a chronic panleukopenia-like syndrome, in that the same cells are destroyed as in panleukopenia.
749. **a** Particles 5 μm in diameter remain in aerosols until they reach the lung.
750. **e** Calicivirus vaccine can protect against upper respiratory infection and pneumonia caused by calicivirus.
751. **d** Infected cats shed calicivirus continuously but shed rhinotracheitis virus intermittently.
752. **b** The virus grows better at temperatures below body temperature.
753. **d** Multivalent vaccines are commonly used. Each multivalent vaccine must be tested for possible interference between multiple components before licensure.
754. **b** Inactivated vaccines are safer for use in pregnant cats than modified-live-virus vaccines.
755. **e** Arbitrarily, 12 weeks has been selected as the cutoff for persistent anemia.
756. **c** Rabies virus, herpesvirus, and morbilliviruses are enveloped and thus are very susceptible to disinfectants.
757. **b** Cats exposed to parvovirus develop antibodies within 6 or 7 days.
758. **c** The half-life of circulating antibodies is 8 to 10 days.
759. **e** The serum neutralization test is very sensitive and specific.
760. **c** This is one way in which virus serotypes are determined.
761. **c** ELISAs can be set up to detect antibody and/or antigen.
762. **c** Canine parvovirus is very resistant to most disinfectants.
763. **e** Although the exact mode of transmission is unclear, cat scratch disease has been associated with cat bites and scratches.
764. **b** Calicivirus is a single-stranded RNA virus that is actively shed and is relatively resistant to disinfectants and adverse environmental conditions.

765. **c** Although Negri bodies do occur in neurons of cats with rabies, histopathologic examination is no longer used routinely to diagnose rabies.
766. **e** The virus is single-stranded, nonenveloped, and resistant to most disinfectants.
767. **c** One cannot determine the time of infection from a single IgG antibody titer.
768. **e** ELISA is used to detect antigen or antibody (positive or negative) but not to measure the titer (antibody level).
769. **c** Indirect fluorescent antibody testing detects virus or antigen within cells but not in fluid samples.
770. **c** The initial FIV test detected anti-FIV antibodies.
771. **e** Feline panleukopenia virus is a single-stranded, nonenveloped DNA virus.
772. **c** All cats with clinical panleukopenia have leukopenia during the early acute phase.
773. **a** Bovine parvovirus is unrelated to feline parvovirus.
774. **c** Household bleach (Clorox) is highly effective against parvovirus.
775. **c** A 1:32 dilution of stock Clorox (bleach) is effective as a disinfecting solution.
776. **b** Modified-live-virus vaccines produce faster protection. One could use an approved intranasal modified-live-virus vaccine as well.
777. **e** Vaccinate as soon as possible. Time is critical.
778. **e** Cats typically do not develop significant illness until 3 to 5 years after FIV infection.
779. **d** Although both are lentiviruses, people cannot contract AIDS from cats.
780. **c** Free-roaming male cats are most commonly infected, typically through bites sustained during fights.
781. **d** Dental disease is not directly related to diseases causing polyuria and polydipsia.
782. **c** Appetite is not necessarily a good indicator of small-bowel versus large-bowel disease.
783. **c** Frank blood in the stool is termed *hematochezia.*
784. **b** Melena is characterized by dark, tarry stools containing digested blood.
785. **a** Ascites is an accumulation of serous fluid in the peritoneal space.
786. **d** Hematuria is blood in the urine.
787. **e** Yellow discoloration of the mucosae and sclerae is termed *icterus* or *jaundice.*
788. **c** These findings are characteristic of shock.
789. **e** This dog's temperature and respiratory rate are abnormally high.
790. **e** This cat is at least 8% dehydrated.
791. **d** A head tile could be caused by damage to the vestibular system, not the spinal cord.
792. **b** Glaucoma is an increased intraocular pressure.
793. **e** Standing to be mounted is characteristic of estrus.
794. **c** Ability to regulate body temperature takes several weeks to develop.
795. **b** Distichiasis is characterized by a double row of eyelashes that impinge on the globe.
796. **d** Epistaxis is a bloody nasal discharge.
797. **c** The tail vein is used for blood collection in cattle but not in small animals.
798. **c** Azotemia is characterized by elevated serum urea nitrogen (BUN) and creatinine levels.
799. **b** The urine of animals with chronic renal failure is typically more dilute than normal (lower specific gravity).
800. **d** Of the tests listed, detection of heartworm antigens using ELISA is most accurate.
801. **a** Thoracic radiographs are useful to assess the degree of disease. Serum chemistry assays are useful to assess liver and kidney function before starting treatment.
802. **d** The bladder must be stabilized to avoid lacerating tissues with the needle.
803. **c** Even using strict aseptic technique, bacteria are likely to be introduced into the bladder during catheterization.
804. **d** Fetal bone calcification is sufficient by 45 days to allow radiographic diagnosis of pregnancy.
805. **e** These findings describe petechial hemorrhages.
806. **d** Thrombocytopenia is the most likely cause of this problem.
807. **c** Shock causes a marked sympathetic response.
808. **b** Stomatitis is characterized by inflammation of the oral mucosa.
809. **a** Examples include uroliths and sialoliths.
810. **d** Colitis is inflammation of the large bowel.
811. **c** Enteritis is inflammation of the small bowel.
812. **e** Coprophagy is the practice of eating feces.
813. **e** Rectal prolapse is characterized by eversion of the rectum out through the anus.

814. **d** Perianal fistulae are draining tracts in the perianal region.
815. **a** Constipation is abnormal accumulation of usually dry feces, making it difficult to defecate.
816. **b** Long-standing constipation leads to accumulation of very dry feces that become very difficult to evacuate.
817. **c** Impaction of the anal sacs commonly causes discomfort, which leads affected dogs to drag their anus along the ground.
818. **c** With regurgitation, food is expelled from the stomach a short time after ingestion. This term may also pertain to backflow of blood through a vessel or valve.
819. **e** Alopecia caused by a hormonal imbalance is not usually pruritic.
820. **e** Muscle pain is not a sign of congestive heart failure.
821. **d** The other tumors listed are relatively common skin tumors.
822. **d** The pelvic limbs are extended, with the femoral head rotated medially.
823. **d** Culture and sensitivity tests are the best way to determine which antibiotic is appropriate for treatment.
824. **c** This 8-week-old puppy is not old enough to develop problems from whipworm infection, because the prepatent period is 3 months.
825. **d** Fenbendazole is effective against whipworms.
826. **c** This cat should be retested after at least 1 month to determine if the infection is active.
827. **b** None of the other organisms typically causes ear infections in dogs.
828. **b** *Isospora* is a common coccidian of young dogs.
829. **e** This is a lungworm.
830. **c** Parainfluenza virus, adenovirus, or herpesvirus may act in concert with the bacterium *Bordetella bronchiseptica.*
831. **d** A 6% solution of sodium hypochlorite is effective.
832. **a** These four diseases are all zoonoses.
833. **d** Demidocisis is more common in purebred dogs.
834. **d** *Microsporum canis* is more common in cats than in dogs.
835. **c** It takes approximately 6 months after infection for microfilariae to appear in the blood.
836. **c** Fenbendazole administration does not prevent heartworm infection.
837. **b** Thiacetarsamide must be given by careful intravenous injection, because perivascular injection causes severe tissue irritation and sloughing.
838. **a** Treated dogs can develop hepatic and renal toxicity.
839. **d** Feline leukemia virus infection may indirectly cause upper respiratory disease through immunosuppression, allowing secondary bacterial infection.
840. **b** One grain equals 65 mg.
841. **b** BID indicates twice daily or every 12 hours. 28 lb = approximately 12.5 kg. A dosage of 2 mg/kg = 2 × 12.5 = 25 mg, given every 12 hours.
842. **a** 55 lb = 25 kg. A dosage of 2 mg/kg = 2 × 25 = 50 mg. A 5% solution contains 5000 mg/dl, or 50 mg/ml. Therefore the dog should receive 1 ml of the 5% furosemide solution.
843. **b** 28 lb = approximately 12.5 kg 0.08 × 12.5 = approximately 1 kg, which, in fluid weight, is equivalent to 1 L (1000 ml). Not mentioned in the question, but also necessary to consider when treating with fluids, are maintenance needs and continuing losses (vomiting, diarrhea).
844. **d** Weight gain in the face of rehydration indicates overhydration. This is the earliest clinical sign. By the time other signs develop, life-threatening overhydration may be occurring.
845. **a** 360 ml ÷ 24 hr = 15 ml/hr. 60 drops = 1 ml. 60 drops × 15 ml = 900 drops. 900 drops ÷ 60 min = 15 drops/min.
846. **c** If the bottle were below the level of the vein, flow would cease.
847. **c** Of those listed, "normal" saline is the only isotonic fluid.
848. **b** The solution contains very small amounts of B vitamins, but a major percentage is dextrose. Dextrose solutions of greater than 10% are too hyperosmolar for safe infusion into peripheral veins. The catheter should be a dedicated line and *never* used for intravenous medication. Frequent monitoring, particularly of blood glucose, packed cell volume (PCV), total protein, and electrolytes, is vital to successful total parenteral nutrition. Strict asepsis must be used; ideally a vented hood should be used to mix solutions in sterile containers not exposed to room air.

849. **c** Warm tap water does not irritate intestinal tissue and effectively hydrates desiccated feces.
850. **c** Anemia is not a complication of enema administration.
851. **b** Splenomegaly is frequently seen in immune-mediated hemolytic anemia and *Hemobartonella* caused by erythrocyte sequestration and destruction. Lymphoma may cause splenomegaly because of the presence of proliferative neoplastic lymphocytes. Patients with bone marrow erythrocyte hypoplasia may also exhibit significant splenomegaly as the result of splenic extramedullary hematopoiesis. Myasthenia gravis is an autoimmune condition affecting muscle motor end plates; it is not associated with splenomegaly.
852. **d** Zinc toxicity has been shown to induce hemolytic disease in dogs. Sources of zinc include ingestion of galvanized wire or kennel cage nuts and pennies produced since 1983. Pennies minted since 1983 have a thin copper coating over zinc as their major metal.
853. **d** Conscious proprioception is a neurologic assessment; it would not be helpful to further assess possible causes of anemia. Fecal examination is appropriate to assess for blood-sucking parasites. Splenic palpation is appropriate to detect splenomegaly, which may be associated with immune-mediated erythrocyte destruction, hemoparasites, or splenic neoplasia leading to possible intraabdominal bleeding. Mucous membrane inspection may reveal petechial hemorrhage, which could be associated with thrombocytopenia and internal bleeding. Urinalysis may reveal hemoglobinuria, which could be associated with intravascular hemolysis.
854. **a** Some poodles may have naturally occurring macrocytosis; mean corpuscular volume (MCV) values may be 80 to 100 fl. Clinicians must be aware of this peculiarity, as it can affect the interpretation of underlying anemia.
855. **a** $[(18 \div 45) \times 18] \div 2 = [0.4 \times 18] \div 2 = 7.2 \div 2 = 3.6$.
856. **b** Immune-mediated hemolytic anemia is often, but not always, associated with marked regenerative anemia. The other listed conditions are typically associated with nonregenerative anemia.
857. **e** Infections are usually associated with an elevated white blood cell count, characterized by a neutrophilia with or without a left shift. In extreme and overwhelming bacterial infections, the neutrophil count can decline and absolute neutropenia can be seen, but this is unusual. Neutropenias are, however, commonly seen in patients with myelophthisis, anticancer chemotherapy administration, parvovirus infection, or endotoxic shock.
858. **a** Hemangiosarcoma is a malignant neoplasm derived from vascular endothelial cells. These tumors are often associated with abnormal blood flow through the tumor. This may lead to erythrocyte fragmentation, platelet aggregation, extensive metastasis, and disseminated intravascular coagulation.
859. **b** Although ehrlichiosis can lead to chronic antigenic stimulation and possible polyclonal gammopathy, this disease has also been associated with monoclonal gammopathy. It can be confused with multiple myeloma; clinicians should be aware of this.
860. **e** Feline leukemia virus and/or feline immunodeficiency virus have been associated with lymphoma, multicentric fibrosarcoma, immunodeficiency, and bone marrow aplasia. Hyperthyroidism has not been associated with underlying retroviral infection.
861. **b** Anticoagulated whole blood should be submitted to the laboratory for a direct Coombs' test. This test detects autoantibodies attached to erythrocytes. Blood is the appropriate sample.
862. **a** A positive antinuclear antibody test is one criterion for diagnosis of systemic lupus erythematosus.
863. **c** Vincristine is not contraindicated in the presence of thrombocytopenia. In fact, it is one of the drugs considered potentially useful in inducing early release of platelets from megakaryocytes. Many cases of immune-mediated thrombocytopenia are treated with vincristine. The other listed drugs suppress platelet production.
864. **a** Cyclophosphamide is metabolized to phosphoramide mustard and acrolein. These metabolic products are likely responsible for uroepithelium irritation, leading to sterile hemorrhagic cystitis and possibly transitional-cell carcinoma of the bladder.

865. **e** Cardiac catheterization is an invasive diagnostic test with very specific and limited indications. It would not be considered for initial evaluation of a patient with a fever of unknown origin. The other listed tests are commonly requested to further search for a cause of unknown fever.

866. **d** Complement is a series of functionally linked proteins that interact with each other to provide many of the effector functions of both inflammation and the humoral immune system. The major functions of complement include cytolysis, opsonization, and activation of inflammation.

867. **a** Venous congestion, hepatic congestion, and splenic congestion are each consistent with right-sided heart failure. Likewise, right-sided heart failure frequently leads to pleural effusion and ascites. Pulmonary congestion and edema, leading to cough, tachypnea, and dyspnea, are classic signs associated with left-sided heart failure.

868. **d** Stress-associated hyperglycemia is not an appropriate differential diagnosis for syncope or intermittent weakness.

869. **b** Sepsis is typically associated with injected, brick-red mucous membranes. Cyanosis may be seen in each of the other listed clinical conditions.

870. **c** Hyperthermia, hypoxia, hypotension, and chocolate intoxication (theobromine intoxication) are each associated with tachycardias. Hypothyroidism, with its associated lowering of the basal metabolic rate, may be associated with bradycardia.

871. **d** Pulmonic stenosis leads to increased right ventricular pressure overload and subsequent ventricular hypertrophy, ventricular dilation, and right atrial enlargement.

872. **e** Cats with acute thromboembolism usually exhibit normoglycemia or stress-associated hyperglycemia.

873. **d** Associated neutropenia would be very unusual. Increased serum lactate dehydrogenase activity is the result of muscle ischemia and subsequent release of this enzyme from muscle tissue. Prerenal azotemia is common. Stress-induced lymphopenia may be seen, as well as disseminated intravascular coagulation.

874. **e** Rarely are the tricuspid or pulmonic valves associated with infectious endocarditis. As a result, thromboemboli would not be distributed to the pulmonary parenchyma. The other conditions (heart murmur, infarction, septic or immune-mediated arthritis, fever) are seen with infectious endocarditis.

875. **b** Congenital patent ductus arteriosus leads to pulmonary vessel overcirculation and results in excessive return of blood to the left atrium and left ventricle. This leads to left atrial and left ventricular enlargement.

876. **e** Thiacetarsamide therapy nearly always is associated with increased liver enzyme activity. Mere elevation of these enzymes, however, is not an indication to discontinue treatment.

877. **c** Pure transudates are associated with very low cell counts (below 2500/μl) and a low protein content (2.5 to 3.0 g/ml). They are usually caused by underlying hypoalbuminemia.

878. **a** Cardiac arrhythmia is the most common clinical complication of pericardiocentesis.

879. **c** Acute nasal trauma is usually not associated with a mucopurulent discharge.

880. **b** *Cryptococcus neoformans* affects cats more frequently than dogs. It enters through the upper respiratory tract and commonly affects the nasal cavity. It is found in the soil and is highly concentrated in pigeon droppings.

881. **d** Intrathoracic collapsing trachea is typically associated with expiratory distress. As the animal makes forced expiratory efforts, intrathoracic pressure increases dramatically, causing the intrathoracic trachea to collapse.

882. **e** The cause of laryngeal paralysis is usually unknown.

883. **c** Hypoadrenocorticism (Addison's disease) is typically associated with hypovolemia, microcardia, and an associated pulmonary vascular under circulation pattern.

884. **b** Pulmonary edema is associated with an alveolar pattern. The other listed diseases are primarily associated with a prominent bronchiolar pattern.

885. **d** *B. dermatitidis* is most frequently transmitted by aerosol infection, not by direct animal-to-animal contact.

886. **b** Hyperadrenocorticism, immune-mediated hemolytic anemia, nephrotic syndrome, and dirofilariasis have each been associated with pulmonary thromboembolic disease.

887. **d** Xerostomia by definition means dry mouth. It would not be associated with excessive salivation (ptyalism).

888. **b** Parvovirus is a single-stranded, nonenveloped DNA virus. Poxvirus, adenovirus, and herpesvirus are double-stranded DNA viruses. Coronavirus is a single-stranded RNA virus.

889. **e** Rectal adenocarcinoma would not cause protein-losing enteropathy.

890. **e** Intestinal lymphangiectasia is a significant cause of protein-losing enteropathy but is not associated with tenesmus or dyschezia.

891. **e** Chronic renal insufficiency is generally associated with normal or reduced renal size.

892. **d** Fibromatous epulis is a benign neoplasm originating from the periodontal stroma. Epulides are often located in the gingiva near incisor teeth. They are typically pedunculated, nonulcerating, and noninvasive neoplasms. They are not known to metastasize.

893. **e** Vitamin K is required for the postribosomal carboxylation of glutamyl residues of factors II, VII, IX, and X. In vitamin K deficiency or antagonism, the liver produces inactive proteins antigenically similar to the active factors. The circulating inactive factors are rapidly converted to active factors following vitamin K administration.

894. **c** Endocrine cells (G cells) in the gastric antrum and duodenum secrete gastrin in response to protein meals and, to a lesser extent, gastric distention. The most important biologic action of gastrin is stimulation of gastric acid secretion by gastric oxyntic (parietal) cells.

895. **d** Cystitis is generally characterized by stranguria and pollakiuria. Owners often believe their pet is demonstrating polyuria, when in fact it is demonstrating pollakiuria.

896. **c** The most common bacterial isolate from canine urine is *Escherichia coli.*

897. **a** Hyperadrenocorticism (Cushing's syndrome) is characterized by each of the items listed, except hypocholesterolemia. In fact, hyperadrenocorticism is typically associated with hypercholesterolemia.

898. **d** Hypercalcemia is observed in hyperparathyroidism.

899. **b** Hyperkalemia prolongs the P-R interval.

900. **c** Azathioprine can induce acute pancreatitis.

NOTES

NOTES

SECTION

7

Nephrology and Urology

K.C. Bovée

Recommended Reading

Berne RM, Levy MN: *Principles of physiology,* ed 2, St. Louis, 1996, Mosby.

Cunningham JG: *Textbook of veterinary physiology,* Philadelphia, 1992, WB Saunders.

Guyton AC, Hall JE: *Textbook of medical physiology,* ed 9, Philadelphia, 1996, WB Saunders.

Osborne C, Finco D: *Canine and feline nephrology and urology,* Baltimore, 1996, Williams & Wilkins.

Reece WO: *Physiology of domestic animals,* ed 2, Baltimore, 1996, Williams & Wilkins.

Swenson MJ, Reece WO: *Dukes' physiology of domestic animals,* ed 11, Ithaca, NY, 1993, Cornell University Press.

Practice answer sheet is on page 299.

Questions

1. *The renal medullary efferent arteriole contains smooth muscle and divides into:*
   a. a single vas rectus surrounding the proximal tubule
   b. multiple vasa recta that penetrate deep into the medulla
   c. a capillary network that absorbs large volumes of fluid from the distal tubule in the cortex
   d. multiple vasa recta that are controlled by the renin-angiotensin system
   e. peritubular capillaries distributed in the cortex and medulla

2. *The rate of blood flow to the renal medulla is important because it influences:*
   a. urine-concentrating capacity and urinary sodium excretion
   b. acid-base balance
   c. the osmolarity of final urine, which is approximately 100 mOsm/L
   d. 50% of blood flow to the kidney
   e. the multiple endocrine functions of the kidney

Correct answers are on pages 176-177.

3. *Autoregulation of renal blood flow is:*
   a. controlled by myogenic tone of the efferent arteriole, dependent on the juxtaglomerular apparatus and angiotensinogen
   b. effective within the range of 70 to 180 mm Hg renal arterial pressure
   c. effective within the range of 30 to 65 mm Hg renal arterial pressure
   d. directly dependent on oxygen extraction by the kidney
   e. controlled by the same factors that control autoregulation of cerebral blood flow

4. *The selective permeability of the glomerular capillary wall to various macromolecules in dogs allows the highest clearance of:*
   a. myoglobin
   b. hemoglobin
   c. albumin
   d. inulin
   e. globulin

5. *The dynamics of glomerular filtration are best characterized by:*
   a. clearance of para-aminohippurate
   b. clearance of creatinine and sodium
   c. the role of mesangial cells
   d. increasing net ultrafiltration pressure throughout the length of the glomerular capillary
   e. increasing plasma oncotic pressure throughout the length of the glomerular capillary

6. *The mean glomerular hydrostatic pressure in dogs is:*
   a. secondary to the glomerular filtration rate and the tone of the efferent arteriole
   b. increased to 80 mm Hg when vasoconstriction of the afferent arteriole is maximal
   c. equal to plasma oncotic pressure
   d. the same as net ultrafiltration
   e. approximately 60 mm Hg and remains unchanged throughout the glomerular capillary

7. *If the renal clearance of creatinine is 20 ml/min for a given animal, one would then expect the clearance of:*
   a. para-aminohippurate to be 100 ml/min
   b. para-aminohippurate to be 250 ml/min
   c. glucose to be the same as for creatinine
   d. inulin to be 50 ml/min
   e. inulin to be approximately the same as for para-aminohippurate

8. *Resorption of sodium in the proximal tubule is normally:*
   a. 65% of the filtered load of sodium
   b. 90% of the filtered load of sodium
   c. closely linked to the renal concentrating mechanism
   d. influenced by aldosterone
   e. 99.9% of the filtered load of sodium

9. *Aldosterone influences tubular transport of sodium and potassium by:*
   a. maintaining high sodium resorption in the proximal tubule
   b. decreasing sodium resorption in the distal tubule
   c. increasing potassium resorption in the proximal tubule
   d. increasing sodium resorption in the distal tubule, representing approximately 5% of the filtered load
   e. enhancing sodium resorption in the distal tubule, representing approximately 30% of the filtered load

10. *What is the primary influence of parathyroid hormone on renal tubular electrolyte transport?*
    a. enhance potassium resorption
    b. decrease calcium resorption
    c. decrease phosphate resorption
    d. enhance bicarbonate resorption and hydrogen ion secretion
    e. enhance sodium resorption of approximately 20% of the filtered load

11. *Which site within the nephron is associated with active transport of chloride?*
    a. cortical collecting duct
    b. distal tubule
    c. descending limb of Henle
    d. proximal straight tubule
    e. diluting segment of the ascending limb of Henle

12. *Which of the following is most likely to activate the renin-angiotensin system?*
    a. extracellular fluid volume depletion
    b. increased renal arterial pressure
    c. decreased sympathetic tone
    d. extracellular fluid volume expansion
    e. a mean arterial pressure of 100 mm Hg

13. *Which of the following is most likely to cause release of atrial natriuretic factor?*
    a. reduced production of antidiuretic hormone
    b. extracellular fluid volume expansion
    c. extracellular fluid volume depletion
    d. renal ischemia
    e. diabetes insipidus

14. *Causes of prerenal azotemia include all the following **except:***
    a. shock
    b. acute hemorrhage
    c. dehydration
    d. acute tubular necrosis
    e. myocardial failure

15. *Which of the following is most consistent with massive proteinuria, hypoalbuminemia, edema and hypercholesterolemia?*
    a. nephrolithiasis
    b. urinary tract infection
    c. nephrotic syndrome
    d. acute renal failure
    e. chronic urinary tract obstruction

16. *Thirty days after 75% nephrectomy, one would expect creatinine clearance to be:*
    a. 20% of normal
    b. 40% of normal
    c. 60% of normal
    d. 95% of normal
    e. 120% of normal

17. *Which species normally has the highest urine specific gravity?*
    a. horses
    b. cattle
    c. pigs
    d. dogs
    e. cats

18. *Concerning glomerulonephritis in dogs, which statement is most accurate?*
    a. It can be effectively controlled with large doses of corticosteroids.
    b. It can be effectively controlled with immunosuppressants.
    c. It can be effectively controlled with anticoagulants and vasoactive amine inhibitors.
    d. It can be effectively controlled with a high-protein diet.
    e. It cannot be effectively controlled with any of the agents listed above.

19. *When performing a urinalysis with the standard dipstick reagent pads for heme pigments, a positive color test indicates:*
    a. intact erythrocytes, free hemoglobin, or free myoglobin
    b. free myoglobin or free hemoglobin only
    c. free hemoglobin only
    d. free hemoglobin or intact erythrocytes only
    e. intact erythrocytes only

20. *White blood cell casts in the urinary sediment are strongly suggestive of:*
    a. glomerulonephritis
    b. amyloidosis
    c. lower urinary tract infection
    d. prostatitis
    e. pyelonephritis

Correct answers are on pages 176-177.

21. *Which type of urolith is most frequently associated with bacterial urinary tract infection?*
   a. cystine
   b. ammonium acid urate
   c. calcium phosphate
   d. calcium oxalate
   e. magnesium ammonium phosphate

22. *After 48 hours of complete lower urinary tract obstruction, one would expect renal blood flow to be approximately:*
   a. 10% of normal
   b. 50% of normal
   c. 90% of normal
   d. normal
   e. essentially zero, resulting in acute tubular necrosis

23. *Which class of antimicrobials is considered to be the most nephrotoxic in domestic animals?*
   a. sulfonamides
   b. tetracyclines
   c. penicillins
   d. aminoglycosides
   e. fluoroquinolones

24. *During progression of chronic renal failure, as the filtered load of sodium changes, one would expect the fractional resorption of sodium to:*
   a. increase to 100%
   b. decrease to approximately 90%
   c. decrease to 20%
   d. remain normal until more than 60% of renal mass is lost
   e. decrease in parallel with glomerular filtration rate

25. *What is the most important cause of the anemia in chronic renal failure?*
   a. insidious blood loss through the gastrointestinal tract
   b. reduced life span of red blood cells
   c. folate deficiency because of increased excretion
   d. inadequate production of erythropoietin
   e. excessive parathyroid hormone

Answers

1. **b** Each efferent arteriole divides into multiple vasa recta, which penetrate the medulla.
2. **a** Slow blood flow through the vasa recta maintains medullary hypertonicity, which allows concentration of urine and sodium excretion.
3. **b** Glomerular filtration rate and renal plasma flow remain fairly constant at a mean systemic blood pressure of 70 to 180 mm Hg via modulation of afferent arteriole resistance.
4. **d** The low molecular weight of inulin allows it to pass through the glomerular membrane as freely as electrolytes and water.
5. **e** As fluid moves out of the capillary and into Bowman's space, plasma proteins become more concentrated and colloid oncotic pressure increases.
6. **e** Hydrostatic pressure within the glomerular capillary remains at about 60 mm Hg.
7. **a** The same amount of creatinine and para-aminohippurate is presented to the glomerulus. Creatinine is filtered, and little or none is secreted by proximal tubular epithelial cells. Para-aminohippurate is filtered and is secreted in large quantities by proximal tubular epithelial cells, increasing its clearance to approximately five times that of creatinine ($5 \times 20 = 100$).
8. **a** Approximately 65% of the filtered sodium is resorbed in the proximal tubule, with approximately 99% resorbed by the end of the tubule.
9. **d** Aldosterone increases resorption of sodium and excretion of potassium.
10. **c** Parathyroid hormone inhibits resorption of phosphate from the proximal tubule.
11. **e** Chloride passes out of the lumen of the ascending loop of Henle by active transport.
12. **a** Dehydration stimulates production of renin and angiotensin II, which stimulates adrenal release of aldosterone, with subsequent increased renal retention of sodium and water.

13. **b** Atrial natriuretic factor is formed by atrial myocytes and is released in response to increased atrial filling (as with volume expansion), causing reduced blood pressure via enhanced sodium excretion.
14. **d** Tubular necrosis is not a prerenal cause of azotemia. All the other answers are prerenal in origin.
15. **c** These abnormalities characterize the nephrotic syndrome.
16. **c** By 30 days after removal of 75% of functional renal tissue, creatinine clearance would rise to approximately 60% of normal through compensatory mechanisms.
17. **e** The specific gravity of feline urine normally is 1.035 to 1.060 but can rise above 1.090.
18. **e** Although various pharmacologic agents and diets have been advocated for management of glomerulonephritis, none is effective.
19. **a** These reagent pads produce a nonspecific reaction to intact erythrocytes, hemoglobin, or myoglobin.
20. **e** Casts comprising white blood cells are formed in the kidney and suggest pyelonephritis.
21. **e** Struvite uroliths are commonly associated with bacterial urinary tract infections.
22. **b** This level of blood flow provides nutrient flow and prevents tubular necrosis.
23. **d** Of the drug classes listed, aminoglycosides have the highest potential for nephrotoxicity.
24. **b** Fractional resorption of sodium rarely falls lower, even when the glomerular filtration rate is 10% of normal, which allows a small population of nephrons to control sodium balance.
25. **d** Insufficient production of erythropoietin by reduced functional renal parenchyma eventually leads to anemia because of decreased erythropoiesis in the bone marrow.

NOTES

NOTES

SECTION

8

Neurology

A.E. Chauvet

Recommended Reading

Braund KG: *Clinical syndromes in veterinary neurology,* ed 2, St. Louis, 1994, Mosby.

Chrisman CL: *Problems in small animal neurology,* ed 2, Baltimore, 1991, Williams & Wilkins.

de Lahunta A: *Veterinary neuroanatomy and clinical neurology,* ed 2, Philadelphia, 1983, WB Saunders.

Ettinger SJ, Feldman ED: *Textbook of veterinary internal medicine,* ed 4, Philadelphia, 1995, WB Saunders.

Oliver JE et al: *Handbook of veterinary neurology,* ed 3, Philadelphia, 1997, WB Saunders.

Practice answer sheet is on page 301.

Questions

1. *Discospondylitis is most commonly caused by infection with:*
   a. *Pseudomonas, Escherichia coli,* or coagulase-positive *Staphylococcus*
   b. *E. coli,* coagulase-positive *Staphylococcus,* or *Brucella canis*
   c. *E. coli,* coagulase-positive *Staphylococcus,* or *Campylobacter*
   d. *Brucella canis, Pseudomonas,* or *Campylobacter*
   e. coagulase-positive *Staphylococcus, Enterobacter,* or *Clostridium*

2. *Hansen type-I intervertebral disk disease characterized by:*
   a. chondroid degeneration of the nucleus pulposus and disk rupture
   b. chondroid degeneration of the annulus fibrosis and disk protrusion
   c. fibrinoid degeneration of the annulus fibrosis and disk rupture
   d. fibrinoid degeneration of the annulus fibrosis and disk protrusion
   e. chondrofibroid degeneration of the nucleus and annulus and disk protrusion

3. *A 3-year-old Rhodesian ridgeback develops sudden onset of paraparesis that is worse in the left pelvic limb. The patient can ambulate with support on the right pelvic limb but not on the left pelvic limb. Reflexes are intact in all limbs. Conscious proprioception is absent in both pelvic limbs and normal in the thoracic limbs. The cutaneous trunci reflex is absent caudal to L3 on the right side and L1 on the left side. The clinical signs have not changed in the past 2 days. The dog shows no pain on palpation of the spine. Where is the lesion most likely located, and what is the most likely cause of these findings?*
   a. T3-L3 myelopathy associated with discospondylitis
   b. T3-L3 myelopathy associated with spinal cord neoplasia
   c. L4-S3 myelopathy associated with intervertebral disk herniation on the left side
   d. T3-L3 myelopathy associated with fibrocartilaginous embolism
   e. T3-L3 myelopathy associated with degenerative myelopathy

4. *Which client is most likely to be affected by granulomatous meningoencephalomyelitis?*
   a. young, intact male, large-breed dog
   b. old, intact female, small-breed dog
   c. middle-aged, spayed, small-breed dog
   d. young, intact female, large-breed dog
   e. castrated, small-breed puppy

5. *Which clinical signs accurately describe cauda equina syndrome?*
   a. dropped tail carriage, decreased pelvic limb reflexes, urinary and fecal incontinence, lumbosacral pain, paraparesis, and pelvic ataxia
   b. dropped tail carriage, increased pelvic limb reflexes, lumbosacral pain, paraparesis, and pelvic ataxia
   c. elevated tail carriage, increased pelvic limb reflexes, urinary and fecal incontinence, paraparesis, and pelvic ataxia
   d. dropped tail carriage, decreased thoracic limb reflexes, urinary and fecal incontinence, paraparesis, and pelvic ataxia
   e. dropped tail carriage, increased limb reflexes in all limbs, urinary and fecal incontinence, lumbosacral pain, paraparesis, and pelvic ataxia

6. *What is the recommended treatment for degenerative myelopathy of German shepherds?*
   a. aminocaproic acid, Karo (corn) syrup, penicillin
   b. aminocaproic acid, vitamin E and B complex daily, exercise every other day
   c. corticosteroids
   d. trimethoprim-sulfa, with pyrimethamine and folic acid supplementation
   e. surgical decompression

7. *During the past 3 days, a 4-year-old spayed poodle developed a progressive right head tilt, circling to the right, and falling to the right. When presented to you, the dog is conscious, with pronounced nonpositional vertical nystagmus in both eyes and opisthotonos. When helped to stand, the dog cannot support weight on its limbs and has decreased conscious proprioception in the left thoracic and left pelvic limbs and absent conscious proprioception in the right thoracic and right pelvic limbs. In what posture was the dog as presented, where is the lesion, and what are the two most likely causes of these findings?*
   a. decerebellate posture; right central vestibular disease; granulomatous meningoencephalomyelitis or neoplasia
   b. decerebrate posture; left central vestibular disease; neoplasia or bacterial infection
   c. Shiff-Sherrington posture; peripheral right vestibular disease; otitis interna or hypothyroidism
   d. decerebellate posture; left central vestibular disease; granulomatous meningoencephalomyelitis or neoplasia
   e. Schiff-Sherrington posture; right central vestibular disease; neoplasia or distemper encephalomyelitis

8. *You suspect that a dog has acquired myasthenia gravis. What is the best diagnostic test to confirm your tentative diagnosis?*
   a. edrophonium chloride (Tensilon) challenge
   b. electromyography
   c. acetylcholine receptor antibody titers
   d. acetylcholine receptor antigen titers
   e. muscle biopsy

9. *An 8-year-old, obese, castrated cat develops weakness in the back legs. The cat is paraparetic and has a plantigrade gait in the pelvic limbs. The withdrawal reflexes are decreased bilaterally. What is the primary differential diagnosis, and what is the most appropriate initial diagnostic procedure?*
   a. diabetic neuropathy; serum glucose assay
   b. diabetic neuropathy; serum albumin assay
   c. myasthenia gravis; muscle biopsy
   d. hepatic encephalopathy; ammonia tolerance test
   e. polyarthritis; arthrocentesis of multiple joints

10. *In what animals is X-linked muscular dystrophy, an inherited disorder, most likely to occur?*
    a. cats and golden retrievers
    b. great Danes and Yorkshire terriers
    c. beagles and coonhounds
    d. pitbulls and pugs
    e. ferrets

11. *Concerning facial nerve paralysis, which statement is most accurate?*
    a. All cases are idiopathic.
    b. Feline cases are idiopathic, but canine cases are usually related to hypothyroidism.
    c. Approximately 75% of canine cases and 25% of feline cases are idiopathic.
    d. The disease is inherited in golden retrievers and cocker spaniels.
    e. It is always associated with Horner's syndrome.

For Questions 12 through 16, select the correct answer from the five choices below.

a. phenobarbital
b. potassium bromide
c. diazepam
d. pentobarbital
e. glucose

12. *Its sedative side effects can be reversed with a high-salt diet.*

13. *Blood levels should be measured 10 to 14 days after initiating therapy.*

14. *Blood levels should be evaluated in any puppy less than 6 months of age with seizures.*

15. *It is often used to control status epilepticus that is unresponsive to diazepam.*

16. *It can cause hepatitis in cats.*

17. *What are the four clinical signs of Horner's syndrome?*
    a. mydriasis, exophthalmos, increased tearing, and blepharospasm
    b. mydriasis, enophthalmos, ptosis, and keratoconjunctivitis sicca
    c. mydriasis, enophthalmos, ptosis, and prolapsed third eyelid
    d. miosis, enophthalmos, ptosis, and blepharospasm
    e. miosis, enophthalmos, ptosis, and prolapsed third eyelid

18. *What is the most common primary brain neoplasm of dolicocephalic dogs?*
    a. astrocytoma
    b. meningioma
    c. schwannoma
    d. choroid plexus papilloma
    e. lymphoma

Correct answers are on pages 183-185.

19. A 10-year-old Labrador retriever develops loss of balance that has progressed over the past 24 hours. The dog cannot walk, rolls to the left, and has hypersalivation, a severe left head tilt, and nonpositional horizontal nystagmus of both eyes, with the fast phase to the right. Conscious proprioception is normal, and the dog is alert and strong. Where is the lesion, and what is the most likely cause of these findings?

a. right central vestibular lesion; meningioma
b. left peripheral vestibular lesion; granulomatous meningoencephalomyelitis
c. right peripheral vestibular lesion; old dog vestibular disease
d. left peripheral vestibular lesion; old dog vestibular disease
e. left central vestibular lesion; trauma

20. Concerning botulism, which statement is most accurate?

a. It causes immune-mediated polyneuropathy; dogs are very susceptible.
b. It inhibits release of acetylcholine at the nerve-muscle junction; dogs are relatively resistant.
c. It destroys acetylcholine receptors; dogs are relatively resistant.
d. It causes degenerative myopathy; dogs are very susceptible.
e. It causes hepatitis with subsequent encephalopathy; dogs are relatively resistant.

21. What is the treatment of choice for tetanus?

a. penicillin and tetanus antitoxin
b. gentamicin and tetanus antitoxin
c. clindamycin and chlorpromazine
d. penicillin; avoid tetanus antitoxin, because it worsens clinical signs
e. gentamicin; avoid tetanus antitoxin, because it worsens clinical signs

22. What is the recommended treatment for central nervous system toxoplasmosis in dogs and cats?

a. clindamycin or sulfonamides
b. clindamycin or oxacillin
c. folic acid supplementation
d. fluconazole or ketoconazole
e. clindamycin, or sulfonamides with pyrimethamine and folic acid supplementation

Questions 23 through 25

You are presented with a dog that developed progressive onset of lameness in the left thoracic limb over the past 4 months. The dog resists weight bearing on the left thoracic limb. The left triceps muscle and distal limb muscles are severely atrophied. The left biceps muscle is slightly atrophied. The left forelimb tends to drag. Conscious proprioception is absent in the left thoracic limb only. The cutaneous trunci reflex is absent on the left side when you pinch the left or right flank. Sensation is absent in the caudal and lateral aspect of the left thoracic limb. In the left thoracic limb,the withdrawal reflex is decreased, the biceps reflex is normal, and triceps reflex is absent. The dog has miosis of the left pupil.

23. Where is the lesion causing these signs?

a. C6-T2 myelopathy
b. left brachial plexus, involving the musculocutaneous nerve
c. left brachial plexus, involving the radial nerve and lateral thoracic nerve
d. left vagosympathetic trunk, just caudal to the head
e. right cerebral cortex

24. Which nerve roots make up the sympathetic pathway to the eye?

a. C6-8
b. C8-T1
c. T3-L3
d. T1-4
e. C1-5

25. What is the most likely cause of these findings?

a. discospondylitis
b. type-II disk disease
c. nerve root tumor
d. trauma
e. myositis associated with toxoplasmosis

Answers

1. **b** Organisms that have been associated with discospondylitis in the dog include *Brucella canis,* coagulase-positive *Staphylococcus, Bacteroides capillosus, Nocardia, Streptococcus canis, Corynebacterium, Escherichia coli, Proteus, Pasteurella, Paecilomyces, Aspergillus,* and *Mycobacterium.*
2. **a** Hansen type-I disk disease is a chondroid degeneration of the nucleus pulposus; type-II disk disease is a fibrinoid degeneration of the annulus fibrosus. Dogs with type-I disk disease usually are small dogs of chondrodystrophic breeds. They demonstrate acute progressive or nonprogressive clinical signs as early as 6 months of age. Dogs with type-II disk disease are usually large-breed dogs with chronic progressive onset of clinical signs starting at middle age. Type-I disk disease usually affects the thoracolumbar and cervical spine, most commonly at C2-3 and T12-13. Type-II disk disease usually affects the caudal cervical spine and lumbosacral spine.
3. **d** The typical presentation of fibrocartilaginous embolism is acute onset of asymmetric signs. The thoracolumbar area is most often affected. The patient can demonstrate pain in the first 24 hours. Signs can progress over the first 24 hours; thereafter, patients are usually nonpainful on spine palpation and clinical signs are stable or improve. Dogs with lower motor neuron signs have a poor prognosis because of irreversible destruction of neuronal cell bodies. Dogs with loss of voluntary motion also do not have a good prognosis because of the severity of the tract involvement.
4. **c** Granulomatous meningoencephalomyelitis is an inflammatory disease thought to be of immune or neoplastic origin. Middle-aged, spayed, small-breed dogs are most commonly affected, as early as 1 year of age. The disease is best diagnosed by cerebrospinal fluid analysis and brain imaging (computed tomography [CT] or magnetic resonance imaging [MRI]). The diagnosis is confirmed by histopathologic examination. The prognosis is poor or guarded because the disease is diagnosed with certainty only after death.
5. **a** Cauda equina syndrome comprises a set of clinical signs that indicate a lesion in the lumbosacral area of the spine. The nerve roots of L4-S3 are often affected (especially L7-S1); the conus medullaris of the spinal cord can also be affected. Clinical signs reflect damage to lower motor neurons controlling pelvic limb, bladder, and rectal function. Pain is often seen because of nerve root irritation or impingement.
6. **b** Degenerative myelopathy is a progressive degenerative or "aging" disease of the spinal cord of middle-aged or old, large-breed dogs. German shepherds are probably overrepresented. The disorder is diagnosed by ruling out other diseases by means of imaging (myelography or MRI) and cerebrospinal fluid analysis. The imaging shows a normal spinal cord; cerebrospinal fluid analysis may indicate an elevated protein level.
7. **a** Decerebrate clients are usually comatose and cannot walk; the lesion is in the midbrain. Decerebellate clients are conscious but cannot walk, the lesion is in the cerebellum or cerebellar peduncles. Dogs with Schiff-Sherrington posture are aware and can walk on the thoracic limbs if "wheelbarrowed"; the lesion is caudal to T2. All three postures are accompanied by opisthotonos when the patient is in lateral recumbency. Vestibular lesions can be localized by remembering that central vestibular disease may cause obtundation, abnormal placing, cerebellar signs, disconjugate nystagmus (and vertical nystagmus in some cases), and abnormalities of cranial nerves other than VIII. The side of the lesion is determined by cerebellar signs and preprioceptive or cranial nerve deficits. If a dog has vestibular signs and none of the above is noted, the dog should be considered to have peripheral vestibular disease until proven otherwise. The side of the lesion is noted by the side of the head tilt, circling, or opposite the fast phase of the nystagmus (for horizonal and rotatory nystagmus).
8. **c** Although edrophonium chloride (Tensilon) challenge helps support the diagnosis of acquired myasthenia gravis, many dogs with other neuromuscular disorders can also show improvement with this test. The muscle biopsy can be negative if sampling is insufficient. Approximately 90% of dogs with acquired myasthenia gravis have a positive or high serum titer for acetylcholine receptor antibodies; this is the most reliable means of confirming acquired myasthenia gravis.

9. **a** A plantigrade gait of the pelvic limbs in cats is almost pathognomonic for diabetic neuropathy. When it is noted, one must take every effort to rule out diabetes mellitus. Remember, however, that many other neuromuscular disorders and L3-S4 myelopathy can cause a plantigrade gait in dogs and cats.
10. **a** Golden retrievers are the dog breed most commonly affected. Cats, usually domestic short-haired cats, are also affected. Because it is an X-linked disorder, males are clinically affected but not females.
11. **c** Facial paresis is common in golden retrievers and cocker spaniels but can occur in any breed. Some clinicians believe the disorder is associated with hypothyroidism, but this has not been proven. The presentation is usually unilateral but may affect both sides eventually. The most common form is idiopathic (75%) in dogs. Many dogs recover spontaneously. In cats, only 25% of cases are idiopathic; middle ear disease must be ruled out, as well as polyneuropathies or other causes.
12. **b** Potassium bromide acts by means of its bromide ion which replaces chloride in the membrane transport. Neurons have a higher affinity for bromide, and thus more bromide enters the cells than chloride. Both are eliminated by the kidneys. There is a competitive excretion in the proximal tubule. When side effects occur, saline infusion or a high-salt diet can accelerate elimination of bromide.
13. **a** The half-life of phenobarbital in dogs and cats is approximately 40 hours. Because it takes at least 5.5 half-lives to reach steady state, at least 10 days (40 hr $\times$ 5.5 = 220 hr) should elapse before trough serum levels are measured.
14. **e** Hypoglycemia is a common cause of seizures of puppies.
15. **d** Pentobarbital is often used to control status epilepticus. It is preferred over thiopental, which is too short acting, and injectable phenobarbital, which is too long acting. Pentobarbital can be infused intravenously by slow drip for maintenance sedation for 24 hours.
16. **c** Diazepam has been reported to induce hepatitis in cats.
17. **c** Horner's syndrome is caused by damage of the sympathetic pathway to the eye. Miosis, enophthalmos, ptosis, and third eyelid prolapse are noted individually (partial Horner's syndrome) or together. Miosis is probably the most common sign.
18. **b** Dolicocephalic breeds are most often affected by meningiomas, whereas brachycephalic breeds are predisposed to gliomas and particularly astrocytomas.
19. **d** This client has no signs supporting central vestibular disease (see answer 7); thus it is peripheral vestibular disease. The lesion is on the side of the circling and tilt. The most common cause of peripheral vestibular disease in older dogs without Horner's syndrome or facial nerve involvement is old dog or idiopathic vestibular disease.
20. **b** Botulism prevents release of acetylcholine packets from the presynaptic membrane of the neuromuscular junction. Myasthenia gravis prevents binding of acetylcholine to the receptor on the postsynaptic membrane. Tick paralysis has the same mechanism as botulism.
21. **a** Tetanus should be treated with penicillin G. Tetanus antitoxin is especially useful early in the disease.
22. **e** Clindamycin is often the drug of choice for treatment of protozoal diseases. Some cats have died after receiving large doses of clindamycin. Sulfonamides and pyrimethamine act in synchrony in the folic acid pathway of the protozoan. Sulfonamide use can lead to keratoconjunctivitis sicca. Because pyrimethamine can cause folic acid deficiency, supplementation with folic acid is necessary.
23. **c** After brachial plexus injury (not avulsion), function remains, especially deep pain. Brachial plexus avulsion refers to complete separation of the nerves; deep pain is absent from areas of the limbs innervated by the affected nerves. Horner's syndrome is noted with injuries of T1-2. Motor function of the cutaneous trunci reflex is affected with injury of the lateral thoracic nerve (C8-T1). The slight biceps atrophy in this dog is probably related to disuse of the limb. The triceps atrophy is probably neurologic, because it is severe and reflexes are absent. The injury in this dog is fairly proximal in the plexus, probably near the spine. The radial nerve (triceps reflex) and lateral thoracic nerve are affected, as well as the sympathetic pathway at the level of the nerve roots or ramus communicans. This is not a myelopathy at C6-T2 because neurologic function of the pelvic limb on the left side is normal.
24. **d** T1-4 contribute to the sympathetic pathway to the eye. T1 provides the most significant contribution.

25. **c** Chronic progressive onset of signs is not characteristic of trauma. Discospondylitis and type-II disk disease would cause myelopathy and not multiple mononeuropathy, as present in this dog. Myositis is a generalized disorder. Nerve root tumors are slow in onset and progress over time. It is not always possible to feel a mass until it is fairly large. Although dogs may manifest pain by their initial lameness and carrying the leg, pain is not often identified by palpation of the axilla.

NOTES

NOTES

SECTION

9

Oncology

S.M. Cotter, E.T. Keller

Recommended Reading

Bonagura JD: *Kirk's current veterinary therapy,* XII, Philadelphia, 1995, WB Saunders.

Ettinger SJ, Feldman EC: *Textbook of veterinary internal medicine,* ed 4, Philadelphia, 1995, WB Saunders.

Hahn KA, Richardson R: *Cancer chemotherapy: a veterinary handbook,* Baltimore, 1994, Williams & Wilkins.

Withrow SJ, MacEwen EG: *Small animal clinical oncology,* ed 2, Philadelphia, 1996, WB Saunders.

Practice answer sheet is on page 303.

Questions

S.M. Cotter

1. *Concerning mammary tumors in dogs, which statement is most accurate?*
   a. About 80% are benign.
   b. The most common metastatic site is bone.
   c. Postoperative chemotherapy significantly decreases the rate of recurrence.
   d. Ovariohysterectomy at the time of tumor removal significantly decreases the rate of recurrence.
   e. Ovariohysterectomy before the first heat period significantly lowers the risk of mammary tumors.

2. *A 12-year-old male German shepherd has had weakness and epistaxis for the past 2 days. You palpate a large splenic mass in the abdomen and aspirate nonclotting bloody fluid from the abdominal cavity. The prothrombin time and partial thromboplastin time are slightly prolonged. The packed cell volume is 28%, total protein level is 7.2 g/dl, and platelet count is 80,000/µl. What is the most likely cause of the bleeding?*
   a. immune-mediated thrombocytopenic purpura
   b. von Willebrand's disease
   c. disseminated intravascular coagulation
   d. hypersplenism
   e. myeloma

Correct answers are on pages 190-191.

3. *All the following may be associated with an elevated packed cell volume* ***except:***
   a. renal tumor
   b. right-to-left cardiac shunt
   c. dehydration
   d. hemorrhagic gastroenteritis
   e. erythroleukemia

4. *A 12-year-old dog is presented for regurgitation of undigested food. Thoracic radiographs show a dilated esophagus and a 5-cm–diameter cranial mediastinal mass. The most likely diagnosis is:*
   a. esophageal carcinoma
   b. lymphoma
   c. thyroid carcinoma
   d. thymoma
   e. systemic mast-cell tumor

5. *Of the following diseases, which two have the best prognosis?*
   a. acute lymphoblastic leukemia and erythroleukemia
   b. acute granulocytic leukemia and cutaneous lymphoma
   c. erythroleukemia and mycosis fungoides
   d. acute granulocytic leukemia and megakaryocytic leukemia
   e. well-differentiated lymphocytic leukemia and polycythemia vera

6. *Which side effect is most likely to occur after use of the respective drugs?*
   a. cystitis from chlorambucil
   b. myelosuppression from L-asparaginase
   c. urticaria from doxorubicin
   d. hepatic necrosis from cyclophosphamide
   e. pancreatitis from vincristine

7. *You are treating lymphoma in a dog using l-asparaginase, vincristine, and cyclophosphamide. Immediately after you infuse the drugs intravenously simultaneously, the dog collapses with pale mucous membranes and vomiting. After 10 to 15 minutes the dog's condition improves. The schedule calls for all three drugs to be given again 3 weeks later. Considering the dog's immediate reaction to the previous treatment, the safest approach for the next treatment would be to:*
   a. omit the vincristine
   b. omit the L-asparaginase
   c. omit the cyclophosphamide
   d. give all the drugs again, but with a 25% reduction in dose for each
   e. give all the drugs at the same dose but as an intravenous drip over 1 hour

8. *In addition to corticosteroids, what drug should be given to a dog with multiple inoperable mast-cell tumors?*
   a. aspirin
   b. cimetidine
   c. propranolol
   d. cyclophosphamide
   e. doxorubicin

9. *A 14-year-old Norwegian elkhound is presented because of lethargy. Physical findings are negative except for moderate splenomegaly. A hemogram shows packed cell volume 32%, white blood cell (WBC) count 95,000/µl, 10% neutrophils, 89% small lymphocytes, and 1% monocytes. The platelet count is 120,000/µl. A bone marrow aspirate shows about 40% small lymphocytes, 20% myeloid cells, and 30% erythroid cells. What is the most likely cause of these findings?*
   a. hypersplenism
   b. hypoadrenocorticism
   c. reactive lymphocytosis
   d. chronic lymphocytic leukemia
   e. acute lymphoblastic leukemia

Questions 10 and 11

10. *While visiting Africa, you find a young adult female shepherd-cross as a stray. You notice vulvar bleeding and palpate an irregular friable mass just inside the vaginal opening. What is the most likely cause of these findings?*

    a. granulomatous vaginitis
    b. vaginal hyperplasia
    c. leiomyosarcoma
    d. squamous-cell carcinoma
    e. transmissible venereal tumor

11. *What treatment is most likely to benefit this dog?*

    a. testosterone
    b. ovariohysterectomy
    c. vincristine
    d. cisplatin
    e. ivermectin

12. *Concerning radiation therapy, which statement is most accurate?*

    a. Sensitivity of cells to radiation increases in the G1 phase of the cell cycle.
    b. Hypothermia combined with irradiation enhances tumor cell kill while minimizing damage to normal tissues.
    c. Hypoxic tumor cells are especially sensitive to radiation.
    d. Adenocarcinomas, osteosarcomas, and fibrosarcomas in dogs and cats are most likely to respond to radiation.
    e. Megavoltage radiation is less likely to cause skin damage than is orthovoltage radiation.

13. *An owner says that her only cat died 1 month ago from feline leukemia virus (FeLV) infection, and she now would like to get a new kitten. The most appropriate advice for her is to:*

    a. wait at least 6 months before obtaining a new kitten
    b. adopt an adult cat rather than a kitten because kittens are more susceptible to FeLV infection
    c. adopt a new kitten with no special precautions
    d. adopt a kitten after having it vaccinated against FeLV infection
    e. first clean the floors with sodium hypochlorite solution (Clorox) and destroy any dishes used by the previous cat

14. *Which of the following is a form of lymphoma that affects the skin?*

    a. reticuloendotheliosis
    b. mycosis fungoides
    c. Marek's disease
    d. myelofibrosis
    e. B cell lymphoma

15. *Which of the following is most often associated with polycythemia?*

    a. renal carcinoma
    b. erythroleukemia
    c. iron overload
    d. testosterone-secreting tumors
    e. mitral insufficiency with early left heart failure

E.T. Keller

16. *Chemotherapy with cyclophosphamide most commonly induces:*

    a. cardiotoxicity
    b. pancreatitis
    c. hemorrhagic cystitis
    d. pulmonary fibrosis
    e. peripheral neuropathy

17. *What is the most effective therapy for long-term control of hypercalcemia in an animal with neoplasia?*

    a. intravenous fluids
    b. diuretics
    c. corticosteroids
    d. antineoplastic therapy
    e. calcitonin

Correct answers are on pages 190-191.

18. *Which tumor is most likely to be associated with hypertension?*
    a. Sertoli-cell tumor
    b. pheochromocytoma
    c. lymphoma
    d. hemangiosarcoma
    e. adenocarcinoma

19. *Initial treatment of multiple metastases is best performed using:*
    a. any well-known chemotherapeutic agent
    b. a combination of doxorubicin, cyclophosphamide, and vincristine
    c. a chemotherapeutic agent effective against the primary tumor
    d. L-asparaginase
    e. resection, followed by whole-body irradiation

20. *In dogs the biologic behavior of hemangiopericytoma is commonly characterized by:*
    a. pulmonary metastases
    b. regional lymph node metastases
    c. local recurrence after resection
    d. moderate recurrence of hypercalcemia
    e. a well-encapsulated, readily excisable mass

21. *Pancytopenia (absence of all three cell lines in the peripheral blood) is most likely to be associated with:*
    a. hemolytic disease
    b. disseminated intravascular coagulation
    c. myelophthisis (infiltration of bone marrow with cancer cells)
    d. gastrointestinal ulcer
    e. initiation of chemotherapy

22. *Which of the following is most likely to be observed in a dog with mast-cell tumors?*
    a. monoclonal gammopathy
    b. elevated serum creatine phosphokinase activity
    c. occult blood in feces
    d. leukocytosis
    e. low urine specific gravity

23. *What is the most important prognostic factor for survival of cats with mammary tumors?*
    a. cat's age
    b. cat's breed
    c. location of affected gland
    d. tumor size
    e. multiple sites of tumors

24. *Which treatment is most appropriate for a 10-year-old female dog with a 3-cm nodule of the fourth left mammary gland?*
    a. observation, with periodic reexamination
    b. cytologic examination of fine-needle aspirates, with observation if it is a benign neoplasm
    c. excisional biopsy, followed by histopathologic examination and further surgery if the surgical margins are not free of tumor cells
    d. chemotherapy, regardless of the tumor type
    e. unilateral radical mastectomy

25. *Which two drugs should* ***not*** *be used in cats because of potentially life-threatening toxic reactions?*
    a. doxorubicin and vincristine
    b. 5-fluorouracil and cisplatin
    c. L-asparaginase and cytosine arabinoside
    d. methotrexate and cyclophosphamide
    e. chlorambucil and prednisone

Answers

1. **e** The beneficial effect is lost partially after the first few estrous cycles and lost totally after 2½ years of age.
2. **c** Disseminated intravascular coagulation frequently occurs in dogs with splenic hemangiosarcoma.
3. **e** All forms of acute leukemia cause myelophthisic anemia.

4. **d** Thymomas are associated with esophageal dilation secondary to myasthenia gravis.
5. **e** Lymphocytic leukemia usually responds to an alkylating agent and corticosteroids. Polycythemia vera responds to phlebotomy and hydroxyurea.
6. **c** The risk of urticaria is lessened by giving the drug slowly intravenously.
7. **b** Intravenous or intraperitoneal L-asparaginase may cause anaphylaxis. The risk of anaphylaxis is reduced if the drug is given intramuscularly or subcutaneously. Once a reaction occurs, it is likely to recur if the drug is given again.
8. **b** Cimetidine is used to inhibit duodenal ulcers, which are likely to form because histamine from the tumor stimulates HCl secretion by the stomach.
9. **d** Chronic lymphocytic leukemia is characterized by a high count of normal lymphocytes.
10. **e** Transmissible venereal tumor is enzootic in Africa, often in young-adult dogs.
11. **c** The cure rate is high after three or four injections given weekly.
12. **e** Megavoltage radiation penetrates skin better than does orthovoltage radiation, allowing it to focus on deeper sites.
13. **c** The virus only lives a few hours to a few days on surfaces in a household after an infected cat leaves the premises.
14. **b** Mycosis fungoides is a T-cell tumor with characteristic histopathologic changes.
15. **a** This tumor secretes erythropoietin.
16. **c** Hemorrhagic cystitis is usually sterile and may be induced by use of this drug.
17. **d** Antineoplastic therapy is most important to control the cause of hypercalcemia.
18. **b** Pheochromocytomas produce epinephrine and norepinephrine, which induce hypertension.
19. **c** The metastatic tumor is most likely, but not always, to respond similarly to the primary tumor.
20. **c** The metastatic rate of hemangiopericytomas is very low; however, they tend to be fairly aggressive locally and recur readily after surgery.
21. **c** The fact that all three cell lines are affected indicates that the bone marrow is involved. Recent initiation of chemotherapy would not cause anemia, because the red blood cell life span is very long. Disseminated intravascular coagulation involves platelets and red blood cells only.
22. **c** Mast-cell tumors may release histamine, which activates histamine receptors of parietal cells in the gastric mucosa. This causes increased gastric acidity and gastric ulceration, which leads to bleeding and positive fecal occult blood.
23. **d** The size of the tumor appears to be the most important prognostic factor. Tumors less than 2 cm in diameter are associated with longer survival times than tumors larger than 2 cm in diameter.
24. **c** Approximately 50% of mammary masses are benign. Excisional biopsy may be curative, but if the histologic examination indicates a malignancy, further excision may be required. Fine-needle aspiration may miss the malignant part of the tumor.
25. **b** 5-Fluorouracil causes neurologic signs and death. Cisplatin causes pulmonary edema and death.

NOTES

NOTES

SECTION

10

Ophthalmology

D.E. Brooks

Recommended Reading

Barnett KC: *Veterinary ophthalmology,* St. Louis, 1996, Mosby.

Gelatt K: *Veterinary ophthalmology,* ed 2, Baltimore, 1991, Williams & Wilkins.

Severin G: *Veterinary ophthalmology notes,* ed 3, Fort Collins, Col, 1995, Author.

Slatter D: *Fundamentals of veterinary ophthalmology,* Philadelphia, 1990, WB Saunders.

Practice answer sheet is on page 305.

Questions

1. *Accommodation of the canine lens for near vision occurs when the:*
   a. ciliary muscle contracts and the zonules relax
   b. ciliary muscle contracts and the zonules are stretched
   c. iris muscles contract and squeeze the lens into a more spheric shape
   d. ciliary muscle relaxes to allow the cornea to alter its shape
   e. iris muscles contract to pull the lens rostrally

2. *Which enzyme is associated with formation of aqueous humor?*
   a. nitric oxide synthetase
   b. serine protease
   c. carbonic anhydrase
   d. sorbitol dehydrogenase
   e. prostaglandin synthetase

3. *Which parasympatholytic mydriatic drug has the shortest duration of effect?*
   a. atropine
   b. tropicamide
   c. homatropine
   d. epinephrine
   e. cyclopentolate

4. *Gonioscopy is a diagnostic technique used for examination of the:*
   a. lens
   b. eyelids
   c. retina
   d. iridocorneal angle
   e. vitreous

5. *Which drug is most effective for treatment of feline herpesviral infection involving the eye?*
   a. trifluorothymidine
   b. flucytosine
   c. mitomycin
   d. apraclonidine
   e. nystatin

6. *Mechanical débridement and use of topical antibiotic solutions are beneficial in treatment of persistent corneal erosions in boxers. What other drug, listed below, is also indicated?*
   a. sodium chloride
   b. dexamethasone
   c. idoxuridine
   d. nystatin
   e. cromolyn sodium

7. *What is the most common eyelid tumor in cats?*
   a. melanoma
   b. squamous-cell carcinoma
   c. meibomian-gland adenoma
   d. mast-cell tumor
   e. fibrosarcoma

8. *Removal of the gland of the third eyelid of dogs with "cherry eye" has been associated with subsequent development of:*
   a. retinal detachment
   b. eversion of the cartilage of the third eyelid
   c. keratoconjunctivitis sicca
   d. squamous-cell carcinoma of the third eyelid
   e. glaucoma

9. *Which breed of dog is most sensitive to the ocular side effects of vaccination against infectious canine hepatitis?*
   a. poodle
   b. Afghan
   c. Labrador retriever
   d. German shepherd
   e. Rottweiler

10. *You detect a brownish black, focal, midstromal corneal lesion in a Persian cat. The lesion does not retain fluorescein dye but stains with rose bengal. What is the most likely diagnosis?*
   a. melanoma
   b. foreign body
   c. corneal sequestrum
   d. corneal dermoid
   e. iris prolapse

11. *The term China eye is a lay term for heterochromia iridis. What is the clinical appearance of the iris in this condition?*
   a. albinotic
   b. blue and white
   c. heavily pigmented
   d. blue
   e. blue and yellow-brown

12. *What term is used to describe the ophthalmoscopic appearance of caudal displacement of the optic nerve in glaucoma patients?*
   a. cupping
   b. atrophy
   c. degeneration
   d. dysplasia
   e. hypoplasia

13. *A dilated, nonresponsive pupil is a clinical sign of:*
   a. iritis
   b. cataracts
   c. glaucoma
   d. episcleritis
   e. iridal cysts

14. *Controlled application of intense cold (cryotherapy) to what part of the eye is useful in managing chronic elevation of intraocular pressure in dogs and cats?*
   a. cornea
   b. ciliary body
   c. iris
   d. lens
   e. choroid

15. *What type of cataract is associated with anterior uveitis and is characterized by a wrinkled anterior capsule?*
    a. incipient
    b. immature
    c. mature
    d. hypermature
    e. intumescent

16. *Which of the following occurs as a result of normal aging of the lens?*
    a. lenticonus
    b. lenticular sclerosis
    c. microphakia
    d. cataracts
    e. persistent tunica vasculosa lentis

17. *Persistent hyperplastic primary vitreous is a congenital defect of the vitreous that is most common in:*
    a. Doberman pinschers
    b. German shepherds
    c. Labrador retrievers
    d. toy poodles
    e. beagles

18. *Which retinal cell is adapted for night vision?*
    a. cone
    b. rod
    c. Müller cell
    d. ganglion cell
    e. amacrine cell

19. *On ophthalmoscopic examination, hyperreflective tapetal regions indicate damage to the:*
    a. choroid
    b. sclera
    c. retina
    d. vitreous
    e. lens

20. *Nyctalopia, or night blindness, is a cardinal sign of:*
    a. optic neuritis
    b. retinal detachment
    c. glaucoma
    d. cataracts
    e. progressive retinal atrophy

21. *A syndrome of vision loss without associated fundic abnormalities has been observed in overweight female dogs. Many affected dogs are also polyuric and polydipsic. This syndrome is known as:*
    a. progressive retinal atrophy
    b. hemeralopia
    c. sudden acquired retinal degeneration
    d. Collie eye anomaly
    e. neuronal ceroid lipofuscinosis

22. *Which clinical sign is* **not** *associated with Horner's syndrome?*
    a. miosis
    b. ptosis
    c. enophthalmos
    d. nictitans protrusion
    e. exophthalmos

23. *A 2-year-old Labrador retriever is presented with acute onset of exophthalmos, pain on opening the mouth, and unilateral nictitans protrusion. The dog has a slight fever and leukocytosis. What is the most likely cause of these signs?*
    a. intraocular neoplasm
    b. glaucoma
    c. orbital neoplasm
    d. orbital cellulitis/abscess
    e. Horner's syndrome

24. *What is the most common primary intraocular tumor of dogs?*
    a. lymphosarcoma
    b. melanoma
    c. mast-cell tumor
    d. adenocarcinoma
    e. astrocytoma

Correct answers are on page 196.

25. *During ophthalmologic examination of a dog, the fundus demonstrates an optic nerve in focus at -6 diopters with the direct ophthalmoscope. The blood vessels appear slightly smaller than normal. What is the most likely cause of these findings?*

   a. retinal detachment
   b. progressive retinal atrophy
   c. glaucoma
   d. normal variation
   e. prior chorioretinitis

Answers

1. **a** When the ciliary muscle is in the contracted state, the lens zonules are relaxed and the eye is accommodated for near vision.
2. **c** Carbonic anhydrase catalyzes formation of carbonic acid from carbon dioxide and water.
3. **b** Tropicamide has the shortest duration of action. Atropine and cyclopentolate have the longest; homatropine is intermediate. Epinephrine is an adrenergic drug.
4. **d** Gonioscopy uses a special corneal lens to examine the iridocorneal angle in glaucoma patients.
5. **a** Trifluorothymidine is the most effective agent against feline herpesvirus. The other drugs listed are not used for antiviral therapy.
6. **a** Five percent NaCl is a hyperosmotic drug used to reduce corneal edema in this condition.
7. **b** Squamous-cell carcinoma is by far the most common feline eyelid tumor.
8. **c** The third eyelid gland produces a large proportion of the tear film in dogs. Surgical removal may be associated with subsequent keratoconjunctivitis sicca.
9. **b** The Afghan and greyhound are most susceptible to side effects of such vaccination.
10. **c** Corneal sequestra are associated with keratoconjunctivitis sicca, herpesvirus infection, entropion (in Persians), and previous corneal ulceration.
11. **d** The iris is blue in China eye.
12. **a** Cupping refers to caudal movement of the laminal cribosa in response to increased intraocular pressure. The other terms are histologic in nature.
13. **c** Glaucoma causes damage to the iris sphincter muscle, resulting in a fixed and dilated pupil.
14. **b** Freezing the ciliary body at multiple sites is beneficial in reducing production of aqueous humor.
15. **d** Hypermature cataracts have a wrinkled anterior capsule because of loss of lens proteins into the anterior chamber. These lens proteins incite anterior uveitis.
16. **b** Aging of the lens results in dehydration and hardening or sclerosis of the lens nucleus.
17. **a** This is a hereditary condition in Doberman pinschers.
18. **b** Rods are for night vision and cones for day vision.
19. **c** Damage that causes thinning to the overlying retina makes it easier to see the tapetal reflection, so it appears brighter than normal, or hyperreflective.
20. **e** Progressive retinal atrophy is characterized by loss of rod cells initially, which causes nyctalopia.
21. **c** Dogs with progressive retinal atrophy are night blind. Hemeralopic dogs are day blind. There are no gender differences in Collie eye anomaly. Neuronal ceroid lipofuscinosis causes neurologic disturbances.
22. **e** Horner's syndrome is caused by loss of sympathetic innervation to the eye. Enophthalmos is caused by loss of adrenergically innervated orbital smooth muscle tone.
23. **d** Orbital abscesses arise suddenly and are very painful. These dogs may be febrile and have elevated white blood cell (WBC) counts.
24. **b** Melanomas are the most common primary intraocular tumor. Lymphosarcoma is more common but is metastatic to the eye of dogs.
25. **c** If the optic nerve is in focus at -6 diopters instead of 0 diopters, it is displaced caudally. Glaucoma is the only answer that could cause this. Progressive retinal atrophy, retinal detachment, or retinitis would cause pallor of the nerve, not cupping. Normal variation would be an optic nerve in focus from 0 to -3 diopters.

SECTION

11

Preventive Medicine

P.C. Bartlett, C.N. Carter, J.D. Hoskins

Recommended Reading

August JR: *Consultations in feline internal medicine,* ed 3, Philadelphia, 1996, WB Saunders.

Bonagura JD: *Kirk's current veterinary therapy,* XII, Philadelphia, 1995, WB Saunders.

Bowman DD: *Georgi's parasitology for veterinarians,* ed 6, Philadelphia, 1995, WB Saunders.

Ettinger SJ, Feldman EC: *Textbook of veterinary internal medicine,* ed 4, Philadelphia, 1995, WB Saunders.

Greene CE: *Infectious diseases of the dog and cat,* ed 2, Philadelphia, 1990, WB Saunders.

Guilford WG et al: *Strombeck's small animal gastroenterology,* Philadelphia, 1996, WB Saunders.

Leib MS, Monroe WE: *Small animal internal medicine,* Philadelphia, 1997, WB Saunders.

Nelson RW, Couto CG: *Essentials of small animal internal medicine,* St. Louis, 1992, Mosby.

Practice answer sheet is on page 307.

Questions

P.C. Bartlett

1. *Concerning vaccination of wild animals against rabies, which statement is most accurate?*
   a. Rabies vaccines are now available and approved for use in pet raccoons and skunks.
   b. Any wild animal can be vaccinated against rabies, as long as it has been adequately domesticated by its owner.
   c. There are no licensed rabies vaccines approved for use in wild animals, with the exception of ferrets.
   d. Rabies vaccines licensed for use in dogs can be used on pet coyotes, foxes, and wolves.
   e. The AVMA does not consider rabies in wild animals to be a real threat in the United States; therefore, vaccination is optional.

2. *What is the appropriate management of a dog or cat that bites a person?*
   a. The animal should be immediately euthanized, regardless of ownership status, and the animal's head sent to the local state health department for rabies examination.
   b. The animal should be confined and observed for 10 days; if any signs of illness arise, a veterinarian should evaluate the animal and report to the health department; if signs of rabies emerge, the animal should be humanely killed and the head sent to the local or state health department for rabies examination.
   c. The animal should be immediately given a rabies booster, confined, and observed for 30 days.
   d. the animal should be simply observed for 10 days and released after examination by a licensed veterinarian.
   e. A copy of the bite report must be given to the local or state health department.

3. *Dogs infected with parvovirus shed large numbers of virus particles and present a significant threat to susceptible animals. Which of the following describes appropriate management of such animals and the environment to protect other dogs from infection?*
   a. Isolate infected dogs from other dogs until 1 week after full recovery, and disinfect the premises with dilute (1:30) chlorine bleach solution.
   b. Dogs routinely shed virus for up to 6 months and should be isolated for at least that period, followed by a thorough detergent cleaning of the environment.
   c. Isolate infected dogs and disinfect the premises only if unvaccinated animals will be in the area.
   d. Isolate infected dogs until they recover, and disinfect the premises with chloroxylenol.
   e. Isolate infected dogs until they are no longer febrile; no environmental disinfection is required, because parvovirus is extremely labile.

4. *Concerning peroxide antiseptics (e.g., hydrogen peroxide), which statement is most accurate?*
   a. They are some of the most effective antiseptics.
   b. They are known for their long-term residual activity.
   c. They provide a mechanical cleansing action via release of oxygen but have only a mild antiseptic action.
   d. They have virtually no use in the medical environment.
   e. Most peroxides are virucidal.

5. *Concerning use of iodophor disinfectants (e.g., povidone-iodine) as surgical scrubs, which statement is **least** accurate?*
   a. Scrubbing of hands and surgical sites with an iodophor reduces bacterial populations for up to 8 hours.
   b. Iodophors are effective against a broad range of bacteria, viruses, and fungi.
   c. Iodophors act as oxidizing agents, although they are less active than chlorine.
   d. Iodophors are known for their action against spores.
   e. Iodophors can irritate the skin.

C.N. Carter

6. *Which of the following is a recognized method of preventing ascariasis in dogs?*
   a. no raw meat in the diet
   b. boiling of all drinking water
   c. treatment of newborn pups with niclosamide
   d. treatment of the postparturient bitch with metronidazole
   e. treatment of the preparturient bitch with fenbendazole

7. *Concerning vaccination and immunity in dogs and cats, which statement is **least** accurate?*
   a. Colostrum-deprived dogs and cats should be given the initial vaccination approximately 2 to 3 weeks earlier than normal.
   b. Maternal antibodies can provide 3 to 6 months of protection against most diseases but can also interfere with development of active immunity from vaccination.
   c. Live agents in vaccines should be attenuated so that they remain antigenic and replicate in the recipient but do not produce illness.
   d. The agents in killed (inactivated) vaccines are immunogenic but do not replicate in the host.
   e. Vaccine failures are most common in very young and very old animals.

8. *A new client with a kitten is asking questions about feline distemper (feline panleukopenia). Which of the following is **least** appropriate in advising this client?*
   a. Two modified-live-virus or three inactivated vaccine doses should be given at 3- to 4-week intervals, beginning at 8 or 9 weeks of age.
   b. Boosters should be given every 2 years if modified-live-virus products are used and annually if inactivated products are used.
   c. Inactivated vaccines should be used in pregnant, immunosuppressed, or diseased animals and in kittens less than 4 weeks of age.
   d. Modified-live-virus products must not be used in kittens less than 4 weeks of age because of the risk of cerebellar degeneration.
   e. Immune serum can give some protection for unvaccinated kittens in the face of exposure.

9. *Concerning prevention and control of borreliosis (Lyme disease), which statement is most accurate?*
   a. Many commercially available vaccines provide good protection.
   b. Immunomodulating drugs work well in preventing borreliosis and should be used when exposure to ticks is probable.
   c. Lifetime prophylactic administration of oxytetracycline to outdoor dogs and people in high-risk occupations provides excellent protection.
   d. It may take up to 24 hours of tick feeding before the *Borrelia* organism is secreted in the tick's saliva.
   e. No progress has been made in developing a borreliosis vaccine, because no species has been found to generate an active immune response.

10. *Which of the following is **least** effective in preventing pseudorabies in dogs and cats?*
    a. Avoid contact with pigs.
    b. Do not feed raw pork to dogs or cats.
    c. Vaccinate with an inactivated product.
    d. Avoid contact with animals with suspected pseudorabies.
    e. Avoid contact with guinea pigs.

11. *An outbreak of tetanus in a veterinary hospital is most likely attributable to:*
    a. bites from an infected animal
    b. inhalation of aerosolized organisms from a convalescing patient
    c. improper sterilization of surgical instruments
    d. indirect transmission via a variety of insects
    e. contact with contaminated fomites

12. *Which of the following is most important in prevention of urolithiasis in cats?*
    a. decreasing the urine volume
    b. reducing urine concentration of calculogenic crystalloids
    c. decreasing the solubility of calculogenic crystalloids
    d. alkalinizing the urine
    e. limiting dietary intake of zinc

Correct answers are on pages 201-202.

13. *Cat scratch disease in people is thought to be caused by* Bartonella henselae. *What is the best advice can you provide clients regarding prevention of this disease in human family members?*
   a. Train children to be gentle with pets to avoid scratching and biting, and declaw cats that will be exposed to children.
   b. Have cats tested serologically every year to identify carriers, and remove them from the household.
   c. Treat cats prophylactically with oxytetracycline to eliminate infection.
   d. Wear protective clothing when around cats.
   e. Euthanize cats that scratch people.

14. *Coccidia are obligate intracellular parasites normally found in the intestinal tract of dogs and cats. Concerning the epizootiology of coccidiosis, which statement is* ***least*** *accurate?*
   a. Coccidiosis is usually seen in conjunction with poor sanitation of premises.
   b. Insect control is important, because cockroaches and flies can act as mechanical vectors of oocysts.
   c. Animals should not be fed uncooked meat.
   d. Coccidiostatic drugs can be given to infected bitches just before or after whelping to help control the spread of infection in puppies.
   e. Coccidial oocysts cannot survive freezing temperatures.

15. *In a state in which no rabies occurred in dogs during the past year, a dog bites a child. During the 10-day rabies observation period, the dog begins acting sick and agitated and showing signs that could be those of rabies or other diseases. What is the most appropriate course of action?*
   a. Euthanize the dog, and send the head to a diagnostic laboratory for rabies testing.
   b. Confirm the diagnosis before euthanizing the dog.
   c. Wait to see if the dog survives the full 10 days; if so, rabies in the bitten child will not be a concern.
   d. Have a sample of the dog's blood tested for a rabies titer.
   e. Wait a few days for clinical signs to more fully develop.

J.D. Hoskins

16. *Dogs or cats being prepared for shipment or entering a boarding facility should be vaccinated how many weeks before the event?*
   a. 16 to 18 weeks
   b. 12 to 14 weeks
   c. 8 to 10 weeks
   d. 4 to 6 weeks
   e. 1 to 2 weeks

17. *At what age should most kittens first be presented for initial immunizations?*
   a. 4 to 6 weeks
   b. 8 to 10 weeks
   c. 12 to 14 weeks
   d. 16 to 20 weeks
   e. 24 to 30 weeks

18. *At what age should most puppies first be presented for initial immunizations?*
   a. 2 to 4 weeks
   b. 8 to 10 weeks
   c. 12 to 16 weeks
   d. 16 to 20 weeks
   e. 24 to 30 weeks

19. *Feline leukemia virus vaccine can be safely administered to kittens as young as:*
   a. 2 weeks of age
   b. 3 weeks of age
   c. 4 weeks of age
   d. 5 weeks of age
   e. 6 weeks of age

20. *The passive antibodies transferred from immune dams to the fetus during gestation may make puppies and kittens unresponsive to vaccination for what period at the beginning of life?*
    a. 3 to 6 weeks
    b. 6 to 8 weeks
    c. 2 to 3 weeks
    d. 6 to 7 days
    e. 10 to 12 days

21. *Which of the following is most likely to cause vaccination failure?*
    a. attenuation of the vaccine components
    b. storage at refrigeration temperatures
    c. no disinfectant used on needles or syringes
    d. wrong strain or type of microbe used to make the vaccine
    e. mixing with a sterile diluent

22. *Which of the following is **least** likely to contribute to vaccination failure?*
    a. vaccination of an anesthetized patient
    b. fever or hypothermia
    c. general debilitation
    d. very young or very old age
    e. use of glucocorticoids or cytotoxic agents

23. *Human errors that may cause vaccination failure include all the following **except:***
    a. vaccinating during estrus
    b. improper mixing of vaccine
    c. incorrect route of administration
    d. storing vaccine at very warm temperatures
    e. vaccinating too frequently

24. *At what age should puppies be given canine distemper-measles vaccine?*
    a. 4 to 6 weeks
    b. 6 to 12 weeks
    c. 14 to 18 weeks
    d. 20 to 24 weeks
    e. 24 to 32 weeks

25. *At what age can puppies safely begin receiving heartworm preventive?*
    a. 1 to 2 weeks
    b. 24 to 30 weeks
    c. 12 to 16 weeks
    d. 6 to 8 weeks
    e. 4 to 5 weeks

Answers

1. **c** Because there are no vaccines licensed for wild animals, the AVMA strongly encourages that states pass laws prohibiting ownership of wild animals and wild animals crossbred to domestic dogs and cats as pets.
2. **b** The 10-day observation period ensures that animals that may have exposed human beings to rabies virus are promptly identified, because virus is shed in the saliva no more than a few days before the onset of clinical signs.
3. **a** Chloroxylenol is not virucidal. Puppies nearing the end of maternal antibody protection (6 to 20 weeks) are at particular risk, because passive antibodies still interfere with vaccination but become inadequate to protect against viral challenge. This is known as the *critical period of susceptibility.*
4. **c** Peroxides are useful for mechanically cleaning purulent, pocketing wounds but have only mild antiseptic qualities. In addition, when the bubbling ends, so does its action.
5. **d** Amphoteric compounds, such as alkalinized glutaraldehyde, are known for their activity against spores. Iodophores are not active against spores.
6. **e** Pups can acquire *Toxocara canis* by transplacental or transmammary transmission. In the last trimester of pregnancy, larvae in tissues are reactivated and migrate to the pups in utero. The larvae are also shed in the milk.
7. **b** Maternal antibodies provide roughly 1 to 3 months' protection against the common infectious diseases.

8. **b** Boosters should be given annually, regardless of use of modified-live or attenuated products, although modified-live-virus products probably provide longer immunity.
9. **d** Borreliosis vaccine has been effective against experimental challenge. Prompt removal of ticks appears to be an effective preventive measure.
10. **e** Guinea pigs are not involved. Attenuated vaccines can cause reactions as serious as natural infection. The newer subunit vaccines being developed for swine may be of great value for pets in the future.
11. **c** Active immunization with tetanus toxoid is not recommended for dogs and cats.
12. **b** To help prevent struvite urolithiasis, restrict dietary intake of magnesium and maintain urine pH at 6.0 or less with methionine or ammonium chloride. If infection is present, perform culture and sensitivity tests and institute appropriate therapy.
13. **b** An indirect fluorescent antibody test is available to determine if a cat has been infected. If this test is positive, the cat's saliva should be cultured to isolate the organism.
14. **e** Coccidial oocysts can survive freezing temperatures. All runs, cages, utensils, and other equipment should be disinfected by steam, immersion in boiling water, or application of 5% ammonia solutions.
15. **a** Euthanize the dog, and send the head to the laboratory for rabies testing. Do not wait to confirm the diagnosis.
16. **e** A period of 1 to 2 weeks is adequate time before shipment or entering a boarding facility for a dog or cat.
17. **b** Eight to ten weeks are the most common age for initial presentation.
18. **b** Eight to ten weeks are the most common age for initial presentation.
19. **e** Kittens 6 weeks of age and older can be safely vaccinated.
20. **c** The maternal antibodies passed in utero can be present in the first 2 weeks of life.
21. **d** The vaccine may contain the wrong strain or type of agent needed for protection of the animal.
22. **a** The other factors listed are more likely to reduce the effectiveness of vaccination.
23. **a** Estrus has no effect on immunization.
24. **b** Check the label of the commercial product.
25. **d** As soon as puppies begin eating solid food, they can safely begin receiving heartworm preventive.

NOTES

SECTION

12

Surgical Diseases

R.M. Bright, P.A. Bushby, J.R. Davidson, J. Harari, D.L. Millis, J.K. Roush

Recommended Reading

Bojrab MJ: *Current techniques in small animal surgery,* ed 4, Baltimore, 1998, Williams & Wilkins.

Ettinger SJ, Feldman EC: *Textbook of veterinary internal medicine,* ed 4, Philadelphia, 1995, WB Saunders.

Fossum TE: *Small animal surgery,* St. Louis, 1997, Mosby.

Guilford WG et al: *Strombeck's small animal gastroenterology,* Philadelphia, 1996, WB Saunders.

Piermattei DL, Flo GL: *Handbook of small animal orthopedics and fracture repair,* Philadephia. 1997, WB Saunders.

Sherding RG: *The cat: diseases and clinical management,* Philadelphia, 1989, WB Saunders.

Slatter DH: *Textbook of small animal surgery,* ed 2, Philadelphia, 1993, WB Saunders.

Swaim SA, Henderson RA: *Small animal wound management,* Baltimore, 1990, Williams & Wilkins.

Practice answer sheets are on pages 309-311.

Questions

DOGS

J.R. Davidson

1. *What is the **least** common oral tumor in dogs?*
   a. acanthomatous epulis
   b. malignant melanoma
   c. squamous-cell carcinoma
   d. fibrosarcoma
   e. osteosarcoma

2. *What is the most effective treatment for malignant oral tumors in dogs?*
   a. resection of neoplastic tissue, along with a 1-cm margin of healthy tissue
   b. radiotherapy using x-rays or gamma rays
   c. immunotherapy with BCG (bacille bilié de Calmette-Guérin)
   d. chemotherapy
   e. cryosurgery

3. *Common complications following hemimandibulectomy include all the following **except:***
   a. drooping of the tongue
   b. sublingual edema or ranula
   c. incision dehiscence
   d. shifting of the mandible
   e. inability to eat for the first 3 to 5 days

4. *Concerning sialoceles, which statement is most accurate?*
   a. Sialoceles are usually caused by trauma to the salivary gland or duct.
   b. A sialocele or salivary mucocele in the sublingual region is termed a *ranula.*
   c. Treatment involves removing the involved gland and removing the sac of accumulated saliva in the tissues, along with its lining.
   d. The mandibular salivary gland is most commonly involved.
   e. Surgery is indicated only if less invasive treatment is unsuccessful.

5. *Concerning esophagotomy, which statement is most accurate?*
   a. Esophagotomy is the treatment of choice for esophageal foreign bodies.
   b. Large doses of corticosteroids should be given following removal of an esophageal foreign body to reduce the chance of stricture formation.
   c. Almost all dogs with esophageal foreign bodies develop some degree of esophagitis.
   d. Animals should be encouraged to drink soon after esophageal surgery to stimulate normal peristaltic activity.
   e. The flow of swallowed saliva tends to flush the esophagus, making it more resistant to infection.

6. *Where do alimentary foreign bodies most commonly lodge?*
   a. pharyngeal esophagus
   b. esophagus, at the thoracic inlet
   c. esophagus, near the base of the heart
   d. esophagus, in the diaphragmatic hiatal region
   e. duodenum

7. *Concerning persistent right aortic arch, which statement is most accurate?*
   a. It is the most common vascular ring anomaly.
   b. It results from persistence of the right sixth aortic arch.
   c. It is characterized by generalized megaesophagus.
   d. It is surgically corrected through a right thoracotomy.
   e. If treated, it has an excellent prognosis.

8. *During surgical correction of gastric dilation-volvulus:*
   a. gastrotomy is often required to empty the stomach
   b. gastropexy is performed between the stomach and left body wall
   c. fluorescein dye is very helpful in assessing gastric viability
   d. partial gastric invagination may be an alternative to partial gastric resection
   e. splenectomy should also be performed if splenic torsion is still present following gastric derotation

9. *Concerning gastric dilation-volvulus, which statement is most accurate?*
   a. The ability to pass a stomach tube indicates that the stomach is not rotated.
   b. The best positioning for abdominal radiography is left lateral recumbency.
   c. When the veterinarian makes an abdominal incision, viewing the omentum overlying the stomach indicates that the stomach is rotated.
   d. Gastropexy is recommended to prevent further episodes.
   e. It only occurs in large and giant-breed dogs.

10. *Concerning intussusceptions, which statement is most accurate?*
    a. They occur most commonly in middle-aged dogs.
    b. Typical signs include vomiting, bloody mucoid diarrhea, and a palpable cylindric abdominal mass.
    c. They occur most commonly in the pylorogastric region.
    d. They should be surgically reduced with traction on the proximal segment of the intussusception.
    e. Food should be withheld for the first 24 to 48 hours after surgery to reduce the risk of recurrence.

11. *What type of system is most effective for draining an effusion associated with generalized peritonitis?*
    a. Penrose drain
    b. closed suction drain
    c. sump-Penrose drain
    d. open peritoneal drainage
    e. continuous suction drain

12. *Concerning perianal fistulae, which statement is **least** accurate?*
    a. They cannot be effectively treated with systemic antibiotics and topical antibiotics or antiseptics.
    b. They occur primarily in German shepherds.
    c. The history may include dyschezia, hematochezia, constipation, pain, and personality changes.
    d. Complications following surgery may include fecal incontinence, anal stricture, and fistula recurrence.
    e. The most common cause is spread of infection from an abscessed anal sac.

13. *Concerning perineal hernias, which statement is most accurate?*
    a. They usually occur between the levator ani and coccygeal muscles.
    b. They are more common in females than in males.
    c. They may require a high-fiber diet and laxatives as adjuncts to surgical therapy.
    d. They rarely recur following surgery.
    e. They have a poor prognosis if fecal incontinence is noted postoperatively.

14. *Concerning portosystemic shunts, which statement is **least** accurate?*
    a. Some dogs develop status epilepticus after ligation of a single extrahepatic shunt.
    b. Postoperative portal hypertension is evidenced by abdominal distention, abdominal pain, or bloody diarrhea.
    c. Animals with moderate portal hypertension following surgery should be treated by expanding the plasma volume with crystalloids and colloids.
    d. The degree of shunt ligation can be determined solely with intraoperative portal venous pressure measurements.
    e. Some affected animals are presented with signs of urinary tract obstruction.

15. *What is the **least** likely postoperative complication of bulla osteotomy through a lateral approach?*
    a. facial nerve paralysis
    b. Horner's syndrome
    c. keratoconjunctivitis sicca
    d. head tilt
    e. hypoglossal nerve damage

16. *Concerning ear surgery for chronic otitis externa, which statement is most accurate?*
    a. Bilateral total ear canal ablation always results in deafness.
    b. Total ear canal ablation is indicated when hypertrophy has produced stenosis of the horizontal canal.
    c. Bulla osteotomy should be avoided unless there is radiographic evidence of otitis media.
    d. Lateral ear resection may result in damage to the zygomatic salivary gland.
    e. Facial nerve paralysis is a complication of lateral ear resection.

Correct answers are on pages 260-275.

17. *Concerning skin grafts in dogs, which statement is **least** accurate?*

   a. Full-thickness grafts have better viability than split-thickness grafts.
   b. An advantage of mesh grafts is that they are flexible, so they can conform to uneven surfaces.
   c. An advantage of mesh grafts is that fluid can drain from beneath the graft.
   d. Split-thickness grafts are less durable and more susceptible to trauma than full-thickness grafts.
   e. Split-thickness grafts may result in an area with sparse hair growth.

18. *What is the primary treatment for acute elbow hygroma?*

   a. providing a well-padded area where the dog can lie
   b. aseptically draining the hygroma with a needle and syringe
   c. placing Penrose drains to allow passive drainage
   d. excision of the affected area
   e. oral corticosteroids and antibiotics

19. *Abnormalities of the upper airway syndrome in brachycephalic dogs include all the following **except:***

   a. stenotic nares
   b. everted laryngeal saccules
   c. elongated soft palate
   d. hypoplastic trachea
   e. tracheal collapse

20. *What is the most common malignant stomach tumor in dogs?*

   a. leiomyosarcoma
   b. squamous-cell carcinoma
   c. adenocarcinoma
   d. fibrosarcoma
   e. gastrinoma

21. *Concerning tracheal collapse, which statement is **least** accurate?*

   a. It is usually seen in toy or miniature dog breeds.
   b. Grade-I tracheal collapse is usually managed medically.
   c. The dorsal tracheal membrane may be plicated in treating dogs with good cartilage development.
   d. The surgical technique of choice is external ring prosthesis.
   e. The cervical portion of the trachea tends to collapse on expiration, whereas the intrathoracic portion of the trachea tends to collapse on inspiration.

22. *What is the preferred approach to repair most traumatic diaphragmatic hernias?*

   a. ventral midline celiotomy
   b. median sternotomy
   c. lateral thoracotomy
   d. transsternal thoracotomy
   e. paracostal abdominal incision

23. *Concerning cesarean section, which statement is most accurate?*

   a. The flank approach is best because it avoids the enlarged mammary glands.
   b. If a placenta is not expelled with each puppy, the uterine horn should be incised to remove any unexpelled placentas.
   c. After surgery, the bitch should remain hospitalized with the puppies overnight to observe for depression, shock, or excessive bleeding.
   d. Avoid performing an en bloc ovariohysterectomy because it entails a longer surgery time than a standard cesarean section.
   e. The hysterotomy incision should be made in the uterine body.

24. *Castration can be used in treatment or prevention of all the following disorders* ***except:***
    a. perianal fistula
    b. perianal adenoma
    c. perineal hernia
    d. benign prostatic hyperplasia
    e. chronic prostatitis

25. *Concerning prostatic neoplasia, which statement is* ***least*** *accurate?*
    a. Both intact and castrated male dogs are at risk.
    b. An affected prostate gland may be enlarged, asymmetric, and painful.
    c. Bacterial prostatitis may occur secondary to prostatic neoplasia.
    d. Transitional-cell carcinoma is the most common prostatic neoplasm.
    e. Metastatic lesions may develop in the pelvis and lumbar vertebrae.

26. *What is the best way to diagnose ectopic ureter?*
    a. clinical signs
    b. positive-contrast urethrogram
    c. positive-contrast cystogram
    d. double-contrast cystogram
    e. excretory urogram

27. *What is the best treatment for a dog with unilateral extramural ectopic ureter that empties into the vagina?*
    a. neoureterocystostomy
    b. ureteral transplantation
    c. nephroureterectomy
    d. ureterotomy
    e. ureteral anastomosis

28. *What is the preferred site for urethrostomy in male dogs?*
    a. prescrotal
    b. scrotal
    c. perineal
    d. antepubic
    e. prepubic

29. *Concerning indwelling urinary catheters, which statement is most accurate?*
    a. They are generally indicated after perineal urethrostomy to prevent stricture formation.
    b. They should be used in conjunction with antibiotics to prevent ascending urinary tract infection.
    c. They can be maintained with a closed collection system to prevent ascending urinary tract infection.
    d. They may be preferable to repeated catheterization in some patients.
    e. They should be placed using the largest-diameter catheter that the urethra can accommodate.

30. *Where is osteochondritis dissecans* ***least*** *likely to occur?*
    a. caudal aspect of the humeral head
    b. medial trochlea of the humeral condyle
    c. medial aspect of the lateral femoral condyle
    d. medial trochlear ridge of the talus
    e. lateral trochlea of the humeral condyle

31. *Concerning fragmented medial coronoid process, which statement is most accurate?*
    a. It is readily identified on a flexed lateral view of the elbow.
    b. It may be induced to resorb with physical therapy or exercise.
    c. It is rarely bilateral.
    d. It is best treated by resection, using a medial approach to the elbow.
    e. It is more common in females than in males.

32. *What is the earliest age at which ununited anconeal process can be diagnosed?*
    a. 6 weeks
    b. 12 weeks
    c. 24 weeks
    d. 28 weeks
    e. 32 weeks

Correct answers are on pages 260-275.

33. *Hypertrophic osteodystrophy is characterized by:*

a. lameness and pain on palpation of the diaphyseal region of long bones
b. unilateral angular deformity of the antebrachium
c. metaphyseal swelling, with pain, fever, and anorexia
d. nonpainful swelling of the metaphyseal region of long bones
e. radiographic changes of the long bones and primary neoplasia in the thoracic cavity

34. *An 8-month-old St. Bernard has hind limb lameness with mild muscle atrophy, hip pain, and a positive Ortolani sign. There is no radiographic evidence of degenerative joint disease. Which treatment is most appropriate at this time?*

a. femoral head and neck ostectomy
b. triple pelvic osteotomy
c. total hip replacement
d. limited activity, with administration of antiinflammatories and chondroprotectives
e. pectineomyotomy

35. *Concerning avascular necrosis of the femoral head, which statement is most accurate?*

a. It usually occurs bilaterally.
b. It is more common in males than in females.
c. It occurs most often in young, large-breed dogs.
d. It is best treated by total hip replacement.
e. It may be heritable.

36. *Which procedure is most appropriate for deepening the trochlear groove in a 7-year-old dog with medial patellar luxation?*

a. trochlear imbrication
b. trochlear chondroplasty
c. tibial tuberosity transposition
d. trochlear wedge resection
e. tibial wedge resection

37. *Concerning mandibular fractures, which statement is **least** accurate?*

a. Restoring normal occlusion is more important than perfect reduction of the fracture fragments.
b. Almost all mandibular fractures are open and contaminated.
c. Mandibular fractures generally heal faster than long bone fractures.
d. Chronic osteomyelitis is a common complication.
e. One objective of repair is early return of jaw function.

38. *Concerning traumatic elbow luxation, which statement is most accurate?*

a. In affected dogs the radius and ulna luxate laterally with respect to the humerus.
b. In affected dogs the antebrachium is carried in internal rotation.
c. Radiographs are not necessary in most cases.
d. Closed reduction provides poor results in most acute cases.
e. After surgical or nonsurgical reduction, the limb should be placed in a Velpeau sling.

39. *In a golden retriever with pelvic trauma, which injuries could be treated conservatively, with good results?*

a. bilateral ischial and pubic fractures, with a minimally displaced right sacroiliac joint luxation
b. unilateral ischial and pubic fractures, with ipsilateral sacroiliac luxation and medial displacement of the ilial shaft
c. bilateral sacroiliac luxations, with minimal displacement and no fractures
d. unilateral ischial and pubic fractures, with an ipsilateral, minimally displaced mid-acetabular fracture
e. unilateral ischial and pubic fractures, with a contralateral, minimally displaced ilial shaft fracture

40. *After reduction of hip luxation, the limb should be maintained in:*
    a. a Velpeau sling
    b. an Ehmer sling
    c. a Robinson sling
    d. a 90-90 flexion sling
    e. a spica splint

41. *Concerning cranial cruciate ligament rupture, which statement is **least** accurate?*
    a. It is usually not associated with major trauma.
    b. Affected dogs are at risk for developing the same problem in the other stifle.
    c. It is often associated with tearing of the lateral meniscus.
    d. Intracapsular or extracapsular techniques may be used to stabilize the joint.
    e. There may be minimal drawer movement in a stifle with partial or chronic cruciate ligament rupture.

42. *A Schroeder-Thomas splint is most appropriate for immobilizing:*
    a. a closed, mid-shaft femoral fracture
    b. an open, mid-shaft humeral fracture
    c. a nondisplaced, distal radial fracture in a toy-breed dog
    d. a closed, oblique tibial fracture in a Labrador retriever puppy
    e. a mandibular fracture

43. *What is the best treatment for a 3-year-old Irish setter with a two-piece, transverse, mid-diaphyseal femoral fracture?*
    a. bone plate
    b. intramedullary pin alone
    c. intramedullary pin and cerclage wire
    d. Schroeder-Thomas splint
    e. external fixator

44. *A 5-month-old puppy is hit by a car and sustains a mid-shaft fracture of the radius. If the dog were to develop an angular limb deformity subsequent to this trauma, what type of deformity is most likely to develop?*
    a. valgus, cranial bowing, and external rotation of the antebrachium because of premature closure of the distal ulnar physis
    b. malarticulation of the elbow joint and limb shortening because of premature closure of the proximal radial physis
    c. valgus and external rotation of the antebrachium because of asymmetric premature closure of the distal radial physis
    d. varus, cranial bowing, and external rotation of the antebrachium because of premature closure of the distal ulnar physis
    e. varus, caudal bowing, and internal rotation of the antebrachium because of premature closure of the proximal ulnar physis

45. *Concerning congenital atlantoaxial luxation, which statement is most accurate?*
    a. It is diagnosed by a lateral radiographic view with the neck in extreme flexion.
    b. It has no breed or gender predisposition.
    c. It may be treated conservatively in dogs with minimal signs, but recurrence is common.
    d. It is usually initiated by moderate to severe trauma.
    e. It may result in tetraparalysis.

46. *Which lesion is **not** associated with "wobbler syndrome"?*
    a. cervical vertebral malformations that cause constant pressure on the cervical spinal cord
    b. spinal cord compression from vertebral malalignment
    c. intermittent spinal cord compression from hypertrophy of the ligamentum flavum
    d. spinal cord compression from intervertebral disk herniation
    e. intermittent spinal cord compression from hypertrophy of the ventral longitudinal ligament

Correct answers are on pages 260-275.

47. *Concerning treatment of a dog with neck pain caused by a ruptured cervical intervertebral disk, which statement is most accurate?*
   a. Surgery should be performed at the first episode of neck pain, before the signs deteriorate.
   b. Surgery should not be performed unless the dog becomes ataxic.
   c. Surgery should not be performed unless the dog loses voluntary motor function.
   d. Surgery should not be performed unless the dog loses deep pain sensation.
   e. Surgery should be performed if the neck pain does not respond to conservative management.

Questions 48 and 49

A 5-year-old male dachshund is presented with sudden onset of hind limb paralysis. Neurologic examination reveals normal cranial nerves and mentation, normal front leg reflexes and motor function, no voluntary motor activity in the hind limbs, normal to increased hind limb reflexes, and positive deep pain perception in the hind limbs.

48. *Based on the neurologic examination, in which spinal cord segment is the lesion most likely located?*
   a. C1-5
   b. C6-T2
   c. T10-L3
   d. T3-L3
   e. L4-S2

49. *What factor is most important in determining a prognosis in this case?*
   a. presence of deep pain in the hind limbs
   b. cranial nerve reflexes
   c. hind limb reflexes
   d. forelimb reflexes
   e. forelimb motor function

50. *Which of the following is most likely to be observed in a dog with an "upper motor neuron bladder"?*
   a. very easy expression of urine from the bladder
   b. constant dribbling of urine
   c. voluntary control of urination
   d. a lesion in spinal cord segment S1-3
   e. increased urethral sphincter tone

J.K. Roush

51. *Which suture pattern provides a continuous inverting closure of hollow organs and does* **not** *expose suture material to the organ lumen?*
   a. Connell
   b. Parker-Kerr
   c. Cushing
   d. vertical mattress
   e. Halsted

For Questions 52 through 56, select the correct answer from the five choices below.

   a. povidone-iodine
   b. chlorhexidine gluconate
   c. hexachlorophene
   d. isopropyl alcohol
   e. sodium hypochlorite

52. *A biguanide hand wash and surgical scrub whose antibacterial action is maintained in the presence of blood*

53. *Sporicidal as well as bactericidal*

54. *Kills bacteria by coagulation of proteins*

55. *Has excellent virucidal action when applied to environmental surfaces but can dissolve blood clots when applied to wounds*

56. *Its cumulative antibacterial action is nullified by alcohol*

Questions 57 through 59

A 6-month-old Rottweiler puppy is presented because of moderate weight-bearing lameness of the left front limb of 2 weeks' duration. There is no history of a traumatic incident. Physical examination findings include pain on flexion of the left elbow joint and effusion in the left elbow joint.

57. *The **least** likely cause of these signs is:*
   a. ununited anconeal process
   b. hypertrophic osteopathy
   c. elbow dysplasia
   d. osteochondrosis of the distal humerus
   e. fragmented medial coronoid process

58. *The diagnostic test most likely to result in definitive diagnosis of the underlying cause of this lameness is:*
   a. thoracic radiography
   b. elbow arthrocentesis
   c. complete blood count and serum chemistry panel
   d. lateral and craniocaudal radiographs of the elbow
   e. bone scintigraphy of the elbow

59. *If the diagnosis is ununited anconeal process, what is the most successful treatment for this disease?*
   a. reattachment of the anconeal process with a bone screw
   b. removal of the anconeal process
   c. cage rest and analgesics for 4 weeks
   d. replacement of the anconeal process with a cortical autograft
   e. reattachment of the anconeal process with cyanoacrylate bone glue

60. *In dogs, osteochondrosis has been reported to affect all the following **except** the:*
   a. temporomandibular joint
   b. coxofemoral joint
   c. vertebrae (spinous process)
   d. elbow joint
   e. scapulohumeral joint

61. *Where is osteochondrosis most commonly located in the stifle and tarsocrural joints of dogs?*
   a. lateral femoral condyle, medial malleolus of the tibia
   b. medial femoral condyle, medial trochlear ridge of the talus
   c. medial femoral condyle, lateral trochlear ridge of the talus
   d. lateral femoral condyle, lateral trochlear ridge of the talus
   e. lateral femoral condyle, medial trochlear ridge of the talus

62. *In dogs, which of the following is **not** a congenital malformation leading to medial patellar luxation?*
   a. lateral bowing of the femur
   b. medial placement of the tibial crest (tibial deformity)
   c. shallow trochlear groove
   d. coxa valga
   e. increased internal tibial rotation

63. *Persistent patellar luxation that **cannot** be manually reduced is classified as:*
   a. grade I
   b. grade II
   c. grade III
   d. grade IV
   e. grade V

64. *Which of the following is generally **not** successful in treatment of medial patellar luxation?*
   a. lateral retinaculum imbrication
   b. trochlear wedge resection
   c. trocheoplasty
   d. tibial crest transposition
   e. patellectomy

Correct answers are on pages 260-275.

65. *Principles of joint arthrodesis include all the following* ***except:***
    a. leaving the joint open postoperatively to drain excess joint fluid
    b. autogenous cancellous bone graft
    c. removal of remaining joint cartilage
    d. placement of the joint at a normal anatomic angle for arthrodesis
    e. rigid fixation across the joint

66. *Which of the following is* ***not*** *a common part of the history of dogs with cranial cruciate ligament rupture?*
    a. obese dogs
    b. injured while actively playing
    c. 8 months old
    d. overactive dog, always jumping and running
    e. large-breed dog

67. *Indications for surgical repair of pelvic fractures include all the following* ***except:***
    a. caudal acetabular fracture, with sciatic nerve entrapment
    b. multiple nondisplaced fractures of the pubis
    c. fractured ilium, with a medially displaced caudal fragment
    d. bilateral sacroiliac luxation
    e. acetabular fracture involving the dorsal acetabular

68. *Which of the following has proven* ***least*** *useful in palliative or definitive treatment of hip dysplasia in dogs?*
    a. total hip replacement
    b. oral ascorbic acid therapy
    c. intertrochanteric varus osteotomy
    d. triple pelvic osteotomy
    e. oral analgesic therapy

69. *A dog with craniodorsal luxation of the right coxofemoral joint may have all the following clinical signs* ***except:***
    a. right greater trochanter is displaced dorsally as compared with the left
    b. palpable crepitation on manipulation of the right hip joint
    c. left hind limb longer than the right when the hind limbs are fully extended
    d. examiner's thumb pushed out of sciatic notch during external femoral rotation ("thumb test")
    e. lameness of the right hind limb

70. *In dogs with avascular necrosis of the femoral head (Legg-Calvé-Perthes disease), the history commonly includes all the following* ***except:***
    a. toy or miniature breed
    b. 3 to 4 years old
    c. no history of trauma
    d. gradual onset with increasing lameness
    e. unilateral or bilateral

71. *In a growing dog, a distal femoral fracture in which the fracture line runs along the distal physis and exits through the distal metaphysis is classified as:*
    a. Salter I
    b. Salter II
    c. Salter III
    d. Salter IV
    e. Salter V

72. *All the following describe correct use of twisted cerclage wire in fracture fixation* ***except:***
    a. two or more full cerclage wires per fracture
    b. wire ends cut off between second and fourth full twists
    c. wire ends bent over
    d. care taken to form symmetric wire twist
    e. ideal fracture configuration is long oblique (obliquity at least two times bone diameter

73. *All the following are successful treatments for coxofemoral luxation* ***except:***
    a. caudal and distal transposition of the greater trochanter
    b. extracapsular suture stabilization
    c. capsulorraphy
    d. transarticular pin fixation
    e. primary suture repair of ligamentum teres

74. *Structures encountered during a medial approach to the mid-shaft tibia include all the following* ***except:***

 a. long digital extensor muscle
 b. medial saphenous vein
 c. superficial peroneal artery
 d. medial saphenous artery
 e. popliteus muscle

75. *Correct positioning of the hind limb to avoid iatrogenic sciatic nerve injury during retrograde intramedullary pinning of the femur is with the:*

 a. coxofemoral joint extended, hind limb abducted
 b. coxofemoral joint flexed, hind limb abducted
 c. coxofemoral joint flexed, hind limb externally rotated
 d. coxofemoral joint extended, hind limb adducted

Questions 76 through 79

A 6-year-old intact male dachshund is presented 6 hours after acute onset of hind limb paresis. The dog had not been observed during the 2 hours before the onset of clinical signs, and the recent history is unknown. The dog is now quadriplegic. Your neurologic examination shows bilaterally hyperreflexive patellar and withdrawal reflexes and hyporeflexive biceps and triceps reflexes. Proprioception is absent in all four limbs. Deep pain is present in all four limbs. Cranial nerve responses are normal.

76. *In what segment of the spinal cord is the lesion most likely located:*

 a. coccygeal (Cy1-10)
 b. lumbosacral (L4-S3)
 c. thoracolumbar (T3-L3)
 d. cervicothoracic (C6-T2)
 e. cervical (C1-5)

77. *Likely differential diagnosis for this dog's neurologic signs include all the following* ***except:***

 a. intervertebral disk rupture
 b. intradural spinal neoplasm
 c. vertebral body fracture
 d. fibrocartilaginous spinal embolism
 e. traumatic vertebral subluxation/luxation

78. *Diagnostic tests that may aid definitive diagnosis of these conditions include all the following* ***except:***

 a. survey radiography of the affected area
 b. myelography
 c. magnetic resonance imaging
 d. computed tomography
 e. spinal ultrasonography

79. *If intervertebral disk rupture at C6-7 is diagnosed in this dog, which of the following is an appropriate surgical therapy?*

 a. right hemilaminectomy
 b. left hemilaminectomy
 c. ventral slot decompression
 d. C6-7 stabilization and arthrodesis
 e. cage rest and corticosteroid therapy

80. *In dogs, which intervertebral disk is* ***least*** *likely to rupture?*

 a. C3-4 (cervical region)
 b. L1-2 (cranial lumbar region)
 c. T12-13 (thoracolumbar region)
 d. T4-5 (thoracic region)
 e. L3-4 (caudal lumbar region)

81. *You are presented with a 10-year-old Labrador retriever with a noncomminuted, closed, transverse fracture of the midshaft femur. Which fracture fixation method would provide the* ***least*** *stable fixation?*

 a. single intramedullary pin
 b. type-I, double-bar external fixator
 c. dynamic compression plate
 d. single intramedullary pin combined with a type-I, single-bar external fixator
 e. multiple (stacked) intramedullary pins

82. *Which of the following is* ***not*** *a general goal of modern internal fracture fixation?*

 a. rigid internal fixation
 b. anatomic fracture reduction
 c. early return of limb function
 d. immobilization of the joints proximal and distal to the fractured bone
 e. aseptic/atraumatic surgical technique

Correct answers are on pages 260-275.

For Questions 83 through 87 select the correct answer from the five choices below.

a. polyglycolic acid
b. polypropylene
c. stainless steel
d. nylon
e. polyglyconate

83. *Nonabsorbable suture material with minimal thrombogenic effects*

84. *Strongest absorbable suture material at implantation*

85. *Nonabsorbable suture material with antibacterial degradation products*

86. *Strongest available suture material*

87. *Absorbable suture material that should not be exposed to the bladder lumen*

88. *All the following are appropriate for treatment of cranial cruciate rupture in a 40-kg Rottweiler* ***except:***

a. "under and over" fascial strip
b. "over the top" fascial strip
c. fibular head transposition
d. imbrication with extracapsular stainless-steel sutures
e. 6 weeks of cage rest

89. *The strongest type of gastropexy used as treatment of gastric dilation-volvulus in dogs is:*

a. circumcostal gastropexy
b. tube gastrostomy
c. belt-loop gastropexy
d. gastrocolopexy
e. gastropexy with scarification of the peritoneum

90. *All the following are accepted general principles of surgical drain placement* ***except:***

a. aseptic drain placement with drain maintained under sterile bandages
b. drains should not exit through incision lines
c. increasing the number of drain lumina decreases wound drainage
d. fewest drains possible placed through the least number of holes
e. drains should be removed when drainage becomes negligible

91. *To serve as universal donors, dogs maintained as on-site blood donors should be* ***negative*** *for which blood allele?*

a. DEA 1
b. DEA 3
c. DEA 4
d. DEA 6
e. DEA 7

92. *All the following are accepted principles of emergency treatment of an open fracture of the midshaft tibia of 24 hours' duration* ***except:***

a. débride immediately and lavage copiously
b. culture before and/or after débridement
c. leave would open and bandage aseptically
d. give broad-spectrum antibiotics before culture and then switch to one effective against isolate organisms
e. apply immediate rigid fixation

93. *The most stable configuration of an external fixation device is:*

a. type I, single bar (unilateral)
b. type I, double bar (unilateral)
c. type II (bilateral, uniplanar)
d. type III (bilateral, biplanar)
e. quadrilateral (unilateral, biplanar)

94. *Which muscle is the only member of the quadriceps group to originate on the ilium?*

a. semitendinosus
b. rectus femoris
c. vastus medialis
d. vastus intermedius
e. vastus lateralis

95. *Which of the following approaches to the elbow is appropriate for repair of a comminuted Y fracture of the distal humerus in a 6-year-old cocker spaniel?*

   a. lateral approach to the lateral humeral epicondyle
   b. olecranon osteotomy (caudal approach to the elbow)
   c. triceps tenotomy (caudal approach to the elbow)
   d. medial approach to the medial humeral epicondyle
   e. caudolateral approach to the elbow joint

96. *You are presented with a 5-year-old Labrador retriever with acute swelling and joint effusion of the right carpus. Radiographs show minimal degenerative changes of the right carpus and soft tissue swelling surrounding the radiocarpal joint. Arthrocentesis and fluid evaluation of the right carpus show the following results: total cell count 150,000 cells/μl, 90% segmented neutrophils, 10% monocytes, mucin clot friable. What is the most likely cause of these findings?*

   a. traumatic arthritis
   b. degenerative arthritis
   c. septic arthritis
   d. systemic lupus erythematosus
   e. rheumatoid arthritis

97. *Which developmental bone disease is confirmed by radiographic findings of a radiolucent linear lesion parallel to the physis of affected bones?*

   a. panosteitis
   b. craniomandibular osteopathy
   c. osteochondrosis
   d. hypertrophic osteodystrophy
   e. retained enchondral bone core

98. *What is an isograft:*

   a. a graft in which the donor tissue is of the same organ type as the recipient site
   b. graft in which the donor and recipient are individuals of different species
   c. graft in which donor and recipient are genetically unrelated individuals of the same species
   d. graft in which tissue is transferred to a new position on the same individual
   e. graft in which donor and recipient are different individuals but genetically identical

99. *Which statement best describes the term osteoconduction as it refers to bone grafting?*

   a. Living cells within the graft and recipient bed are induced to differentiate and produce bone by a stimulatory factor from the graft.
   b. The bone graft acts as a scaffold and is incorporated by creeping substitution.
   c. New bone is deposited by viable osteocyte precursors within the graft.
   d. The bone graft is revascularized through inosculation (growth of new vessels into former existing vessel lumina).
   e. Bone morphogenic protein acts to increase osteoclast resorption and stimulates bone production by osteoblasts.

100. *Concerning limb amputation in dogs, which statement is **least** accurate?*

   a. Hind limb amputation is best accomplished by coxofemoral disarticulation for optimal postoperative cosmetic results.
   b. Forequarter amputation is the preferred method for front limb amputation.
   c. Mid-femoral amputation is adequate for lesions distal to the stifle.
   d. Forelimb amputation by scapulohumeral disarticulation results in a less favorable cosmetic appearance because of scapular muscle atrophy.
   e. Forelimb amputation by mid-humeral osteotomy produces acceptable results.

Correct answers are on pages 260-275.

CATS

R.M. Bright

101. *Which antimicrobial is most effective for chemoprophylaxis in a cat undergoing colotomy?*
   a. trimethoprim-sulfa
   b. penicillin
   c. tetracycline
   d. clindamycin
   e. second-generation cephalosporin

102. *The most common type of dehydration that must be corrected before any surgical procedure is:*
   a. hypotonic dehydration (low serum sodium)
   b. isotonic dehydration (normal serum sodium)
   c. Addison-type dehydration (high potassium, low sodium)
   d. isotonic dehydration with hypokalemia
   e. hypertonic dehydration with hypernatremia

103. *In cats, chronic vomiting associated with pyloric outflow obstruction is likely to cause:*
   a. metabolic alkalosis with hyperkalemia and normochloremia
   b. metabolic alkalosis with hypokalemia and hypochloremia
   c. metabolic acidosis with hyperkalemia and normochloremia
   d. metabolic acidosis with hypokalemia and hypochloremia
   e. respiratory acidosis with compensatory metabolic alkalosis

104. *The fluid of choice for correcting dehydration and metabolic alkalosis before surgical treatment of pyloric stenosis is:*
   a. lactated Ringer's solution
   b. 0.9% saline
   c. hypertonic (7%) saline
   d. 5% dextrose
   e. 10% dextrose

105. *The most common electrolyte disturbance seen in cats after bilateral thyroidectomy is:*
   a. hypokalemia from the aggressive fluid therapy necessary in these cats
   b. hypocalcemia
   c. hypercalcemia
   d. hyperkalemia
   e. hypernatremia

106. *The surgical approach for closure of a patent ductus arteriosus is via:*
   a. the left fourth intercostal space
   b. the left seventh intercostal space
   c. the right fourth intercostal space
   d. median sternotomy
   e. transsternal thoracotomy

107. *Which of the following is* ***not*** *an indication for emergency repair of a diaphragmatic hernia (herniorrhaphy)?*
   a. hemopneumothorax
   b. incarcerated intestine within the rent
   c. severe respiratory failure from viscera encroaching on the lungs
   d. stomach entrapment within the thorax, with enlarging gas accumulation
   e. persistent cyanosis despite oxygen and fluid therapy

108. *In treatment of chronic frontal sinusitis in cats, the frontal sinuses can be obliterated using:*
   a. a cancellous bone graft
   b. a fat graft implant
   c. a musculocutaneous graft
   d. temporalis muscle (free graft)
   e. synthetic mesh (polypropylene)

109. *What is the most likely source of intrathoracic hemorrhage following median sternotomy?*
   a. the internal thoracic artery
   b. the bronchoesophageal artery
   c. the intercostal arteries
   d. the marrow of split sternebrae
   e. the subclavian artery

110. *To facilitate removal of the left caudal lung lobe, which structure attaching the lung lobe to the mediastinal pleura should be severed?*
   a. hilar-mediastinal band
   b. diaphragmatic tendon
   c. pulmonary ligament
   d. sternopericardial ligament
   e. pneumopericardial ligament

111. *Lymphangiography to diagnose chylothorax is best performed by placing a catheter in a mesenteric lymphatic via:*
   a. the right ninth intercostal space
   b. the left ninth intercostal space
   c. a midline ventral abdominal incision
   d. a right paracostal incision
   e. a left paracostal incision

112. *Thoracic duct leakage of chyle into the pleural cavity is thought to be most often related to:*
   a. thymoma
   b. lung lobe torsion
   c. cardiomyopathy
   d. thoracic duct obstruction/lymphangiectasia
   e. thoracic duct tear secondary to trauma

113. *In cats, one of the most severe postoperative complications associated with repair of a chronic diaphragmatic hernia is:*
   a. liver failure
   b. renal infarcts
   c. atrial fibrillation
   d. pulmonary edema
   e. hemorrhage from the diaphragmatic wound

114. *The structure that can be used in lieu of a synthetic mesh implant to repair caudal thoracic wall defects following en bloc resection of tumors is:*
   a. the pericardium made into an advancement flap
   b. the diaphragm used as an advancement flap
   c. an intercostal muscle flap
   d. a bone allograft
   e. the rhomboideus muscle belly

115. *The agent of choice for anesthetic induction and maintenance of cats undergoing surgery for correction of a portosystemic shunt is:*
   a. methoxyflurane
   b. halothane
   c. ether
   d. thiamylal sodium
   e. isoflurane

116. *What muscle is associated with laryngeal paralysis secondary to trauma of the recurrent laryngeal nerve during thyroidectomy?*
   a. thyropharyngeal
   b. cricothyroideus dorsalis
   c. arytenoideus ventralis
   d. cricoarytenoideus dorsalis
   e. intrinsic adductor muscles of the larynx

117. *The most medially located muscle that is separated bluntly on ventral approach to the trachea is the:*
   a. sternothyroideus
   b. sternohyoideus
   c. sternocephalicus
   d. cleidomastoideus
   e. thyrohyoideus

Correct answers are on pages 260-275.

118. *Which of the following is most likely to contribute to postoperative aspiration pneumonia in a cat subjected to surgery for correction of severe pyloric outflow disease caused by a benign or neoplastic tumor?*

a. concurrent megaesophagus caused by vagal nerve involvement by the tumor
b. gastric retention of fluids
c. dysphagia
d. impingement on the diaphragm by the distended stomach
e. postoperative use of a vagolytic agent

119. *In cats, megacolon is most commonly associated with:*

a. an extraluminal mass, such as adenocarcinoma
b. an intraluminal mass, such as a foreign body
c. unknown factors
d. lumbosacral trauma
e. pelvic fractures

120. *In cats, oral surgery is done primarily to treat which type of tumor?*

a. fibrosarcoma
b. osteosarcoma
c. lymphosarcoma
d. squamous-cell carcinoma
e. malignant melanoma

121. *A foreign body lodged in the thoracic esophagus between intercostal spaces 2 and 3 is best approached via:*

a. the right sixth intercostal space
b. the left fourth intercostal space
c. the right second or third intercostal space
d. the left second or third intercostal space
e. median sternotomy

122. *An oronasal defect created by partial maxillectomy is most often repaired/closed with a:*

a. lingual-facial rotating flap
b. buccal flap
c. hard palate rotating flap
d. free graft with microvascular technique
e. bilateral hard palate mucosal overlay

123. *In hemimandibulectomy for treatment of oral neoplasia, where is the mandibular artery encountered and ligated?*

a. lateral aspect of the temporomandibular joint
b. on the buccal mucosa just caudal to the third premolar
c. between the mylohyoid and geniohyoid muscles
d. as it enters the medial aspect of the caudal end of the mandible
e. on the lateral aspect of the digastricus muscle, running parallel with the mandible

124. *If a squamous-cell carcinoma involves the middle segment of the mandible but has not metastasized to the lungs or lymph nodes, what is the most appropriate surgical procedure to decrease the chances of tumor recurrence?*

a. bilateral rostral mandibulectomy
b. hemimandibulectomy
c. segmental mandibulectomy with a cortical bone graft
d. complete mandibulectomy
e. excision of the mass, limited to soft tissue structures overlying the hemimandible

125. *In a cat with suspected esophageal foreign body, a contrast esophagogram also reveals contrast material in the trachea. Preoperative planning for treatment of this cat should consider the possibility of encountering:*

a. an esophagotracheal fistula
b. pneumomediastinum
c. mediastinitis
d. an oronasal fistula
e. stricture of the esophagus

126. *What is the most likely cause of regurgitation in a cat 4 to 8 weeks after ovariohysterectomy?*
   a. megaesophagus caused by the residual effects of preanesthetic drugs
   b. megaesophagus caused by transient generalized esophageal hypomotility
   c. esophageal stricture secondary to reflux esophagitis
   d. dysautonomia caused by a vagal nerve disorder
   e. hypersensitivity to the food given at home because it is different from that given in the hospital

127. *The layer of the esophagus that is the most likely to retain sutures is the:*
   a. surrounding adventitia
   b. mucosa
   c. submucosa
   d. smooth muscle layer
   e. skeletal muscle

128. *As seen through the right third intercostal space at thoracotomy, the large blood-filled structure running transversely over the esophagus is the:*
   a. confluence of the external and internal jugular veins
   b. major deep thoracic artery branching from the bronchoesophageal artery
   c. azygos vein
   d. left subclavian vein
   e. thymus vein, seen only in cats under 1 year of age

129. *A surgical technique designed to correct spraying or inappropriate urination in cats is:*
   a. perineal urethrostomy
   b. scrotal urethrostomy
   c. transection of the ischiourethralis musculature
   d. ischiocavernosus myectomy
   e. muscle sling technique to reposition the course of the penile urethra

130. *During laparotomy in an icteric cat from Florida, you find extensive scar tissue around the bile ducts. The most likely cause of this scar tissue is:*
   a. toxoplasmosis
   b. liver fluke *(Platynosomum)*
   c. hepatic amyloidosis
   d. hepatic lipidosis
   e. portosystemic shunt with secondary biliary lithiasis

131. *In cats, granulomatous masses found during surgical exploration of the nasal cavity are most likely associated with:*
   a. histoplasmosis
   b. cryptococcosis
   c. blastomycosis
   d. coccidioidomycosis
   e. aspergillosis

132. *A unilateral chain mastectomy includes removal of which lymph node lying dorsal to the fifth mammary gland?*
   a. pudendal
   b. superficial perineal
   c. inguinal
   d. pudendoepigastric
   e. popliteal

133. *The paired artery and vein that must be located, isolate, ligated, and transected during removal of the fifth mammary gland in cats is the:*
   a. caudal superficial epigastric
   b. pudendoepigastric
   c. caudal deep epigastric
   d. inguinal
   e. external pudendal

134. *A surgical incision into the respiratory tract is classified as:*
   a. clean
   b. clean-contaminated
   c. contaminated
   d. dirty
   e. purulent

Correct answers are on pages 260-275.

135. *During exploration of the nasal cavity, the turbinate structures located most caudal and contiguous with the cribriform plate are the:*

a. maxilloturbinates
b. ethmoturbinates
c. cribroturbinates
d. septoturbinates
e. sinonasal turbinates

136. *A common postoperative complication of rhinotomy in cats is:*

a. weakness of the rear quarters
b. pyothorax
c. subcutaneous emphysema
d. pneumothorax
e. Horner's syndrome

137. *Although rare, which pleural-related problem may be associated with rhinotomy in cats?*

a. hydrothorax
b. pneumothorax
c. chylothorax
d. pyothorax
e. pleuritis

138. *In nasopharyngeal polyps involve the osseous bullae, which surgical treatment is recommended?*

a. soft palate splitting and traction on the pharyngeal component
b. bulla osteotomy via a lateral approach
c. bulla osteotomy following total ear ablation
d. ventral bulla osteotomy
e. intraoral approach to each bulla

139. *Surgical management of laryngeal paralysis in cats includes:*

a. ventriculocordectomy and arytenoidopexy via a ventral approach
b. bilateral arytenoidopexy
c. partial laryngectomy and vocal fold removal
d. bilateral "tie-back" procedure
e. vocal cord removal and partial amputation of the epiglottis

140. *A traumatic tear of the cranial portion of the thoracic trachea is approached surgically via:*

a. a ventral midline caudal cervical approach, with cranial traction on the trachea
b. thoracotomy through the left third intercostal space
c. thoracotomy through the right third intercostal space
d. a transsternal approach between the third and fourth sternebrae
e. median sternotomy

141. *The most important complicated related to use of tracheostomy tubes in cats is:*

a. subcutaneous emphysema
b. pneumomediastinum
c. laryngeal paralysis caused by recurrent laryngeal nerve entrapment
d. obstruction of the tube with mucus
e. serous drainage from the skin wound

142. *Tracheal stenosis secondary to anastomosis of two tracheal segments is most often caused by:*

a. poor perfusion of the tracheal segments
b. tension across the suture line
c. use of nonabsorbable sutures
d. bacteria in the lumen of the trachea
e. sutures placed too far apart

143. *The tracheostomy incision* ***least*** *likely to result in tracheal stricture is:*

a. longitudinal paramedian incision involving six tracheal rings
b. longitudinal midline incision involving six tracheal rings
c. transverse incision between tracheal rings 4 and 5
d. longitudinal paramedian incision involving tracheal rings 3 through 6
e. midline incision creating a triangular opening

144. A thoracic wall chondrosarcoma is best treated surgically by:

a. "fillet" excision of the mass to the level of the rib cage
b. resection of the mass and associated rib
c. en bloc excision involving one rib cranial and one rib caudal to the extent of the mass
d. wide en bloc excision involving a minimum of four ribs
e. electrosurgical resection, followed by cryosurgery

145. Thoracic wall defects repaired with a mesh implant sometimes do not have enough muscle to overlay the mesh and fill the defect. Which technique can be used to fill the remaining defect?

a. diaphragmatic advancement flap
b. omental pedicle flap
c. rib rotation
d. ox fascia implant
e. rotational muscle flap using iliopsoas muscle

146. When using synthetic mesh to repair a thoracic wall defect, it is best to place it:

a. as an extrapleural single-layer onlay implant
b. as a double-layer onlay implant
c. intrapleurally, with the edges doubled over
d. between the layers of muscle adjacent to the defect
e. overlying the muscle and subcutaneous tissue initially used to close the defect

147. Correction of a salivary mucocele manifested as a cervical swelling requires removal of the:

a. parotid gland
b. lacrimal and parotid glands
c. monostomatic and polystomatic portions of the mandibular salivary gland
d. mandibular and parotid glands
e. sublingual and mandibular glands

148. Which salivary gland is most often associated with a salivary mucocele?

a. mandibular
b. sublingual
c. parotid
d. acromial
e. zygomatic

149. Which vessels serve as important landmarks for the skin incision used in the lateral approach to salivary-gland resection?

a. sublingual and submandibular arteries
b. parotid and maxillary veins
c. submaxillary and facial veins
d. maxillary and linguofacial veins
e. deep mandibular and superficial lacrimal veins

150. In what areas is a salivary mucocele likely to be manifested?

a. sublingual, pharyngeal, and cervical
b. cervical, subauricular, and intermandibular
c. retrobulbar, pharyngeal, and cervical
d. sublingual, cervical, and sublaryngeal
e. retrolaryngeal, retropharyngeal, and sublingual

151. A term used to describe a salivary mucocele located ventral to the tongue is:

a. linguoma
b. frenulocele
c. ranula
d. myoglossal cyst
e. thyroglossal duct cyst

152. Omental patching techniques used to reinforce primary suture lines have been described for use primarily in:

a. adrenalectomy
b. partial splenectomy
c. partial hepatectomy
d. enterotomy and end-to-end anastomosis
e. choleenterostomy

153. The portion of the gastrointestinal tract that is used as a serosal patch to reinforce primary closure of the bowel is the:

a. ileum
b. cecum
c. greater curvature of the stomach
d. jejunum
e. ascending colon

Correct answers are on pages 260-275.

154. *Intestinal malabsorption with diarrhea and malnutrition that may follow resection of a large portion of the small intestine is called the:*

a. Zollinger-Ellison syndrome
b. Branham reflex
c. steatorrhea complex
d. short-bowel syndrome
e. lymphangiectasia

155. *Removal of the ileocolic valve may result in malabsorption and diarrhea. This is most likely related to:*

a. bacterial overgrowth
b. disruption of lymphatic drainage
c. increased possibility of eosinophilic enteritis
d. decreased transit time of ingesta coursing through the small and large bowels
e. increased intestinal motility

156. *Two segments of esophagus can be anastomosed with a horizontal mattress suture pattern, which is:*

a. an everting suture pattern
b. an inverting suture pattern
c. an approximating suture pattern
d. a simple appositional suture pattern
e. a "crushing" suture pattern

157. *Cushing or Lembert sutures used to close a gastrotomy incision are an example of:*

a. an inverting suture pattern
b. an everting suture pattern
c. a simple continuous suture pattern
d. an approximating suture pattern
e. a "crushing" suture pattern

158. *A pancreatic mass and an ulcer involving the duodenum are most likely associated with:*

a. an insulinoma
b. the Zollinger-Ellison syndrome (gastrinoma)
c. an islet-cell tumor of the pancreas
d. a hepatoma
e. exocrine pancreatic insufficiency

159. *When doing some routine blood tests in a cat before surgery for resection of an intestinal mass in cats, you detect hypercalcemia. This finding is most likely related to:*

a. adenocarcinoma
b. leiomyosarcoma
c. lymphosarcoma
d. plasmacytoma
e. leiomyoma

160. *After resection of an intestinal adenocarcinoma, the average survival time is approximately:*

a. 4 to 6 months
b. 4 to 6 weeks
c. 1 year
d. 2 to 3 years
e. 1 week

161. *At exploratory laparotomy on a cat, you find an intestinal lesion that is both nodular and diffuse. This lesion is most likely:*

a. a leiomyosarcoma
b. an adenocarcinoma
c. a carcinoid
d. lymphosarcoma
e. an adenomatous polyp

162. *A cat with a complete mid-duodenal obstruction has frequent episodes of profuse vomiting. Before surgery to remove the obstruction, the cat should be treated to correct:*

a. respiratory acidosis with compensatory metabolic alkalemia
b. metabolic acidosis
c. metabolic alkalosis
d. respiratory alkalosis with compensatory metabolic acidemia
e. metabolic alkalosis with compensatory respiratory acidemia

163. *The muscle in the cervical region that is most often used to reinforce esophageal suture lines is the:*

a. sternobrachialis
b. sternocephalicus
c. cleidomastoideus
d. sternothyroideus
e. sternohyoideus

164. *Esophageal strictures caused by esophagitis following surgery or general anesthesia usually are located:*
   a. in the mid-cervical region
   b. in the mid-thoracic region
   c. just cranial to the diaphragm
   d. just caudal to the cricopharyngeal muscle (upper esophageal sphincter)
   e. at the thoracic inlet

165. *The most common vascular ring anomaly causing regurgitation in cats is:*
   a. aberrant left subclavian artery
   b. right subclavian artery originating from the aorta
   c. double aorta
   d. persistent right aortic arch
   e. right caudal vena cava

166. *Most hiatal hernias are:*
   a. axial-type sliding hernias
   b. related to gastroesophageal intussusceptions
   c. related to type-II esophageal hypoplasia
   d. strangulating hernias
   e. paraesophageal hernias

167. *Sometimes a fundoplication procedure is necessary to prevent gastroesophageal reflux associated with hiatal hernia. The fundoplication procedure recommended for use in cats is the:*
   a. Ellison 270-degree fundoplication
   b. Markhaun 180-degree fundoplication
   c. Leonardi fundoplication
   d. Nissen 360-degree fundoplication
   e. Boerma fundoplication

168. *The most common indication for gastrotomy in cats is:*
   a. gastric parasitism *(Physaloptera)*
   b. neoplasia
   c. gastric ulcers
   d. chronic hypertrophic pyloric gastropathy
   e. foreign bodies

169. *The most common sign related to pyloric stenosis in cats is:*
   a. ptyalism
   b. anorexia
   c. emesis
   d. abdominal pain
   e. hematemesis

170. *The surgical procedure that uses an antral flap to increase the diameter of the pyloric outflow tract is the:*
   a. Heineke-Mikulicz pyloroplasty
   b. Y-U pyloroplasty
   c. Fredet-Ramstedt pyloroplasty
   d. Finney pyloroplasty
   e. MacPherson submucosal resection/sliding flap technique

171. *The Gambee suture pattern used in intestinal surgery is:*
   a. everting
   b. continuous
   c. approximating
   d. inverting
   e. crushing

172. *Which set of criteria is used to assess the viability of small intestine involved in intussusception?*
   a. serosal texture, venous congestion, color
   b. color, arterial pulsations, venous congestion
   c. peristalsis, arterial pulsations, venous congestion
   d. decreased bowel contractility when occluding the portal vein (Bella-Wein reflex), serosal texture, venous congestion
   e. color, peristalsis, arterial pulsations

173. *The invaginated portion of the bowel in an intussusception is called the:*
   a. intussusceptum
   b. intussuscipiens
   c. inverted segment
   d. invaginatiens
   e. inaperistalicum

Correct answers are on pages 260-275.

174. The portion of the bowel most commonly involved in intussusception is the:

a. duodenocolic segment
b. distal jejunum
c. transverse/proximal colon
d. ileocolic valve area
e. duodenojejunal function

175. In cats, adenocarcinomas most often involve which portion of the gastrointestinal tract?

a. duodenum
b. ileum
c. jejunum
d. stomach
e. distal colon

176. The surgical procedure of choice for relieving chronic constipation associated with idiopathic megacolon is:

a. segmental colectomy
b. removal of a longitudinal strip of colon to decrease lumen diameter
c. multiple colotomy incisions
d. colopexy
e. subtotal colectomy

177. The microbes of most concern in colorectal surgery are:

a. gram-positive aerobes
b. gram-negative enterics
c. anaerobes and gram-positive aerobes
d. gram-negative enterics and anaerobes
e. anaerobes only

178. The antimicrobial of choice for perioperative use in colotomy is:

a. metronidazole
b. erythromycin
c. neomycin
d. second-generation cephalosporin
e. ampicillin

179. The most important postoperative complication related to liver biopsy or lobectomy is:

a. liver abscess
b. bile leakage peritonitis
c. vomiting
d. hemorrhage
e. arteriovenous fistula

180. In animals with a portosystemic shunt, the sign seen far more frequently in affected cats than in affected dogs is:

a. emesis
b. ascites
c. ptyalism
d. head pressing
e. diarrhea

181. Ascites during the early postoperative period following occlusion of a portosystemic shunt suggests:

a. right-sided heart failure
b. endotoxemia
c. peritonitis
d. hypoglobinemia
e. portal hypertension

182. When evaluating the portal vein for anomalous shunts to the systemic circulation, the surgeon should know that the vein normally contributing the most blood to portal flow is the:

a. caudal mesenteric vein
b. cranial mesenteric vein
c. gastric vein
d. splenic vein
e. pancreaticoduodenal vein

183. In normal cats, intraoperative portal vein pressure is approximately:

a. 8 to 10 cm H_2O
b. 20 to 40 cm H_2O
c. 8 to 10 mm Hg
d. 1 to 2 mm Hg
e. 3 to 5 mm Hg

184. As a preoperative measure, the blood ammonia level in cats with a portosystemic shunt is best reduced by:

a. periodic phlebotomy
b. administration of ammonium chloride
c. administration of sodium bicarbonate and lactulose
d. administration of penicillin G and feeding a low-protein diet
e. administration of lactulose and neomycin and feeding a low-protein diet

185. Which drug should be avoided preoperatively in a cat with ascites and encephalopathy associated with a portosystemic shunt?

a. injectable penicillin G
b. prednisolone
c. furosemide
d. lactulose
e. neomycin

186. The most important anatomic feature to be considered during partial or complete pancreatectomy is the:

a. major papilla
b. minor papilla
c. common bile duct
d. common blood supply with the duodenum
e. splenic vein draining the left lobe

187. One day after exploratory laparotomy, a cat develops acute abdominal pain localized to the cranial right quadrant of the abdominal cavity and vomiting. These signs are most likely related to:

a. pyelonephritis
b. hepatic hematoma
c. pancreatitis
d. intestinal volvulus
e. ileus

188. The cranial thyroid artery is the primary blood supply to each lobe of the thyroid gland. From which artery does this vessel arise on the left side?

a. internal carotid artery
b. common carotid artery
c. sternohyoideus artery
d. supracervical artery
e. ventral psoas artery

189. In cats the most serious complication following bilateral thyroidectomy is:

a. hypocalcemia
b. hyperkalemia
c. hemorrhage from the major arterial supply
d. hypercalcemia
e. laryngeal paralysis secondary to recurrent laryngeal nerve trauma

190. In cats the most important ***disadvantage*** *related to the intracapsular technique of thyroidectomy is:*

a. hypoparathyroidism and hypocalcemia
b. hemorrhage
c. recurrence of hyperthyroidism
d. recurrent laryngeal nerve damage
e. thrombosis of the cranial thyroid artery

191. Clinical signs of hypocalcemia that may develop following bilateral thyroidectomy usually occur within:

a. 30 minutes
b. 1 to 3 hours
c. 7 to 10 days
d. 24 to 72 hours
e. 3 weeks

192. Careless application of a tourniquet to the limb during onychectomy may result in:

a. ulnar neuropraxis
b. temporary radial nerve paralysis
c. permanent branchial nerve damage
d. permanent median nerve paralysis
e. severance of the ulnar nerve

193. Which nerve is most likely to become entrapped during surgery to repair a proximal femoral fracture or pelvic fracture?

a. obturator nerve
b. perineal nerve
c. internal pudendal nerve
d. external pudendal nerve
e. ischiatic nerve

Correct answers are on pages 260-275.

194. *Fibrosarcoma involving the scapula is best treated with:*

a. limb-sparing techniques, including resection of the tumor mass followed by cisplatin therapy
b. cisplatin injections into the major artery leading to the scapula
c. amputation of the limb
d. wide en bloc excision with 3-cm margins
e. en bloc excision and hyperthermia

195. *A cat develops ureteral obstruction after erroneous ureteral ligature during ovariohysterectomy. This cat is likely to lose 80% of the ipsilateral kidney's function within:*

a. 48 hours
b. 4 to 6 hours
c. 30 to 35 days
d. 1 week
e. 2 weeks

196. *How long (total time) can the renal artery be occluded during nephrolithotomy without damage to the kidney?*

a. 3 to 5 minutes
b. 20 to 25 minutes
c. 2 hours
d. 1 hour
e. 5 hours

197. *If the paired fan-shaped muscle covering the crus of the penis is not excised during perineal urethrostomy, urethral obstruction may recur. This muscle is the:*

a. retractor penis
b. rectococcygeus
c. sacrotuberous
d. bulbocavernosus
e. ischiocavernosus

198. *In male cats with complete urethral obstruction, the most common metabolic derangements that must be corrected before urethrostomy are:*

a. metabolic alkalosis, hyperkalemia, and azotemia
b. metabolic acidosis, hyperkalemia, and azotemia
c. metabolic acidosis, hyperkalemia, and azotemia
d. respiratory alkalosis, hyperkalemia, and hypernatremia
e. hypernatremia, metabolic acidosis, and hyperchloremia

199. *An inverting suture pattern suitable for closure of a cystotomy incision is the:*

a. Gambee
b. simple continuous
c. continuous mattress
d. Lembert
e. simple interrupted crushing

200. *During perineal urethrostomy, the most caudal extent of the pelvic urethra is located by finding the:*

a. corpus cavernosus muscle
b. prostate gland
c. ischiourethralis muscle
d. bulbourethral glands
e. bulbocavernosus muscle

201. *The most common and serious complication following perineal urethrostomy is:*

a. urethral stricture
b. urinary incontinence
c. fecal incontinence
d. rectal prolapse
e. urine scalding

202. *Extensive damage or stricture of the urethra is best treated definitively with:*

a. tube cystostomy
b. urine diversion via a Stamey prepubic catheter
c. urethral metal prosthesis
d. marsupialization of the bladder
e. antepubic urethrostomy

203. Vulvar bleeding persisting after 3 weeks postpartum is most likely associated with:

a. excessive use of oxytocin
b. endometritis
c. hyperestrogenism
d. subinvolution of placental sites
e. postpartum hypocalcemia

204. In cats, empiric antimicrobial therapy following ovariohysterectomy for pyometra should be directed against which commonly isolated organism?

a. *Staphylococcus aureus*
b. *Staphylococcus epidermidis*
c. *Streptococcus pyogenes*
d. *Escherichia coli*
e. *Pseudomonas aeruginosa*

205. Of the following antibacterials, which is the best choice for perioperative use in a cat with pyometra?

a. erythromycin
b. metronidazole
c. tetracycline
d. cefoxitin
e. clindamycin

206. Unilateral ablation of the ear canal is most often performed in treatment of:

a. end-stage otitis externa
b. middle-ear infection
c. neoplasia
d. chronic yeast infection
e. traumatic avulsion of the base of the ear

207. When incised, which tunic differentiates a "closed" castration from an "open" castration?

a. visceral vaginal tunic
b. double vaginal tunic
c. spermatic tunic
d. parietal vaginal tunic
e. parietal testicular tunic

208. Which of the following is most helpful in determining if a male cat is bilaterally cryptorchid and still producing androgenic hormones?

a. urine spraying behavior
b. territorial behavior
c. presence of fully developed spines on the penis
d. no history of urethral obstruction
e. prominent retractor penis muscle on palpation

209. Following vasectomy, a tomcat may have viable sperm in its ejaculate for up to:

a. 50 days
b. 15 days
c. 3 days
d. 6 months
e. 1 year

210. Which ligament of the female reproductive tract courses caudally along the free edge of the mesometrium and through the inguinal canal and, when broken down, allows better exteriorization of the uterine body during ovariohysterectomy?

a. suspensor ligament
b. proper ligament
c. uteroovarian ligament
d. round ligament
e. broad ligament

211. If a prolapsed uterus is corrected via laparotomy and the owner wishes the cat to remain intact for breeding purposes, the most appropriate course of action is to:

a. perform a unilateral hysterectomy to decrease uterine volume so prolapse is less likely to recur
b. perform a unilateral ovariohysterectomy
c. perform a hysterocolopexy
d. suture the uterine body or each uterine horn to the lateral body wall
e. place pursestring sutures (nonabsorbable) in the vaginal vault via episiotomy

Correct answers are on pages 260-275.

212. *Which surgical procedure is designed to enlarge the vulvar opening?*

a. hysterotomy
b. vaginotomy
c. episiotomy
d. celiotomy
e. stomostomy

213. *The surgical procedure of choice for treatment of a mammary tumor present in one gland is:*

a. simple mastectomy, with removal of lymph nodes nearest the affected gland
b. resection of the tumor mass only (lumpectomy)
c. regional mastectomy
d. ovariohysterectomy
e. ipsilateral chain mastectomy, with regional lymph node removal

214. *Which four components form the "module of wound repair"?*

a. tissue macrophage, lymphocyte, monocyte, and granulocyte
b. tissue macrophage, fibroblast, granulocyte, and capillary bud
c. capillary bud, tissue macrophage, plasmacyte, and granulocyte
d. tissue macrophage, capillary bud, prostaglandins, and granulocyte
e. leukotrienes, prostaglandins, serotonin, and histamine

215. *The cell that directs events in early would repair, such as fibroplasia and angiogenesis, is the:*

a. small lymphocyte
b. granulocyte
c. macrophage
d. plasma cell
e. fibroblast

216. *The specialized cells responsible for wound contraction are the:*

a. fibrilloblasts
b. macrophages
c. myofibroblasts
d. monofibroblasts
e. chondrofibroblasts

217. *Stretching and thinning of the skin surrounding a contracted wound are called:*

a. bolstered growth
b. epithelial migration
c. intussusceptive growth
d. collagenolysis
e. epidermolytic migration

218. *The mineral sometimes given to help mobilize vitamin A from the liver in an effort to stimulate wound epithelialization following corticosteroid therapy is:*

a. magnesium
b. copper
c. zinc
d. calcium
e. manganese

219. *A pedicle graft that incorporates a direct cutaneous artery and vein is the:*

a. circular flap graft
b. random pedicle flap
c. direct cutaneous flap
d. rotating flap
e. axial-pattern flap

220. *An example of a compound or composite flap for reconstructive surgery is the:*

a. axial-pattern flap
b. myocutanous flap
c. sliding H-pattern flap
d. random-pattern flap
e. thoracic pouch flap

D.L. Millis

221. *Which structures run through the supracondylar foramen and should be avoided when repairing a fracture of the distal humerus in cats?*
    a. radial nerve and brachial artery
    b. median nerve and brachial artery
    c. ulnar nerve and brachial artery
    d. radial nerve and cephalic vein
    e. median nerve and cephalic vein

222. *Which cat breed has a greater prevalence of cryptorchidism than other breeds?*
    a. Persian
    b. Siamese
    c. domestic long hair
    d. Devon Rex
    e. Burmese

223. *An otherwise healthy 7-month-old female cat has moderate swelling of the mammary glands. What is the most likely cause of these findings?*
    a. mammary gland adenocarcinoma
    b. mastitis
    c. mammary gland abscess
    d. mammary hypertrophy-fibroadenoma complex
    e. fibrosarcoma

224. *What is the **least** appropriate suture pattern for closing a cystotomy incision?*
    a. Lembert
    b. simple interrupted
    c. Cushing
    d. Connell
    e. horizontal mattress

225. *Which of the following is **least** likely to be found in a male cat with urethral obstruction?*
    a. azotemia
    b. vomiting
    c. hypokalemia
    d. cardiac arrhythmia
    e. metabolic acidosis

226. *Which clinical feature in cats is **not** associated with polyarthritis caused by bacterial L-forms?*
    a. a positive culture for mycobacteria
    b. subcutaneous swellings and fistulous tracts
    c. radiographic evidence of articular cartilage destruction, periosteal bone proliferation, and cystlike metaphyseal defects
    d. degenerate neutrophils in synovial fluid
    e. initial involvement of the carpi and tarsi

227. *Which antibiotic is most appropriate for treatment of polyarthritis caused by bacterial L-forms in cats?*
    a. penicillin
    b. amoxicillin
    c. tetracycline
    d. cephalexin
    e. ampicillin

228. *What is the most common postsurgical complication following ventral bulla osteotomy for treatment of middle ear polyps in cats?*
    a. draining tracts
    b. dysphagia
    c. otitis interna
    d. Horner's syndrome
    e. recurrence of the polyp

229. *When performing bulla osteotomy in cats, the risk of iatrogenic Horner's syndrome may be reduced by taking special care to avoid the:*
    a. parasympathetic nerves as they course through the petrous temporal bone and the middle ear canal
    b. sympathetic nerves as they course through the petrous temporal bone and the middle ear canal
    c. facial nerve as it courses ventral to the external ear canal
    d. parasympathetic nerves as they course through the inner ear
    e. sympathetic nerves as they course through the inner ear

Correct answers are on pages 260-275.

230. *Which drug is best for preoperative treatment of sinus tachycardia in a hyperthyroid cat?*

a. quinidine
b. lidocaine
c. enalapril
d. digoxin
e. propranolol

231. *A cat exhibits restlessness, weakness, face rubbing, twitching, and muscle tremors 48 hours after bilateral thyroidectomy. What is the most likely cause of these findings?*

a. acute hypothyroidism
b. hypercalcemia
c. hypocalcemia
d. hypermagnesemia
e. hypomagnesemia

232. *When performing a thyroidectomy in a cat, special care should be taken to avoid damage to the:*

a. external parathyroid gland, which is usually located on the cranial pole of the thyroid gland
b. external parathyroid gland, which is usually located on the caudal pole of the thyroid gland
c. internal parathyroid gland, which is usually located within the cranial pole of the thyroid gland
d. internal parathyroid gland, which is usually located within the caudal pole of the thyroid gland
e. contralateral thyroid gland

233. *Which vessel should* ***not*** *be ligated during colectomy in cats?*

a. caudal mesenteric artery
b. celiac artery
c. middle colic artery
d. right colic artery
e. cranial rectal artery

234. *Concerning linear foreign bodies in cats, which statement is* ***least*** *accurate?*

a. Conservative management may be used in some cases.
b. The most common location for fixation of the linear foreign body is the base of the tongue.
c. An upper gastrointestinal study using barium should be performed to detect intestinal perforation.
d. An abnormal intestinal gas and fluid pattern and intestinal plication may be seen on radiographs.
e. The leukogram may be normal at the time of presentation.

235. *When placing an intramedullary pin in retrograde fashion for repair of a fracture of the midshaft femur, how should the limb be positioned to minimize the risk of damage to the sciatic nerve?*

a. adduct the femur and flex the coxofemoral joint
b. adduct the femur and extend the coxofemoral joint
c. abduct the femur and flex the coxofemoral joint
d. abduct the femur and extend the coxofemoral joint
e. adduct and medially rotate the femur

236. *Which technique is* ***least*** *appropriate for surgical management of traumatic separation of the proximal femoral epiphysis in a cat?*

a. femoral head and neck excision
b. fixation with a screw placed in lag fashion
c. fixation with two Kirschner-wires placed divergently
d. fixation with a screw placed in neutral fashion and a single Kirschner-wire
e. fixation with hemicerclage wire

237. Which bacteria are most commonly isolated from cats with septic arthritis caused by a bite wound from another cat?

a. staphylococci, streptococci, and anaerobes
b. *Nocardia* and anaerobes
c. *Escherichia coli*, staphylococci, and anaerobes
d. *Pasteurella*, streptococci, and anaerobes
e. staphylococci, *E. coli*, and streptococci

238. A 2-year-old male cat exhibits lameness, fever, swollen tarsi and carpi, and moderate periarticular periosteal proliferations. What is the most likely cause of these findings?

a. chronic progressive polyarthritis
b. rheumatoid arthritis
c. systemic lupus erythematosus
d. polyarthritis caused by *Mycoplasma* infection
e. polyarthritis caused by calicivirus infection

239. Fractures of which pelvic bones are usually managed conservatively?

a. ilium and sacroiliac
b. acetabulum and ilium
c. ischium and acetabulum
d. ilium and acetabulum
e. pubis and ischium

*240. Which technique is **not** recommended for treatment of coxofemoral luxation in cats?*

a. closed reduction, followed by application of an Ehmer sling if the joint is stable
b. femoral head and neck excision
c. closed reduction and stabilization with a De Vita pin
d. open reduction and capsulorrhaphy
e. open reduction and stabilization with a toggle pin

241. Following closed reduction of elbow luxation, which external coaptation device should be applied?

a. Velpeau sling
b. spica splint
c. Robert Jones bandage
d. Ehmer sling
e. Robinson sling

242. Following perineal urethrostomy for treatment of urethral obstruction caused by feline urologic syndrome, approximately what percentage of cats subsequently develop urinary tract infection after the urethrostomy site has healed?

a. 2%
b. 8%
c. 25%
d. 60%
e. 90%

243. A 9-year-old cat has a pink mass on one side of the oropharynx, ventral to the soft palate. What is the most likely cause of this finding?

a. tonsillar squamous-cell carcinoma
b. lymphosarcoma
c. fibrosarcoma
d. malignant melanoma
e. bacterial tonsillitis

244. A 9-month-old cat exhibits depression, seizures, ptyalism, diarrhea, polyuria, and polydipsia. What is the most likely cause of these findings?

a. meningioma
b. renal lymphosarcoma
c. idiopathic epilepsy
d. portosystemic shunt
e. toxoplasmosis

*245. Which clinicopathologic finding is **least** likely to be found in a cat with a portosystemic shunt?*

a. erythrocyte microcytosis and poikilocytosis
b. elevated blood urea nitrogen concentration
c. ammonium biurate crystalluria
d. elevated plasma ammonia concentration
e. elevated postprandial serum bile acid concentration

Correct answers are on pages 260-275.

DOGS AND CATS

J. Harari

246. *The most common cause of degenerative osteoarthritis of the canine stifle joint is:*

   a. medial patellar luxation
   b. lateral patellar luxation
   c. rupture of the cranial cruciate ligament
   d. rupture of the caudal cruciate ligament
   e. lateral meniscal tear

247. *Which Putnam classification of medial patellar luxation is characterized by femoral and tibial bone deformations, persistent lameness, and inability to manually reduce the luxation?*

   a. grade I
   b. grade II
   c. grade III
   d. grade IV
   e. grade V

248. *In repairing patellar luxations, what is the name of the technique in which the trochlear groove is deepened and covered by a triangular osteochondral fragment?*

   a. lateral imbrication
   b. retinacular plication
   c. derotation suture
   d. tibial tuberosity transplantation
   e. wedge recession

249. *The stifle joint is classified as:*

   a. a condylar joint
   b. a ball-and-socket joint
   c. an ellipsoid joint
   d. a hinge joint
   e. a plane joint

250. *What is the most common concurrent injury in dogs with cranial cruciate ligament rupture?*

   a. medial patellar luxation
   b. medial meniscal tear
   c. lateral meniscal tear
   d. gastrocnemius tendon avulsion
   e. long digital extensor tendon avulsion

251. *Rupture of the cranial cruciate ligament is characterized clinically by:*

   a. external tibial rotation
   b. cranial drawer motion of the tibia
   c. caudal drawer motion of the tibia
   d. valgus deviation of the stifle joint
   e. varus deviation of the stifle joint

252. *Medial luxation of the patella in dogs is most appropriately treated with:*

   a. a partial medial meniscectomy
   b. a medial relief incision and lateral tightening procedures
   c. a lateral relief incision and medial tightening procedures
   d. a partial patellectomy
   e. intraarticular corticosteroid injections

253. *Which of the following is an extracapsular repair for rupture of the cranial cruciate ligament?*

   a. fabella to tibial tuberosity derotation suture
   b. fascia lata autograft
   c. medial one third of the patellar tendon autograft
   d. middle one third of the patellar tendon autograft
   e. lateral one third of the patellar tendon autograft

254. *In general, surgical treatments for repair of cranial cruciate ligament injury are classified as:*

   a. extracapsular and intracapsular procedures
   b. arthrodesis or amputation procedures
   c. corrective osteotomy procedures
   d. limb-lengthening procedures
   e. limb-shortening procedures

255. Lateral luxation of the patella in large dogs is often associated with:

a. lateral meniscal tear
b. lateral collateral ligament injury
c. avulsion of the tibial tuberosity
d. medial meniscal tear
e. hip dysplasia

256. The surgical approach that provides the greatest exposure to organs in the thoracic cavity is via:

a. lateral intercostal thoracotomy
b. rib resection
c. rib pivot
d. median sternotomy
e. ventral celiotomy and incision through the diaphragm

257. The most common surgical approach for treatment of a patent ductus arteriosus or persistent right aortic arch is:

a. left fourth intercostal thoracotomy
b. right fourth intercostal thoracotomy
c. median sternotomy
d. left tenth rib resection
e. right tenth rib pivot

258. A pathognomonic sign of a persistent right aortic arch is:

a. fever
b. machinery murmur
c. postprandial regurgitation at weaning
d. caudal paresis
e. thoracic pain

259. The most common congenital cardiac anomaly in dogs is:

a. persistent right aortic arch
b. ventricular septal defect
c. tetralogy of Fallot
d. patent ductus arteriosus
e. aortic stenosis

260. The most common congenital cardiac defect in cats is:

a. ventricular septal defect
b. cardiomyopathy
c. patent ductus arteriosus
d. persistent right aortic arch
e. pulmonic stenosis

261. The most common congenital cardiac anomaly in dogs that produces cyanosis is:

a. cardiomyopathy
b. tetralogy of Fallot
c. pulmonic stenosis
d. pulmonic insufficiency
e. aortic stenosis

262. Treatment for patent ductus arteriosus requires:

a. ligation of the ductus
b. β-adrenergic blockers
c. a low-protein diet
d. arterial embolectomy
e. cardiac path grafting

*263. Which of the following is **not** an appropriate treatment for chylothorax?*

a. thoracostomy tube drainage
b. pleuroperitoneal shunting
c. pleurodesis
d. short- and medium-chain fatty acid dietary supplementation
e. long-chain fatty acid dietary supplementation

264. Instability of a thoracic chest wall segment, associated with trauma, that causes paradoxic chest motions is called:

a. flail chest
b. hemothorax
c. pneumothorax
d. peritoneopericardial hernia
e. chylothorax

Correct answers are on pages 260-275.

265. *An abnormal patent communication between an artery and a vein is termed:*

a. hemangioma
b. hemangiosarcoma
c. arteriovenous fistula
d. Eck's fistula
e. arterioma

266. *Neoplasia of the spleen is best treated by:*

a. irradiation
b. chemotherapy
c. arterial bypass procedures
d. splenectomy
e. debulking procedures

267. *A large dog with sudden, gaseous abdominal distention associated with exercise after eating most likely has:*

a. rectal prolapse
b. infectious hepatitis
c. splenic rupture
d. esophageal neoplasia
e. gastric dilation-volvulus

268. *The most common neurologic disorder in small animals is:*

a. cervical vertebral instability
b. spinal cord neoplasia
c. intervertebral disk disease
d. diskospondylitis
e. atlantoaxial subluxation

269. *Which of the following is **not** an appropriate treatment for lumbosacral stenosis in dogs?*

a. analgesics
b. vitamin E/selenium injections
c. antiinflammatories
d. dorsal laminectomy
e. foraminotomy

270. *A thoracolumbar spinal cord lesion associated with disk herniation produces:*

a. upper motor neuron lesions of the hind limbs
b. lower motor neuron lesions of the hind limbs
c. cervical pain
d. upper motor neuron lesions of the front limbs
e. lower motor neuron lesions of the front limbs

271. *Progressive cervical vertebral instability in Doberman pinschers requires:*

a. cervical disk fenestration
b. cervical decompression and stabilization
c. cervical facetectomy
d. chemonucleolysis of the cervical disks
e. vitamin E/selenium and dimethyl sulfoxide injections

272. *A progressive, nonpainful condition that causes hind limb paresis in German shepherds is:*

a. lumbosacral stenosis
b. lumbosacral instability
c. thoracolumbar disk herniation
d. degenerative myelopathy
e. cervical vertebral instability

273. *In dachshunds, the most common site of intervertebral disk disease is:*

a. C1-2
b. T1-2
c. T12-13
d. L1-2
e. L7-S1

274. *Which of the following lesions is **not** involved in the "brachycephalic airway syndrome"?*

a. eustachian tube dilation
b. stenotic nares
c. elongated soft palate
d. everted laryngeal saccules
e. hypoplastic trachea

275. *Which of the following is **not** a likely complication of laryngeal surgery?*

a. scar formation
b. inhalation pneumonia
c. laryngeal edema
d. cervical ventroflexion
e. dyspnea

276. *The most common surgical approach for debulking of the nasal cavity is termed:*
   a. dorsal craniotomy
   b. dorsal rhinotomy
   c. ventral rhinotomy
   d. ventral sinotomy
   e. ventral laryngotomy

277. *Which surgical procedure can provide immediate relief of upper airway obstruction?*
   a. ventriculocordectomy
   b. arytenoidectomy
   c. tracheostomy
   d. thoracostomy
   e. pneumonectomy

278. *An abnormal communication between the mouth and nasal sinuses is termed:*
   a. arteriovenous shunt
   b. oronasal fistula
   c. odontoplastic diverticulum
   d. sinopharyngeal tube
   e. brachygnathism

279. *Osteochondritis dissecans is* ***not*** *usually associated with which joint:*
   a. shoulder
   b. elbow
   c. carpus
   d. stifle
   e. hock

280. *Surgical treatment for osteochondritis dissecans involves:*
   a. cancellous bone autografts
   b. arthrodesis of the affected joint
   c. cartilage flap removal and curettage of subchondral bone
   d. joint stabilization with an external fixator
   e. synovectomy

281. *A young, rapidly growing, large dog is being fed a high-energy diet and has forelimb lameness associated with the elbow joint. Which lesion is likely to require surgical intervention in this dog?*
   a. panosteitis
   b. retained cartilaginous cores
   c. fragmented medial coronoid process
   d. medial meniscal tear
   e. epiphysitis

282. *Traumatic hip luxation occurs most commonly in which direction:*
   a. craniodorsal
   b. caudoventral
   c. caudodorsal
   d. lateral
   e. cranioventral

283. *Which of the following is a surgical treatment for traumatic hip luxation?*
   a. intramedullary pinning
   b. tension-band wiring
   c. cerclage wiring
   d. bone plating
   e. De Vita pinning

284. *Which physeal injury (based on the Salter-Harris classification) has the* ***poorest*** *prognosis for recovery?*
   a. type I
   b. type II
   c. type III
   d. type IV
   e. type V

285. *In repair of epiphyseal fractures, what is the primary aim of surgical intervention?*
   a. bone alignment
   b. articular cartilage congruency
   c. periosteal stripping
   d. physeal compression
   e. physeal distraction

Correct answers are on pages 260-275.

286. *An intramedullary pin used for repair of a long bone fracture provides:*

a. interfragmentary compression
b. rotational stability
c. metaphyseal compression
d. tension-band stabilization
e. axial alignment

287 *Which orthopedic device provides the greatest degree of compression across a fracture line?*

a. dynamic compression plate
b. Kirschner wires
c. intramedullary pins
d. cerclage wire
e. external skeletal fixation

288. *Primary bone union is most likely to occur in a fracture being treated with:*

a. bone plate and screws
b. hemicerclage and full cerclage wires
c. multiple intramedullary pins
d. external fixator
e. plaster cast

289. *Which condition should be treated before orthopedic surgery in a trauma patient?*

a. fracture phalanges
b. fractured, nondisplaced ribs
c. muscle bruising
d. ruptured urinary bladder
e. epistaxis

290. *Which lesion could cause depression, poor growth, and central nervous system disorders in a young dog being fed a high-protein diet?*

a. patent ductus arteriosus
b. persistent right aortic arch
c. portosystemic shunt
d. persistent urachus
e. congenital megaesophagus

291. *Surgical treatment for unilateral ectopic ureter consists of:*

a. urinary diversion using a segment of ileum
b. perineal urethrostomy
c. prepubic urethrostomy
d. cystopexy
e. ureteral reimplantation

292. *In obese female dogs, chronic perivulvar dermatitis associated with redundant tissue can be treated with:*

a. episiotomy
b. episioplasty
c. ovariohysterectomy
d. vaginotomy
e. typhlectomy

293. *Which of the following is most appropriate for treatment of a transverse mid-shaft radial fracture in a large dog?*

a. intramedullary pinning
b. cerclage wires
c. external skeletal fixator
d. Kirschner pins
e. Robert Jones bandage

294. *At what time should prophylactic antibiotics be given to prevent surgical wound infections?*

a. 1 to 2 days before surgery
b. 1 week before surgery
c. 12 hours after surgery is terminated
d. 1 to 2 hours after surgery is terminated
e. immediately before surgery

295. *The highest concentrations of antibiotics in serum, plasma, and tissues are achieved when prophylactic antibiotics are given:*

a. orally
b. intravenously
c. intramuscularly
d. subcutaneously
e. topically in lavage fluid

296. *In a dog with hypoglycemia, you identify a solitary pancreatic tumor during laparotomy. The most likely cause of this dog's hypoglycemia is:*

    a. diabetes insipidus
    b. hemangioma
    c. acute hemorrhagic pancreatitis
    d. chronic fibrosing pancreatitis
    e. insulinoma

297. *To reduce swelling and provide temporary fracture stability, which device should be applied to a tibial fracture in a dog?*

    a. external fixator
    b. Schroeder-Thomas splint
    c. Robert Jones bandage
    d. Mason meta splint
    e. padded limb bandage

298. *Which drug is useful for treatment of spinal cord swelling caused by the trauma of disk herniation?*

    a. aspirin
    b. phenylbutazone
    c. acetaminophen
    d. dexamethasone
    e. acepromazine

299. *Chronic obstipation associated with megacolon in cats is effectively treated by:*

    a. staphylectomy
    b. colopexy
    c. colectomy
    d. cystotomy
    e. gastropexy

300. *Chronic multifocal abscessation around the anus and base of the tail in German shepherds is termed:*

    a. perianal fistulae
    b. perineal hernia
    c. stud tail
    d. circumanal metaplasia
    e. pilonidal cysts

P.A. Bushby

301. *A 6-month-old female Irish setter is presented to your clinic with a 3-day history of vomiting. Following physical examination, laboratory workup, and abdominal radiographs, you confirm a diagnosis of intestinal obstruction from a radiopaque foreign body. For surgical exploration and correction of this problem, what is the most appropriate incisional approach?*

    a. ventral abdominal midline, xyphoid to umbilicus
    b. ventral abdominal midline, umbilicus to pubis
    c. ventral abdominal midline, xyphoid to pubis
    d. right paramedian, xyphoid to pubis
    e. right paramedian, umbilicus to pubis

302. *You are performing a surgery to remove an intestinal foreign body from a 6-month-old female Irish setter. You find the foreign body in the distal jejunum. Visual inspection reveals that the intestine proximal (cranial) to the foreign body is distended. Palpation suggests that the intestinal contents are fluid and gas. The foreign body is rough and irregular. The intestines at the site of the foreign body are intact but discolored. On digital manipulation, the serosa at the site of the lesion begins to tear but does not bleed. The most appropriate course of action is to:*

    a. digitally manipulate the foreign body proximally and then perform an enterotomy
    b. digitally manipulate the foreign body distally and then perform an enterotomy
    c. perform an enterotomy at the site of the foreign body
    d. perform an intestinal resection of devitalized intestine, including removal of the foreign body and anastomosis of viable intestine
    e. flush the lumen of the distal intestine with sterile saline to move the foreign body proximally and then perform an enterotomy

Correct answers are on pages 260-275.

303. *In performing an intestinal resection and anastomosis, you remember that the blood supply to the remaining intestine is critical. To ensure adequate blood supply to the remaining intestine, you must make your intestinal incisions at an angle. Which of the following is most likely to maintain an adequate blood supply to remaining intestine?*

a. leave the mesenteric surface longer than the antimesenteric
b. leave the antimesenteric surface longer than the mesenteric
c. leave the mesenteric and antimesenteric surfaces the same length
d. leave the medial surface longer than the lateral surface
e. leave the proximal surface longer than the distal surface

304. *Which suture pattern is most appropriate for closure of the small intestine in a dog after intestinal resection?*

a. Cushing
b. Bunnell
c. Parker-Kerr
d. simple interrupted
e. vertical mattress

Question 305

You are presented with a 6-year-old male poodle with acute onset of caudal paresis. Physical examination reveals abnormalities only in the nervous system. Neurologic examination reveals the following:

Mental Status: alert, with no abnormalities noted
Cranial Nerves: no abnormalities noted
Posture and Gait: paraplegia

Postural Reactions:

	Left Front	*Left Rear*	*Right Front*	*Right Rear*
Wheelbarrowing	2	0	0	2
Ext Post Thrust	2	0	0	2
Hemiwalk	2	0	0	2
Consc Proprio	2	0	0	2
Hopping	2	0	0	2

Spinal Reflexes:

	Left Front	*Left Rear*	*Right Front*	*Right Rear*
Biceps	2	—	—	2
Triceps	2	—	—	2
Patellar	—	3	3	—
Cranial Tibial	—	3	3	—
Gastrocnemius	—	3	3	—
Flexor	2	2	2	2
Anal Sphincter	—	2	2	—
Panniculus	absent caudal to thoracolumbar area			

Sensation: hyperesthesia over thoracolumbar area, superficial pain absent caudal to thoracolumbar area, deep pain present in all four limbs

305. *Which neurologic pathway is most likely affected?*

a. upper motor neuron to the front limbs
b. upper motor neuron to the rear limbs
c. lower motor neuron to the front limbs
d. lower motor neuron to the rear limbs
e. upper motor neuron to all four limbs

306. *A 6-year-old male poodle is presented to your clinic with acute onset of caudal paresis. Radiographs confirm intervertebral disk protrusion at L1-2. You plan to perform a decompressive hemilaminectomy combined with intervertebral disk fenestration. After making the incision in the skin, subcutaneous tissue, and thoracolumbar fascia, you must elevate the epaxial muscles off one side of the vertebra. Starting dorsally, you perform subperiosteal elevation of these muscles. You must continue this dissection until you find what landmark?*

a. dorsal spinous processes
b. articular processes
c. transverse spinous processes
d. ventral spinous processes
e. accessory process

307. *You wish to perform spinal decompression in a 6-year-old male poodle with spinal cord compression associated with intervertebral disk disease. Radiographs confirm on intervertebral disk rupture at L1-2. Assuming normal anatomy, what is the most appropriate landmark to use during surgery to identify the first lumbar vertebra (L1)?*
   a. the last rib
   b. dorsal spinous process of L1
   c. L1 is the anticlinal vertebra
   d. T10 and count backward to L1
   e. L1 has a large ventral process off the transverse spinous process

308. *You are performing a hemilaminectomy on a 6-year-old male poodle with an intervertebral disk rupture that is causing spinal compression of L1-2. You begin your decompression at the L2-3 articular processes and proceed cranially. You find intervertebral disk material under the spinal cord at L1-2 and carefully remove the material. You must determine the most cranial and caudal extent for your decompression. Which of the following is most helpful in making that decision?*
   a. condition of the dura mater
   b. absence of cord swelling
   c. presence of epidural hematoma
   d. absence of intervertebral disk material
   e. presence of epidural fat

309. *Surgical castration of cats requires:*
   a. one incision in the prescrotal skin
   b. two incisions in the scrotum
   c. two incisions in the prescrotal skin
   d. one incision in the scrotum
   e. scrotal ablation

310. *Surgical castration of dogs requires:*
   a. one incision in the prescrotal skin
   b. two incisions in the scrotum
   c. two incisions in the prescrotal skin
   d. one incision in the scrotum
   e. scrotal ablation

311. *For ovariohysterectomy in a cat, the skin incision is made:*
   a. caudally from the umbilicus
   b. from the umbilicus to the pubis
   c. cranially from the umbilicus
   d. midway between the umbilicus and pubis
   e. midway between the xyphoid and umbilicus

312. *For ovariohysterectomy in a dog, the skin incision is made:*
   a. caudally from the umbilicus
   b. from the umbilicus to the pubis
   c. cranially from the umbilicus
   d. midway between the umbilicus and pubis
   e. midway between the xyphoid and umbilicus

313. *You are performing a perineal urethrostomy in a 7-year-old castrated cat to correct recurrent urinary obstruction. You remember that the bulbourethral glands are a critical landmark for determining the site of the new urethral orifice. What is the anatomic basis for slitting the dorsal wall of the urethra to the location of the bulbourethral glands?*
   a. It is located at the junction of the vascular and avascular urethra.
   b. It represents the site of least hemorrhage.
   c. It represents the site of control of urinary continence.
   d. Proximal to this point, the urethra is narrowed.
   e. It is located at the junction of the pelvic and penile urethra.

314. *In transplantation of the ureter into the urinary bladder, what is the purpose of tunneling through the bladder wall so the ureter passes obliquely through the bladder wall?*
   a. increases surface area for healing of ureter to bladder
   b. minimizes stricture by increasing ureteral lumen diameter
   c. minimizes backflow of urine by acting as a one-way valve
   d. prevents hydronephrosis by facilitating urine flow
   e. encourages emptying of the ureter because of muscular action of the bladder

Correct answers are on pages 260-275.

315. *Concerning the relationship between skin incisions and skin tension lines in dogs, which statement is most accurate?*

a. Incisions parallel to tension lines decrease healing time.
b. Incisions perpendicular to tension lines decrease healing time.
c. Incisions perpendicular to tension lines decrease the chance of dehiscence.
d. Incisions parallel to tension lines decrease the chance of dehiscence.
e. Skin tension lines have no relationship to wound healing or closure.

316. *In closure of the urinary bladder following cystotomy, sutures must* ***not*** *penetrate the lumen of the bladder. Why is this so?*

a. Sutures in the bladder lumen increase the chance of ascending urinary tract infection.
b. Sutures in the bladder lumen increase the chance of urine leakage into the abdomen.
c. Sutures in the bladder lumen increase the chance of cystic calculi formation.
d. Sutures in the bladder lumen impede healing.
e. Sutures in the bladder lumen increase the chance of bladder dehiscence.

317. *You are presented with a 3-year-old, 30-kg dog with a large (12-cm-long) laceration of the skin on the right side in the midthoracic region. The dog had been missing for 3 days, and the owners are not sure what happened. On physical examination you detect a significant amount of debris in the wound. You judge the laceration to be at least 2 days old (if not older). Your goal is to minimize infection, scarring, and healing time. Which plan of management would best accomplish your goals?*

a. Clean and débride the wound, implant a drain, and suture the wound.
b. Clean, débride, and suture the wound.
c. Leave the wound open to heal by granulation.
d. Clean and débride the wound and leave open to heal by granulation.
e. Give oral broad-spectrum antibiotics and clean, débride, and suture the wound.

318. *Your associate performed an ovariohysterectomy on a 6-month-old Irish setter last week. He is out of the office today, and the owners are now returning the dog for suture removal. On examination you note serosanguineous drainage from the suture line. On closer inspection you palpate an obvious defect in the abdominal wall, with what you believe is small intestine palpable under the skin. What is the most appropriate course of action?*

a. As long as the skin incision is healed, remove the sutures and send the dog home; this situation should pose no problem.
b. Leave the skin sutures intact, manipulate the abdominal contents back into the abdominal cavity, place a belly band around the animal, and reexamine the dog in 1 week.
c. Leave the skin sutures intact, manipulate the abdominal contents back into the abdominal cavity, place a belly band around the animal, hospitalize the dog for 1 week of cage rest, and recheck after that time.
d. Hospitalize the animal for surgery to repair the defect in the abdominal wall.
e. Leave the sutures in place, send the dog home, and recheck in 1 week.

319. *In an adult dog, the amount of callus formed in healing of a fractured long bone is:*

a. inversely proportional to the degree of stability of the fractured site
b. directly proportional to the amount of hemorrhage at the time for fracture
c. dependent on the age of the animal
d. inversely proportional to the amount of soft tissue injury associated with the fracture
e. directly proportional to the amount of soft tissue injury associated with the fracture

320. *Concerning bone healing and callus formation in a fracture repaired with an intramedullary pin versus with a plate and screws, which statement is most accurate?*

a. Callus formation with either stabilization technique is essentially the same.
b. With an intramedullary pin, healing occurs primarily by periosteal bridging callus, whereas with the plate and screws, healing occurs primarily by medullary bridging callus.
c. With an intramedullary pin, healing occurs by periosteal, intercortical, and medullary bridging callus, whereas with the plate and screws, healing occurs primarily by medullary bridging callus.
d. With an intramedullary pin, healing occurs by periosteal, intercortical, and medullary bridging callus, whereas with the plate and screws, healing occurs primarily by intercortical bridging callus.
e. With an intramedullary pin, healing occurs by intercortical bridging callus, whereas with the plate and screws, healing occurs primarily by medullary bridging callus.

321. *You are repairing a closed comminuted femoral fracture in a 2-year-old, 20-kg male mongrel dog. A butterfly fragment, 2 cm long and entirely devoid of blood supply, is present at the midshaft of the femur. What is the most appropriate course of action?*

a. The fragment should be discarded; with no blood supply, the risk of bone sequestration far outweighs the value of including the fragment in the repair.
b. The fragment should be discarded; the best approach to management of a comminuted fracture is removal of small fragments and stabilization of the proximal and distal fragments of the femoral shaft.
c. The fragment should be placed loosely in the defect during the repair; it will revascularize and contribute to callus formation.
d. The fragment should be incorporated into the repair and secured in place, it will function as a cancellous bone graft during healing.
e. The fragment should be incorporated into the repair and secured in place; it will function as an autogenous bone graft during healing.

322. *In the surgical approach to the left hemithorax for repair of a patent ductus arteriosus, which muscle is **not** encountered?*

a. cutaneous trunci
b. latissimus dorsi
c. serratus dorsalis
d. serratus ventralis
e. scalenus

323. *You are performing resection and anastomosis of a section of cervical esophagus. The preferred method of closure is a:*

a. two-layer closure, with one layer in the mucosa/submucosa and the second layer in the muscularis/adventitia
b. two-layer closure, with one layer in the mucosa and the second layer in the submucosa
c. single-layer crushing suture passing full-thickness through the wall of the esophagus
d. single-layer closure, with sutures not entering the esophageal lumen
e. three-layer closure, with one layer in the mucosa, and the second in the submucosa, and third in the muscularis

324. *Surgical correction and prevention of recurrence of salivary mucoceles generally involve excision of the:*

a. cyst and mandibular salivary gland
b. cyst and sublingual salivary gland
c. parotid and mandibular salivary glands
d. parotid and mandibular salivary glands
e. mandibular and sublingual salivary glands

Correct answers are on pages 260-275.

325. *Cushing and Connell suture patterns are used primarily for closure of hollow organs. Which of the following best differentiates between Cushing and Connell sutures?*

a. Cushing sutures are everting, whereas Connell sutures are inverting.
b. Connell sutures enter the lumen, whereas Cushing sutures do not enter the lumen.
c. Cushing sutures are absorbable, whereas Connell sutures are nonabsorbable.
d. Connell sutures are interrupted, whereas Cushing sutures are continuous.
e. Cushing sutures parallel the incision line, whereas Connell sutures are perpendicular to the incision line.

326. *Alteration of the luminal diameter of the pylorus is advocated for surgical correction of pyloric stenosis in dogs. Which technique is **not** appropriate for surgical management of pyloric stenosis?*

a. Heller's myotomy
b. Fredet-Ramstedt myotomy
c. Heineke-Mikulicz procedure
d. Finney procedure
e. Y-V pyloroplasty

327. *You have performed an enterotomy through a longitudinal incision in the jejunum of an 8-kg dog. As you begin to close the enterotomy, you suspect that there may be a significant reduction in lumen diameter. What is the most appropriate course of action?*

a. Perform a resection and anastomosis at the site of the enterotomy.
b. Suture the longitudinal enterotomy transversely.
c. Suture the enterotomy longitudinally using an everting suture pattern.
d. Do not worry about the reduction in diameter; the intestine will expand to normal diameter during healing.
e. Make sure that the enterotomy incision is at a 60-degree angle to the longitudinal axis of the intestine.

328. *To minimize the risk of leakage of intestinal contents into the abdomen after single-layer closure of an enterotomy of the small intestine in a dog, you should:*

a. wrap the involved intestine in omentum
b. wrap the involved intestine in mesentery
c. oversew the enterotomy with a second layer of sutures
d. place a Penrose drain in the abdomen at the site of the enterotomy
e. oversew the enterotomy with a second layer of sutures and wrap the involved intestine in omentum

329. *Brachycephalic dogs may develop upper airway obstruction because of one or more anatomic abnormalities. Which abnormality **cannot** be corrected surgically?*

a. elongated soft palate
b. laryngeal collapse
c. tracheal hypoplasia
d. stenotic nares
e. everting laryngeal saccules

330. *A 9-month-old golden retriever has been lame on its right forelimb for approximately 3 weeks. The dog is bearing weight only partially on the right forelimb and shows pain on extension of the right shoulder. What is the most likely cause of this dog's lameness?*

a. panosteitis
b. osteochondritis dissecans
c. ununited anconeal process
d. fragmented coronoid process
e. scapulohumeral luxation

331. *Accidental wounds can be classified as open or closed. Which of the following is considered a closed wound?*

a. contusion
b. abrasion
c. laceration
d. incision
e. puncture

332. *Assuming identical environmental conditions and identical risks of contamination, which wound is most at risk of infection?*
   a. contusion
   b. abrasion
   c. laceration
   d. incision
   e. puncture

333. *A 6-year-old, 32-kg male mongrel dog is presented to your clinic 6 days after being involved in a fight with another dog. The dog has a three-cornered laceration on the left lateral thoracic wall with a 4-cm horizontal tear and a 6-cm vertical tear in the skin. You find the skin flap to be necrotic and discover purulent discharge from the wound. Your goal is to manage the infection and minimize scarring. Which of the following would best meet these goals?*
   a. Clean and débride the wound, implant a drain, and suture the wound.
   b. Clean, débride, and suture the wound.
   c. Leave the wound open to heal by granulation.
   d. Clean and débride the wound, and leave it open to heal by granulation.
   e. Clean and débride the wound, leave it open until healthy granulation appears, and then suture the wound.

334. *Which of the following accurately describes an allograft?*
   a. The recipient and donor sites are on the same animal.
   b. The recipient and donor sites are on genetically different animals of the same species.
   c. The recipient and donor are on animals of different species.
   d. The recipient and donor are identical twins.
   e. The recipient and donor are F1 hybrids produced by crossing inbred strains.

335. *In declawing a cat (oncychectomy), the surgeon must be careful to prevent regrowth of the claw. This is done by removing the:*
   a. entire third phalanx
   b. germinal cells in the ungual process
   c. germinal cells in the ungual crest
   d. digital pad
   e. bilateral dorsal ligaments

336. *You are planning for correction of patent ductus arteriosus in a 6-month-old mongrel dog. The most appropriate site for the thoracotomy is the:*
   a. right fourth intercostal space
   b. left fourth intercostal space
   c. right sixth intercostal space
   d. left sixth intercostal space
   e. ventral midline sternum

337. *You are planning for a correction of a persistent right aortic arch (PRAA) in a 6-month-old mongrel dog. The most appropriate site for the thoracotomy is the:*
   a. right fourth intercostal space
   b. left fourth intercostal space
   c. right sixth intercostal space
   d. left sixth intercostal space
   e. ventral midline sternum

338. *What is the primary objective in surgical management of persistent right aortic arch?*
   a. Establish normal patency of the thoracic esophagus.
   b. Prevent shunting of blood from pulmonary vessels to the aorta.
   c. Prevent shunting of blood from the aorta to pulmonary vessels.
   d. Establish normal patency of the aorta.
   e. Prevent eventual congestive heart failure.

Correct answers are on pages 260-275.

339. *Sialoliths are relatively rare in dogs. They are usually found in the ducts of the parotid salivary glands. Which of the following most accurately represents appropriate surgical management of unilateral parotid sialolithiasis?*

a. Excise the involved parotid salivary gland, and leave the stone in the duct.
b. Incise the duct through a ventral cervical incision, remove the stone, and leave the wound open to drain.
c. Incise the duct through a lateral cervical incision, remove the stone, and leave the wound open to drain.
d. Incise the duct through a lateral cervical incision, remove the stone, and suture the wound.
e. Incise the duct through a oral incision, remove the stone, and leave the wound open to drain.

340. *A 4-year-old female Irish setter with a history of regurgitation for 3 days has an irregularly shaped radiopaque foreign body in the caudal thoracic esophagus. You elect to perform a thoracic esophagotomy for removal of the foreign body. The most appropriate location for the thoracic approach is the:*

a. right fourth intercostal space
b. right eighth intercostal space
c. left fourth intercostal space
d. left eighth intercostal space
e. ventral midline sternum

341. *A 6-year-old male basset hound is presented to your clinic with acute onset of restlessness, salivation, retching without vomition, and abdominal distention. You confirm gastric dilation/torsion. In management of this patient, which of the following is* ***least*** *appropriate?*

a. treatment of shock
b. correction of acid-base and electrolyte imbalances
c. gastropexy
d. pyloroplasty
e. gastrotomy

342. *The preferred approach for percutaneous hepatic biopsy is:*

a. transthoracic, with needle entry at the right seventh intercostal space
b. transthoracic, with needle entry at the left seventh intercostal space
c. with needle entry at the left caudal costochondral junction
d. transabdominal, with needle entry at the right caudal costochondral junction
e. transthoracic, with needle entry at the right twelfth intercostal space

343. *The appropriate site of trocar insertion for bone marrow aspiration in a 20-kg mongrel dog is the:*

a. tuber ischii
b. tibial crest
c. sternum
d. iliac crest
e. greater tubercle of the humerus

344. *Which of the following is an indication for partial splenectomy, as opposed to total splenectomy?*

a. splenic tumor confined to one end of the spleen
b. splenic rupture confined to one end of the spleen
c. splenic torsion
d. gastric torsion
e. generalized splenic trauma

345. *Concerning classification of intervertebral disk disease, which statement is most accurate?*
   a. Chondroid metaplasia occurs in young chondrodystrophoid dogs and may result in extensive mechanical rupture of one or more disks.
   b. Chondroid metaplasia occurs primarily in old chondrodystrophoid dogs and may result in extensive mechanical rupture of one or more disks.
   c. Chondroid metaplasia occurs in nonchondrodystrophoid dogs and results in partial rupture of the annular band.
   d. Massive ruptures of the disk are generally associated with fibroid metaplasia in chondrodystrophoid dogs.
   e. Massive ruptures of the disk are generally associated with fibroid metaplasia in nonchondrodystrophoid dogs.

346. *The surgeon confronted with a patient with cervical intervertebral disk disease must choose among medical management, or a combination of these techniques. Which of the following is the most appropriate candidate for fenestration only?*
   a. a 2-year-old chondrodystrophoid dog with radiographic evidence of nuclear mineralization and no clinical signs
   b. a 1-year-old chondrodystrophoid dog with radiographic evidence of nuclear mineralization and protrusion, with intermittent hyperesthesia
   c. a 2-year-old nonchondrodystrophoid dog with radiographic evidence of mineralized disk material in the spinal canal and hyperesthesia with motor deficits
   d. a 6-year-old nonchondrodystrophoid dog with radiographic evidence of mineralized disk material in the spinal canal and motor and sensory deficits
   e. a 10-year-old chondrodystrophoid dog with radiographic evidence of mineralized disk material in the spinal canal and hyperesthesia with motor deficits

347. *A 12-year-old cocker spaniel is presented to your clinic with a history of vomiting and anorexia. You confirm bilateral renal calculi with significant impairment of renal function and elect to remove the calculi by nephrotomy. This procedure involves:*
   a. incision of the renal pelvis to expose the calculi in the pelvis
   b. removal of one pole of the kidney to expose the calculi in the pelvis
   c. longitudinal incision through the renal parenchyma to expose the calculi in the pelvis
   d. surgical removal of the kidney
   e. transverse incision through the renal parenchyma to expose the calculi in the pelvis

348. *An 8-year-old male beagle with stranguria and hematuria has radiopaque calculi in the urinary bladder and in the urethra just caudal to the os penis. What is the most appropriate management of this dog?*
   a. urethrotomy to remove urethral calculi and dietary management to dissolve the cystic calculi
   b. urethrostomy at the site of urethral calculi and cystotomy
   c. urethrostomy at the site of the urethral calculi and dietary management to dissolve the cystic calculi
   d. dietary management to dissolve all the calculi
   e. back flush of the urethral calculi into the bladder for removal of all calculi by cystotomy

349. *Forces acting on a fractured long bone have been classified as rotational, bending, shearing, or appositional. Which fixation technique is most likely to neutralize all these forces?*
   a. compression plate
   b. single intramedullary pin
   c. multiple intramedullary pins
   d. lag screw fixation
   e. cerclage wire

Correct answers are on pages 260-275.

350. *Forces acting on a fracture long bone have been classified as rotational, bending, shearing, or appositional. Which fixation technique is* ***least*** *likely to overcome rotational forces?*

a. compression plate
b. single intramedullary pin
c. multiple intramedullary pins
d. lag screw fixation
e. hemicerclage wire

351. *A 1-year-old mongrel dog is brought to your clinic immediately after being hit by a car. Radiographs confirm a diaphragmatic hernia on the left side, with abdominal contents in the thoracic cavity. The most common surgical approach for repair of this type of hernia is:*

a. thoracotomy through the left fourth intercostal space
b. thoracotomy through the eighth intercostal space
c. left paracostal approach
d. left paramedian approach
e. ventral abdominal midline approach

352. *Five days previously, you spayed a 6-month-old mongrel dog through a ventral abdominal midline approach. Today the dog is presented to your clinic with a breakdown of the abdominal closure. The skin suture line is intact, but you palpate an incisional hernia in the abdominal wall. Which statement describes appropriate surgical correction of this incisional hernia?*

a. A skin incision should be made lateral to the original incision, and the edges of the linea alba should be débrided before closure.
b. An elliptic skin incision should be made excising the tissue bordering the original incision line, and the edges of the linea alba should be débrided before closure.
c. The original incision should be opened, and the linea alba stripped of any adhesions but not débrided before closure.
d. The original incision should be opened, the linea alba stripped of any adhesions, and the edges of the skin incision should be débrided before closure.
e. An elliptic incision should be made in the skin encompassing the original skin incision, and a second elliptic incision should be made in the linea alba encompassing the original linea incision before closure.

353. *Surgical repair of a perineal hernia may incorporate all the following structures* ***except*** *the:*

a. rectococcygeus muscle
b. coccygeus muscle
c. levator ani muscle
d. external anal sphincter
e. internal obturator muscle

354. *Perineal hernia is most likely to occur in:*

a. an 8-month-old male Boston terrier
b. a 2-year-old female poodle
c. a 4-year-old mongrel dog
d. a 6-year-old female cocker spaniel
e. a 12-year-old male collie

355. *In surgical correction of patent ductus arteriosus with a left-to-right shunt, the surgeon must be extremely cautious during the dissection necessary to pass ligatures around the ductus. What is the reason for this caution?*

a. The ductus arteriosus is generally dilated, weakened, and at risk of tear or rupture.
b. The aorta is generally dilated, weakened, and at risk of tear or rupture.
c. The pulmonary artery is generally dilated, weakened, and at risk of tear or rupture.
d. The subclavian artery is generally dilated, weakened, and at risk of tear or rupture.
e. The vagus nerve passes deep to the ductus arteriosus and must be avoided.

356. *Which of the following most accurately describes the proper technique for retrograde placement of an intramedullary pin for stabilization of an irregular oblique midshaft femoral fracture?*

a. The pin is inserted at the trochanteric fossa and directed distally, crosses the fracture site, and is secured in the distal cancellus bone.
b. The pin is inserted at the site of the fracture and directed distally to protrude from the femur at the stifle. The chuck is reversed and the pin driven proximally, crossing the fracture site and lodging in the proximal cancellous bone.
c. The leg is held in a normal weight-bearing position and slightly abducted. The pin is inserted at the fracture site and directed proximally to protrude from the femur at the trochanteric fossa. The chuck is reversed and the pin is driven distally, crossing the fracture site to lodge in the distal cancellous bone.
d. The leg is held in a normal weight-bearing position and slightly adducted. The pin is inserted at the fracture site and directed proximally to protrude from the femur at the trochanteric fossa. The chuck is reversed and the pin is driven distally, crossing the fracture site to lodge in the distal cancellous bone.
e. The hip is extended maximally and the leg slightly adducted. The pin is inserted at the fracture site and directed proximally to protrude from the femur at the trochanteric fossa. The chuck is reversed and the pin is driven distally, crossing the fracture site to lodge in the distal cancellous bone.

357. *Screws should be placed through the center of bone fragments to ensure maximal compression. What is the effect if a screw is placed eccentrically rather than centrally in bone fragments?*

a. Fragments are distracted rather than compressed.
b. Shearing forces impair fracture reduction.
c. Rotational forces impair fracture reduction.
d. Bending forces deform the bone.
e. There is no adverse effect.

358. *A plate used to bridge a diaphyseal defect is referred to as a:*

a. tension-band plate
b. neutralization plate
c. double-hooked plate
d. dynamic compression plate
e. buttress plate

359. *A plate that converts distractional forces into compressive forces is considered a:*

a. tension-band plate
b. neutralization plate
c. double-hooked plate
d. dynamic compression plate
e. buttress plate

360. *A 6-year-old mongrel dog is presented with a nonunion fracture of the mid-shaft right femur. The original transverse fracture had been treated with a single intramedullary pin 4 months previously. The pin was removed after 10 weeks, and the animal has been very lame since then. Radiographs reveal callus formation and a persistent fracture gap. There is no evidence of infection. What is the most appropriate treatment protocol?*

a. compression plating, with or without cancellous bone grafting
b. compression plating, with cortical bone grafting
c. débridement of the ends of the nonunion with rongeurs, cancellous bone grafting, and compression plating
d. tension-band plating, with or without cancellous bone grafting
e. intramedullary pin fixation, with cancellous bone grafting

361. *Concerning management of animals with osteomyelitis and nonhealing of a fracture treated with an orthopedic implant, which statement is most accurate?*

a. All orthopedic implants should be removed from the site until the infection is eliminated; at that time the fracture should be rigidly stabilized.
b. If the orthopedic implants are providing rigid stability to the fracture, they should be left intact.
c. Bone plats should be removed, but intramedullary pins should remain in place.
d. Intramedullary pins should be removed, but bone plates should remain in place.
e. All internal fixation devices should be removed and replaced with external fixation devices.

362. *Physeal fractures have been classified by Salter and Harris. A transverse fracture through the region of cartilage hypertrophy is considered a:*

a. Salter-I fracture
b. Salter-II fracture
c. Salter-III fracture
d. Salter-IV fracture
e. Salter-V fracture

363. *A transverse fracture through the region of cartilage hypertrophy and extending into the metaphysis is considered a:*

a. Salter-I fracture
b. Salter-II fracture
c. Salter-III fracture
d. Salter-IV fracture
e. Salter-V fracture

364. *A fracture that crushes the chondroblastic cell layer is considered a:*

a. Salter-I fracture
b. Salter-II fracture
c. Salter-III fracture
d. Salter-IV fracture
e. Salter-V fracture

365. *A 5-month-old German shepherd sustains a Salter-V fracture of the distal ulnar epiphysis. What is the most likely complication?*

a. nonunion caused by limited blood supply to the distal radius
b. nonunion caused by rotational forces
c. radius curvis caused by premature closure of the ulnar physis
d. radius curvis caused by premature closure of the radial physis
e. osteomyelitis caused by sequestration

366. *After a 5-year-old mongrel dog is hit by a car, you confirm a fracture of the left humeral diaphysis at the junction of the middle and distal thirds. Which nerve is most likely to be injured when the fracture occurs or during surgical repair?*

a. humeral nerve
b. lateral cutaneous brachial nerve
c. musculocutaneous nerve
d. radial nerve
e. ulnar nerve

367. *A 6-month-old sheltie is presented to your clinic with a fracture of the lateral condyle of the right humerus. The fracture line extends from the articular surface through the epiphysis and into the metaphysis. Which treatment offers the greatest chance for return of full function?*

a. closed reduction and a coaptation splint
b. open reduction and a single intramedullary pin
c. open reduction and a bone plate
d. open reduction and cancellous bone screws
e. open reduction and full-pin splintage

368. *A 4-year-old pointer is presented to your clinic with a comminuted fracture of the left acetabulum. Which approach provides the best exposure for repair of this fracture by plating?*

a. trochanteric osteotomy
b. gluteal "roll-up" procedure
c. separation of the vastus lateralis and rectus femoris muscles
d. ventral approach to the hip
e. dorsal intergluteal incision

369. *The most definitive indication of cranial cruciate ligament rupture in a dog is:*

a. the Ortolani sign
b. the cranial drawer sign
c. the caudal drawer sign
d. non-weight-bearing lameness
e. the Balani sign

370. *What type of meniscal damage is most likely to occur in conjunction with rupture of the cranial cruciate ligament?*

a. tear of the caudal body of the medial meniscus
b. tear of the cranial body of the medial meniscus
c. tear of the caudal body of the lateral meniscus
d. tear of the cranial body of the lateral meniscus
e. tear of the intermeniscal ligament

371. *A noninflammatory, nonneoplastic proliferative bone disease with a predilection for endochondral bone is:*

a. hypertrophic osteodystrophy
b. osteochondritis dissecans
c. panosteitis
d. hypertrophic osteoarthropathy
e. craniomandibular osteopathy

372. *A young growing dog is presented to you with a history of shifting-leg lameness of 3 weeks' duration. Physical examination reveals pain on compression of the long bones. The most likely cause of these signs is:*

a. hypertrophic osteodystrophy
b. osteochondritis dissecans
c. panosteitis
d. hypertrophic osteoarthropathy
e. craniomandibular osteopathy

373. *A dog with a fragmented coronoid process is best treated by:*

a. external immobilization with a cast and cage rest
b. removal of the process via medial arthrotomy
c. stabilization with a bone screw
d. removal of the process via lateral arthrotomy
e. dietary supplementation with calcium and limited exercise

374. *You review a radiograph of a dog's fractured femur. Multiple fracture lines converge on one point. This fracture is appropriately classified as:*

a. oblique
b. spiral
c. segmental
d. comminuted
e. bicondylar

375. *You review the radiograph of a dog's fractured tibia. The cortex on one side of the bone is broken, and the other is bent. This fracture is appropriately classified as a:*

a. fissure fracture
b. greenstick fracture
c. physeal fracture
d. comminuted fracture
e. compacted fracture

376. *Which fracture is best treated with a tension-band wire?*

a. avulsion fraction of the olecranon
b. compression fracture of the distal femoral physis
c. spiral fracture of the humeral diaphysis
d. segmental fracture of the femoral diaphysis
e. greenstick fracture of the distal ulnar metaphysis

Correct answers are on pages 260-275.

377. *Concerning the difference between osteochondrosis and osteochondritis dissecans, which statement is most accurate?*

a. Osteochondrosis is an abnormality of endochondral ossification, with asymmetric maturation into bone. Osteochondritis dissecans is a sequel to osteochondrosis in which a cartilaginous flap pulls loose from underlying bone.
b. Osteochondrosis is an abnormality of nutrition to the articular cartilage. Osteochondritis dissecans occurs when the articular cartilage becomes inflamed and separates from the underlying bone.
c. Osteochondrosis is a developmental defect of bone. Osteochondritis dissecans refers specifically to osteochondrosis of the humeral head.
d. Osteochondrosis does not result in a cleft that separates cartilage from bone, whereas osteochondritis dissecans does.
e. Osteochondrosis must be treated surgically, whereas osteochondritis dissecans can be treated with antiinflammatories and cage rest.

378. *Most coxofemoral luxations in dogs are the result of vehicular trauma. Which type of coxofemoral luxation is most common in dogs?*

a. lateral
b. caudoventral
c. craniodorsal
d. caudodorsal
e. ventral

379. *While performing small intestinal resection and anastomosis in a cat, you discover that the proximal segment of bowel has a diameter of approximately 20% greater than that of the distal segment of bowel. The easiest way to solve this problem is to:*

a. perform an end-to-side anastomosis
b. perform a side-to-side anastomosis
c. cut the distal segment of the intestine at a more oblique angle
d. perform a Bilroth-2 anastomosis

380. *An 8-month-old St. Bernard puppy is rushed to your clinic as an emergency at 11 PM. The owners saw the dog swallow a marble 1.5 cm in diameter. What is the most appropriate course of action?*

a. Make radiographs to confirm the presence of the foreign body; then administer general anesthesia and remove the foreign body with a gastroscope.
b. Make radiographs to confirm the presence of the foreign body; then administer general anesthesia and remove the foreign body by gastrotomy or enterotomy.
c. Administer apomorphine to induce vomiting.
d. Hospitalize the dog for observation.
e. Send the dog home, and instruct the owners to watch for vomiting or lack of appetite.

381. *During intestinal resection the mucosa frequently everts from the cut surfaces of the intestinal wall. What is the most appropriate way to manage such mucosal eversion in a small-breed dog?*

a. Suture the intestine with an inverting pattern.
b. Trim the everted mucosa with a scissors before suturing.
c. Suture the mucosal layer first, and then oversew the serosal layer.
d. Repeat the resection to remove bowel segment with the everted mucosa.
e. Suture the intestine with a modified Bunnell-Meyer pattern.

Question 382

A 4-year-old mongrel dog develops acute onset of neurologic signs. Physical examination reveals abnormalities only in the nervous system. Neurologic examination reveals the following:

Mental Status: alert, with no abnormalities noted
Cranial Nerves: no abnormalities noted
Posture and Gait: paraplegia

Postural Reactions:

	Left Front	*Left Rear*	*Right Front*	*Right Rear*
Wheelbarrowing	0	0	0	0
Ext Post Thrust	0	0	0	0
Hemiwalk	0	0	0	0
Consc Proprio	0	0	0	0
Hopping	0	0	0	0

Spinal Reflexes

	Left Front	*Left Rear*	*Right Front*	*Right Rear*
Biceps	1	—	—	1
Triceps	1	—	—	1
Patellar	—	1	1	—
Cranial Tibial	—	1	1	—
Gastrocnemius	—	1	1	—
Flexor	1	1	1	1
Anal Sphincter	—	1	1	—
Panniculus	absent caudal to thoracolumbar area			

Sensation: superficial pain absent in all four limbs, deep pain present in all four limbs.

382: *Which neurologic pathway is most likely affected?*

a. upper motor neuron to all four limbs
b. upper motor neuron to the rear limbs, lower motor neuron to the front limbs
c. lower motor neuron to all four limbs
d. lower motor neuron to the rear limbs, upper motor neuron to the front limbs
e. upper motor neuron to the front limbs

Questions 383 and 384

A 2-year-old female poodle suddenly refuses to stand or walk. Physical examination reveals abnormalities only in the nervous system. Neurologic examination reveals the following:

Mental Status: alert, with no abnormalities noted
Cranial Nerves: no abnormalities noted
Posture and Gait: paraplegia

Postural Reactions:

	Left Front	*Left Rear*	*Right Front*	*Right Rear*
Wheelbarrowing	0	0	0	0
Ext Post Thrust	0	0	0	0
Hemiwalk	0	0	0	0
Consc Proprio	0	0	0	0
Hopping				

Spinal Reflexes

	Left Front	*Left Rear*	*Right Front*	*Right Rear*
Biceps	3	—	—	3
Triceps	3	—	—	3
Patellar	—	3	3	—
Cranial Tibial	—	3	3	—
Gastrocnemius	—	3	3	—
Flexor	3	3	3	3
Anal Sphincter	—	3	3	—
Panniculus	absent caudal to thoracolumbar area			

Sensation: hyperesthesia over thoracolumbar area, superficial pain absent caudal to thoracolumbar area, deep pain present in all four limbs.

383. *Which neurologic pathway is most likely affected?*

a. upper motor neuron to all four limbs
b. upper motor neuron to the rear limbs, lower motor neuron to the front limbs
c. lower motor neuron to all four limbs
d. lower motor neuron to the rear limbs, upper motor neuron to the front limbs
e. lower motor neuron to the front limbs

Correct answers are on pages 260-275.

384. What is the most likely location of the lesion causing neurologic signs in this dog?

a. brain stem
b. C1-4 segment of the spinal cord
c. C5-T2 segment of the spinal cord
d. T2-L3 segment of the spinal cord
e. L3-S2 segment of the spinal cord

385. Which anatomic landmarks best help determine vertebral location during ventral decompressive surgery in a dachshund with a ruptured intervertebral disk at the C3-4 spinal cord segment?

a. wings of the atlas and ventral tubercle
b. wings of the atlas and ventral protuberance of the transverse spinous process of C7
c. wings of the atlas and ventral protuberance of the transverse spinous process of C6
d. ventral tubercle of C6 and wings of C1
e. intervertebral disk space of C1-2 and ventral protuberance of the transverse spinous process of C7

*386. Which of the following is **not** appropriate for hemostasis in castration of a cat?*

a. tying the vas deferens to the venous plexus on each side
b. tying the venous plexus on itself
c. ligating the venous plexus with absorbable suture
d. pulling the vas deferens and venous plexus until they stretch and break
e. applying hemostatic clips to the venous plexus

387. Concerning ovariohysterectomy in dogs, which statement is most accurate?

a. The left ovary is located farther cranially in the abdominal cavity than the right ovary, increasing the difficulty in exteriorizing the left ovary.
b. The right ovary is located farther cranially in the abdominal cavity than the left ovary, increasing the difficulty in exteriorizing the right ovary.
c. The ovaries are freely movable, but the cervix is difficult to exteriorize.
d. The ovarian arteries are small and rarely require ligation.
e. The uterine arteries are small and rarely require ligation.

388. To maximize the chances of future fertility in an adult dog, the incision for cesarean section should be made:

a. in the dorsal wall of the uterine body
b. in the ventral wall of the uterine body
c. in the ventral wall of the uterine horn containing more pups
d. in the dorsal wall of the uterine horn containing more pups
e. transversely in the ventral wall of the uterine body, extending from one horn to the other

389. Concerning perineal urethrostomy, which statement is most accurate?

a. A stent should be placed in the new urethral orifice to minimize the risk of stricture formation.
b. A stent is generally contraindicated because of the increased risk of ascending infection and interference with healing.
c. An indwelling urethral catheter is indicated until primary healing occurs.
d. The urethra should be flushed daily for the first 3 days to prevent clot formation that could cause urinary obstruction.
e. Topical corticosteroids should be applied to the suture line to minimize the risk of stricture.

390. While performing an ovariohysterectomy, your associate releases the stump of the right ovarian pedicle before it is ligated. He reaches into the abdomen with a hemostat and is about to clamp all the tissue in the vicinity of the bleeder. You stop him from doing this because of the risk of damage to the:

a. right ureter
b. caudal pole of the right kidney
c. caudal vena cava
d. pancreas
e. right ovary

391. *You have previously diagnosed a left-sided perineal hernia in an 11-year-old mongrel dog. For financial reasons the owners have delayed surgical repair. The dog is now presented to your clinic with a 24-hour history of anuria and distention in the left perineal area. You suspect that the urinary bladder has herniated into the perineal defect. Which technique will allow you to manually return the bladder to its normal anatomic position while preparing the animal for primary correction of the hernia?*

a. urethral catheterization to remove urine
b. administration of a diuretic to facilitate urine production
c. perineal incision over the bladder
d. caudoventral compression of the abdomen
e. cystocentesis to remove urine

392. *Which of the following is **not** an appropriate site for urethrostomy in dogs?*

a. preputial
b. prescrotal
c. scrotal
d. perineal
e. prepubic

393. *Dogs with portal vascular anomalies have a high incidence of which type of cystic calculi?*

a. cystine
b. struvite
c. ammonium urate
d. calcium oxalate
e. silica

394. *The Zepp procedure and modifications of the Zepp procedure have been used in management of chronic otitis externa refractory to medical therapy. Which of the following best describes the Zepp procedure?*

a. resection of the pinna to improve ventilation
b. resection of the lateral cartilaginous wall of the vertical ear canal, with formation of a ventral cartilaginous flap
c. ablation of the external ear canal
d. resection of the ventral cartilaginous wall of the horizontal ear canal
e. resection of the cartilaginous wall of the vertical and horizontal ear canals, with formation of cartilaginous flaps

395. *Drainage of the middle ear in animals with chronic or recurrent middle ear infections is best achieved via:*

a. myringotomy
b. pharyngeal bulla osteotomy
c. penetration of the tympanic membrane and ventral floor of the bulla with a Steinmann pin
d. Zepp procedure
e. ventral bulla osteotomy

396. *Surgical correction of a patent ductus arteriosus requires:*

a. resection of the ductus arteriosus
b. ligation of the ductus arteriosus
c. transection of the ductus arteriosus
d. anastomosis of the ductus arteriosus
e. transposition of the ductus arteriosus

397. *Surgical correction of a persistent right aortic arch requires:*

a. resection of the ligamentum arteriosus
b. ligation of the ligamentum arteriosus
c. transection of the ligamentum arteriosus
d. anastomosis of the ligamentum arteriosus
e. transposition of the ligamentum arteriosus

398. *Concerning traumatic diaphragmatic hernias in dogs, which statement is most accurate?*

a. The muscular portion of the diaphragm is more frequently torn than the central tendon.
b. The prevalence of left-sided hernias is significantly greater than the prevalence of right-sided hernias.
c. The spleen is the abdominal organ that most commonly herniates into the thorax.
d. Traumatic diaphragmatic hernias represent an emergency situation requiring immediate surgical correction.
e. Surgical correction of traumatic diaphragmatic hernias is not indicated unless signs of respiratory distress are evident.

Correct answers are on pages 260-275.

399. *In routine ovariohysterectomy of dogs, exteriorizing the ovaries is facilitated by:*

a. transection of the ovarian pedicle
b. stretching or breaking the suspensory ligament
c. extending the skin incision caudally
d. incision of the broad ligament
e. retraction of the colon on the left side and the duodenum on the right side

400. *A perineal hernia is most likely to occur in a:*

a. 4-year-old intact female beagle
b. 10-year-old spayed collie
c. 12-year-old intact male boxer
d. 4-year-old castrated sheltie
e. 16-year-old intact female Boston terrier

401. *How would you classify the suture material polydioxanone?*

a. synthetic nonabsorbable
b. synthetic absorbable
c. natural nonabsorbable
d. natural absorbable
e. monofilament nonabsorbable

402. *How would you classify the suture material polypropylene?*

a. synthetic nonabsorbable
b. synthetic absorbable
c. natural nonabsorbable
d. natural absorbable
e. monofilament nonabsorbable

403. *How would you classify the suture material chromic catgut?*

a. synthetic nonabsorbable
b. synthetic absorbable
c. natural nonabsorbable
d. natural absorbable
e. monofilament nonabsorbable

404. *Which suture material produces the* **least** *tissue reaction?*

a. chromic catgut
b. plain catgut
c. polyglycolic acid
d. polyester fiber
e. stainless steel

405. *Which suture material produces the most tissue reaction?*

a. chromic catgut
b. plain catgut
c. polyglycolic acid
d. polyester fiber
e. stainless steel

406. *Which suture pattern is considered everting?*

a. Cushing
b. simple continuous
c. vertical mattress
d. cross mattress
e. Ford interlocking

407. *Which suture pattern is considered inverting?*

a. Cushing
b. simple continuous
c. vertical mattress
d. cross mattress
e. Ford interlocking

408. *In a 1-year-old, 12-kg mongrel dog, which condition is most appropriately treated with a Schroeder-Thomas splint?*

a. irregular oblique mid-shaft fracture of the humerus
b. fracture of the distal femoral epiphysis
c. craniodorsal coxofemoral luxation
d. comminuted mid-diaphyseal tibial fracture
e. avulsion fracture of the olecranon

409. *A 3-year-old female golden retriever is brought to your clinic with a severely comminuted, highly unstable fracture of the left radius. Which of the following would provide the best temporary immobilization while you prepare for surgical repair?*

   a. Schroeder-Thomas splint
   b. fiberglass cast
   c. Velpeau bandage
   d. Ehmer sling
   e. Robert Jones bandage

410. *The Heineke-Mikulicz procedure has been recommended for surgical management of pyloric stenosis. Which of the following best describes this procedure?*

   a. longitudinal incision through all layers of the pylorus, except the mucosa
   b. longitudinal incision through all layers of the pylorus, sutured transversely
   c. Y-shaped incision in the pylorus, sutured as a V
   d. gastroduodenostomy
   e. longitudinal incision through all layers of the pylorus, with the mucosa sutured longitudinally

411. *The goal of surgical correction of an elongated soft palate is to have the caudal border of the soft palate located:*

   a. 1 cm caudal to the tip of the epiglottis
   b. at the tip of the epiglottis
   c. 1 cm rostral to the tip of the epiglottis
   d. at the level of the lateral saccules
   e. at the level of the fourth upper premolar

412. *A 12-month-old German short-haired pointer is presented to your clinic with left forelimb lameness of 6 months' duration. You suspect osteochondritis dissecans, and radiographs reveal a defect in the caudal aspect of the left humeral head. What is the most appropriate treatment for this dog?*

   a. cage rest for 2 months
   b. administration of corticosteroids as needed
   c. surgical exploration of the joint and curettage of the lesion, with removal of any joint mice
   d. surgical exploration of the joint, with removal of any joint mice
   e. intraarticular injection of corticosteroids, combined with cage rest

413. *In a 10-month-old German shepherd with acute onset of right forelimb lameness, radiographs reveal panosteitis. What is the most appropriate treatment for this dog?*

   a. daily administration of antiinflammatory dosages of corticosteroids for 2 months
   b. excision of the anconeal process
   c. culture of bone marrow aspirates, with administration of appropriate antibiotics
   d. reevaluation after 2 months of cage rest
   e. administration of aspirin as needed

414. *In routine elective surgery of small animals, which of the following does* ***not*** *increase the likelihood of wound infection?*

   a. prolonged operative time
   b. administration of corticosteroids
   c. crushing muscle tissue with hemostats
   d. rough handling of tissues
   e. good hemostasis

Questions 415 and 416

A dog sustained a laceration of the right metatarsal area 15 minutes previously. The owner presents the dog and has the leg wrapped in a tee shirt that is now soaked with blood. On removing the shirt, you find bright red blood spurting from the wound under pressure.

415. *In regard to source and time of occurrence, how is this dog's hemorrhage classified?*

   a. arterial, primary
   b. venous, primary
   c. capillary, primary
   d. arterial, intermediate
   e. venous, intermediate

Correct answers are on pages 260-275.

416. *You plan to repair the laceration. Before closing the wound, you must stop the hemorrhage. What is the most appropriate way to stop the hemorrhage from this wound, without likelihood of recurrence?*

a. crushing the vessels with hemostats
b. ligating any bleeders
c. applying a tourniquet
d. applying astringents
e. applying gentle manual or digital pressure

Questions 417 and 418

A cat is admitted for elective surgery. After making the skin incision, you note that blood oozes from the subcutaneous tissue under very low pressure.

417. *In regard to source and time of occurrence, how is this cat's hemorrhage classified?*

a. arterial, primary
b. venous, primary
c. capillary, primary
d. venous, intermediate
e. capillary, intermediate

418. *Before proceeding with the surgery, you decide to stop the bleeding. What is the most appropriate way to stop the hemorrhage at the surgical site, without likelihood of recurrence?*

a. crushing the vessels with hemostats
b. ligating any bleeders
c. applying an ice pack
d. applying astringents
e. applying gentle manual or digital pressure

419. *Properly placing subcutaneous sutures during closure of a routine skin incision is most likely to:*

a. improve hemostasis
b. decrease skin apposition
c. decrease dead space
d. improve strength of the healed wound
e. decrease contamination of the wound

420. *A dog sustains a skin laceration but is not presented for treatment until 24 hours later. The 4-inch wound exposes subcutaneous tissue only. How is this wound classified?*

a. clean
b. clean-contaminated
c. contaminated
d. dirty
e. necrotic

421. *Concerning function of electrosurgical units, which statement is most accurate?*

a. No current passes through the patient's body.
b. Current is concentrated at the active electrode.
c. Current is concentrated at the passive electrode.
d. Heat is produced in the transformer.
e. Heat is concentrated at the passive electrode.

422. *Why is a linen surgical drape considered contaminated if it becomes wet during a surgical procedure?*

a. Fluid diminishes the antibacterial action of the drape.
b. The fluid may contain disinfectants.
c. Fluid on the skin rinses away the disinfectant solutions.
d. Capillary action can draw bacteria through the material of the drape.
e. The space between threads of the drape increases with wetting.

423. *During a routine celiotomy, you discover a fatty structure adhered to the peritoneal surface of the linea alba, just cranial to the umbilicus. What is this structure?*

a. ligamentum arteriosus
b. falciform ligament
c. greater omentum
d. lesser omentum
e. gastrohepatic ligament

424. *In nephrectomy the ipsilateral ureter should be ligated and transected:*
   a. as close to the bladder as possible
   b. as close to the renal pelvis as possible
   c. at the midpoint of the ureter
   d. 4 cm distal to the renal pelvis
   e. 4 cm proximal to the ureterovesicular junction

425. *Cryosurgery has been advocated as treatment for perianal fistulae, superficial tumors, and other lesions in small animals. The most common cryogenic agent used in veterinary medicine is:*
   a. nitrous oxide
   b. freon
   c. liquid nitrogen
   d. liquid helium
   e. carbon dioxide

426. *During cryosurgery the frozen tissue is termed an ice ball. Not all tissue within the ice ball dies. Which tissue in the ice ball becomes necrotic after cryosurgery?*
   a. the most superficial two thirds of the tissue
   b. tissue that reaches -20° C or colder
   c. tissue in direct contact with the cryogen
   d. the most poorly perfused tissue
   e. the inner one third of the ice ball

427. *Laser surgery has predictable effects on soft tissue. In relation to the tip of the laser instrument, which area of tissue shows reversible changes?*
   a. zone of vaporization
   b. zone of carbonization
   c. zone of coagulation
   d. zone of edema
   e. zone of necrosis

428. *When using laser surgical instruments, the surgeon must carefully avoid "collateral" thermal injury. Collateral thermal injury is best avoided by:*
   a. using a carbon dioxide laser
   b. setting the laser at high power (60 to 100 watts)
   c. holding the instrument perpendicular to the tissue
   d. setting the laser at low power (20 to 40 watts)
   e. quickly making the incision

429. *In the surgical approach to the* ***right*** *kidney, what structure can be used to help retract the abdominal contents and facilitate visualization of the kidney?*
   a. spleen
   b. omentum
   c. descending colon
   d. descending duodenum
   e. broad ligament

430. *In the surgical approach to the* ***left*** *kidney, what structure can be used to help retract the abdominal contents and facilitate visualization of the kidney?*
   a. spleen
   b. omentum
   c. descending colon
   d. descending duodenum
   e. broad ligament

431. *Different tissues have differing reactions to cryosurgery. The factor that most influences a tissue's reaction to application of cold is:*
   a. proximity to major blood vessels
   b. amount of intracellular and extracellular water
   c. metabolic rate
   d. degree of perfusion
   e. surface area subjected to application of cold

432. *Which procedure is most effective in management of a descemetocele?*
   a. conjunctival flap
   b. third eyelid flap
   c. superficial keratectomy
   d. transposition of the parotid duct
   e. corneal eburnation

Correct answers are on pages 260-275.

433. *An untreated skin wound heals by a process of granulation, contraction, and reepithelialization. This type of healing is best termed:*

a. first-intention healing
b. second-intention healing
c. third-intention healing
d. fourth-intention healing
e. delayed primary closure

434. *In treatment of keratoconjunctivitis sicca, which surgical technique maintains corneal hydration?*

a. transplantation of the mandibular duct
b. transplantation of the zygomatic duct
c. transplantation of the parotid duct
d. conjunctival flap
e. superficial keratectomy

435. *In routine application of a bone plate for fixation of a long-bone fracture, how many screws should anchor the plate proximal and distal to the fracture line?*

a. at least one screw proximally and two distally
b. at least two screws proximally and one distally
c. at least three screws proximally and three distally
d. at least four screws proximally and two distally
e. at least five screws proximally and five distally

436. *A cat is presented to you with a laceration several days old. You elect to débride the wound, let it granulate for several days, and only suture the wound closed when all evidence of infection is gone. This type of wound healing is referred to as:*

a. first-intention healing
b. second-intention healing
c. third-intention healing
d. fourth-intention healing
e. primary closure

437. *In performing a paramedian abdominal approach in a dog, you enter the abdomen through an incision 1 cm to the right of the linea alba. In this approach the fibers of what muscle must be separated?*

a. external abdominal oblique
b. internal abdominal oblique
c. scalenus
d. rectus intermedius
e. rectus abdominis

438. *A cat is presented to your clinic with upper motor neuron signs to the rear limbs and lower motor neuron signs to the front limbs. What do these signs indicate?*

a. generalized neurologic disease
b. a lesion at C5-T2
c. a lesion at T2-L3
d. lesions at C1-5 and L4-S3
e. lesions at C5-T2 and L4-S3

439. *A dog is presented to your clinic with lower motor neuron signs to the rear limbs and upper motor neuron signs to the front limbs. What do these signs indicate?*

a. generalized neurologic disease
b. a lesion at C5-T2
c. a lesion at T2-L3
d. lesions at C1-5 and L4-S3
e. lesions at C5-T2 and L4-S3

440. *Which suture pattern is **not** considered appositional?*

a. simple interrupted
b. cross mattress
c. Ford interlocking
d. simple continuous
e. Connell

441. *A 5-year-old pointer is brought to your clinic with a craniodorsal luxation of the left coxofemoral joint. You attempt closed reduction. Which of the following should be applied after closed reduction of a coxofemoral luxation?*

a. Schroeder-Thomas splint
b. fiberglass cast
c. Velpeau bandage
d. Ehmer sling
e. Robert Jones bandage

442. *A 7-year-old mongrel dog is brought to your clinic with a fracture of the left scapula. The fracture parallels the spine of the scapula. Which of the following should be applied in initial management of this fracture?*

   a. Schroeder-Thomas splint
   b. fiberglass cast
   c. Velpeau bandage
   d. Ehmer sling
   e. Robert Jones bandage

443. *Which suture pattern is most appropriate for closure of the uterine stump after ovariohysterectomy for pyometra?*

   a. Cushing
   b. Bunnell
   c. Parker-Kerr
   d. simple interrupted
   e. vertical mattress

444. *Which technique does **not** help stabilize the stifle joint after rupture of the cranial cruciate ligament?*

   a. Paatsama technique
   b. over-the-top technique
   c. cranial transposition of the fibular head
   d. tibial crest transplantation
   e. imbrication of the lateral joint capsule

445. *Cushing and Lembert suture patterns are used primarily for closure of hollow organs. Which of the following most accurately describes the difference between Cushing and Lembert sutures?*

   a. Cushing sutures are everting, whereas Lembert sutures are inverting.
   b. Cushing sutures enter the lumen, whereas Lembert sutures do not enter the lumen.
   c. Cushing sutures are absorbable, whereas Lembert sutures are nonabsorbable.
   d. Lembert sutures are interrupted, whereas Cushing sutures are continuous.
   e. Cushing sutures parallel the incision line, whereas Lembert sutures are perpendicular to the incision line.

446. *Neurologic signs associated with rupture of intervertebral disks between T2 and T10 are very rare in dogs. Why is this so?*

   a. The dorsal longitudinal ligament prevents dorsal rupture.
   b. The disks from segment T2 to T10 do not degenerate.
   c. The intercapital ligaments prevent dorsal rupture.
   d. There are no disks from segment T2 to T10.
   e. The ventral longitudinal ligament prevents dorsal rupture.

447. *A 2-year-old mongrel dog is presented to your clinic with a luxation between the third sacral vertebra and first coccygeal vertebra. The dog has no voluntary motion of the tail and no deep pain sensation in the tail but exhibits extreme pain on manual elevation of the tail. Urinary and bowel function remains normal. What is the most appropriate treatment for this animal?*

   a. amputation of the tail at the site of the luxation
   b. amputation of the tail at the junction of the third and fourth coccygeal vertebrae
   c. open reduction of the luxation and stabilization with a plate
   d. open reduction of the luxation and stabilization with pins and wires
   e. conservative therapy consisting of corticosteroids and cage rest

448. *For repair of a mid-diaphyseal femoral fracture, the fascia lata is incised and the femur is exposed by retraction of the:*

   a. rectus femoris and biceps femoris
   b. vastus lateralis and biceps femoris
   c. rectus femoris and vastus lateralis
   d. vastus intermedius and rectus femoris
   e. vastus intermedius and biceps femoris

449. *For removal of a gastric foreign body, the stomach should be incised in an avascular area:*

   a. midway between the greater and lesser curvatures of the stomach
   b. of the lesser curvature of the stomach
   c. of the greater curvature of the stomach
   d. of the pylorus
   e. of the cardia

Correct answers are on pages 260-275.

450. *In routine surgery of the urinary bladder and stomach, use of "stay" or retention sutures is recommended. Which of the following most accurately describes a "stay" suture?*

a. suture place to prevent other sutures from slipping
b. suture placed to allow atraumatic manipulation of tissue
c. nonabsorbable suture that is not removed from the tissue
d. suture that is not removed from the tissue but that is eventually absorbed
e. suture placed to oversew the primary suture line

Answers

1. **e** Osteosarcoma is least likely to affect the mouth of dogs.
2. **a** Excision is the most effective treatment. Acanthomatous epulis may respond to radiation, but the other malignant tumors have a poor response to radiation alone. Immunotherapy is generally ineffective for oral tumors. Chemotherapy is generally ineffective for oral tumors. Cryosurgery may be curative for benign oral neoplasms and palliative for nonresectable malignant oral neoplasms.
3. **e** Most dogs can eat soft food within 24 hours after surgery. Drooping of the tongue occurs from disruption of the support to the tongue base and is often transient. It may be prevented by cheiloplasty at the time of surgery. Edema or ranula can occur and is usually transient. Incision dehiscence can occur as a result of self-trauma, excessive use of cautery during surgery, or excessive suture line tension. Mandibular drift can result in impaction of the lower canine into the hard palate, necessitating blunting of the tooth, or extraction in severe cases.
4. **b** The etiology is unknown, and there is usually no history of trauma. The accumulated saliva should be drained, and redundant tissue will regress. The lining of this area is nonepithelial and nonsecretory, so it does not need to be removed. The sublingual gland is most commonly involved. Surgery is the treatment of choice.
5. **c** The first choice is esophagoscopy. The second choice is advancing the foreign body into the stomach and then letting it dissolve or retrieving it via a gastrotomy. Esophagotomy is avoided because it is the most invasive treatment. Corticosteroids have not been shown to reduce stricture formation and may increase the chance of perforation. Oral food and water should be withheld to decrease mechanical trauma and encourage healing. Saliva is contaminated by oral bacterial flora.
6. **d** Most studies agree that most foreign bodies lodge in the hiatal region, although one study says the cervical esophagus is the most common site.
7. **a** Persistent right fourth aortic arch is characterized by megaesophagus cranial to the anomaly at the heart base. The approach is a left fourth intercostal thoracotomy to cut the ligamentum arteriosum crossing from the pulmonary artery to the aorta. Overall mortality from spontaneous death or euthanasia is 40% within the first few weeks after surgery.
8. **d** Gastrotomy is rarely required and is generally avoided because of the risk of abdominal contamination. Gastropexy is performed between the antral region of the stomach and the right body wall. Fluorescein is unreliable and may result in false-positive diagnosis of gastric ischemia from subserosal hemorrhage. Splenectomy is only indicated if the spleen is necrotic.
9. **c** The ability or disability to pass a stomach tube gives no information about the position of the stomach. Radiographs should be made with the dog in right lateral recumbency to distinguish gastric volvulus from gastric dilation. The stomach can become dilated after gastropexy, but it cannot rotate. Gastric dilation-volvulus has been reported in cats and small-breed dogs.
10. **b** Puppies and kittens have a much higher incidence of intussusceptions than adults. Most intussusceptions occur in the enterocolic region. The intussusceptum is "milked" from the intussuscipiens with minimal traction on the proximal segment. Early return to oral feeding is encouraged to stimulate normal gastrointestinal motility and avoid postoperative ileus.
11. **d** Open drainage is preferred.
12. **e** The cause is unknown. The anal sacs are often secondarily infected but may not be the source of the problem.

13. **c** Perineal hernias usually occur between the levator ani and external anal sphincter. Perineal hernias are common in males and rare in females. Recurrence rates vary between 31% and 45%. Postoperative incontinence may be temporary or permanent. Fecal incontinence persists when the pudendal nerves have been extensively damaged bilaterally, but these animals may still be acceptable pets if the stool is formed and the dog is taken outside frequently.
14. **d** The degree of shunt ligation should be based on portal venous pressure, central venous pressure, and such clinical criteria as bowel color and motility.
15. **e** Hypoglossal nerve damage may be a complication of the ventral approach but not the lateral approach.
16. **b** The middle and inner ears may still be functional. Radiographs often do not demonstrate otitis media, so bulla osteotomy should be performed in all cases of total ear canal ablation and considered in any cases with chronic otitis externa. (More than 50% of dogs with chronic otitis externa have coexisting middle ear disease.) Lateral ear resection may damage the parotid salivary gland. Facial nerve paralysis is a complication of total ear canal ablation.
17. **a** Full-thickness grafts are more likely to fail.
18. **a** Recurrent local trauma causes hygromas. This can be ameliorated with padded bandages or providing a padded surface to lie on. Drainage is only successful if the trauma ceases. Surgery may be indicated if conservative management fails or the hygroma is secondarily infected.
19. **e** Affected dogs do not have a collapsed trachea.
20. **c** Adenocarcinomas are the most common malignant stomach tumor in males 8 years of age and older.
21. **e** Just the opposite is true. The cervical portion of the trachea tends to collapse on inspiration, whereas the intrathoracic portion of the trachea tends to collapse on expiration.
22. **a** A midline laparotomy incision may be extended to a sternotomy for better exposure. The ninth intercostal approach may be used, but it requires knowing which side of the diaphragm is torn and does not allow thorough exploration of the abdominal cavity. An approach between the seventh and eighth ribs allows good exposure of the diaphragm but is more painful than laparotomy and does not allow exploration of the abdominal organs. A paracostal approach would not provide adequate exposure in most cases.
23. **e** Midline celiotomy is preferred because it provides the best exposure, is most familiar, and does not require incising muscle. Try to "milk" the placenta out, but leave it if it is firmly adhered. Have the owner watch to be sure it is expelled postoperatively, but do not incise the uterine horn. The bitch and her litter should be sent home as soon as possible, so she can be in a familiar environment. En bloc ovariohysterectomy may be performed if the owners want the bitch to be spayed. It is faster than cesarean section but requires more nonsterile assistants to recover the entire litter at one time.
24. **a** Castration offers no benefit in treating or preventing recurrence of perianal fistulae.
25. **d** Adenocarcinoma is the most common prostatic neoplasm.
26. **e** Urinary incontinence is the most common clinical sign, and is not specific for ectopic ureter. A contrast urethrogram is useful to identify urethral lesions. Cystograms are useful for identifying lesions of the bladder.
27. **b** Neoureterocystostomy is performed when the ureter runs within the bladder wall. Nephroureterectomy is a last resort. If the ectopic ureter can be corrected, hydroureter or hydronephrosis may resolve. Ureterotomy is primarily used to remove urinary calculi from the ureter. Ureteral anastomosis is useful for repairing a traumatized ureter.
28. **b** The urethra is more superficial and wider in this area. It is also surrounded by less cavernous tissue. Urine scald is less of a problem here than with perineal urethrostomy.
29. **d** Indwelling urinary catheters increase the likelihood of stricture formation. Concurrent use of antibiotics generally leads to infection with antibiotic-resistant organisms. A closed collection system delays onset of infection but does not prevent it. Smaller-diameter catheters are least likely to cause physical injury.
30. **e** Osteochondritis dissecans is least likely to affect the lateral trochlea of the humeral condyle.
31. **d** A fragmented coronoid process is rarely identified radiographically. Degenerative joint disease associated with a fragmented coronoid process may be treated conservatively with rest and antiinflammatories, but the fractured process is not resorbed. Fragmented coronoid process is often bilateral. Although resection is somewhat controversial, it is generally regarded as the treatment of choice if the fracture is diagnosed early. Fragmented coronoid process is more common in males than in females.

32. **c** The anconeal process normally fuses with the ulna at 16 to 24 weeks of age.
33. **c** The signs listed in answer a are consistent with panosteitis. Unilateral limb deformities are usually a result of trauma. The changes listed in answer e are consistent with hypertrophic osteopathy.
34. **b** Femoral head ostectomy is a salvage procedure and is only done as a last resort. A dog with a positive Ortolani sign and minimal degenerative joint disease should be evaluated as a candidate for a triple pelvic osteotomy. This dog is too young for a total hip replacement. Medical management would be acceptable, but triple pelvic osteotomy is recommended over this. Pectineomyotomy may help temporarily if the pectineus muscles are taut, but it is not a long-term solution.
35. **e** An incomplete autosomal recessive mode of inheritance has been suggested. Avascular necrosis of the femoral head (Legg-Calvé-Perthes disease) is usually unilateral and affects males and females with equal frequency. It is commonly seen in toy and miniature breeds and is treated by femoral head and neck ostectomy. Total hip replacement appliances are not available for toy breeds.
36. **d** The techniques listed in answers a and e do not exist. Trochlear chondroplasty can only be performed in young dogs, usually less than 6 months of age. Tibial tuberosity transposition is used to align the quadriceps mechanism.
37. **d** Chronic osteomyelitis is rare. Oral tissues readily eliminate infection.
38. **a** The affected limb is held with the elbow flexed and the antebrachium abducted and in external rotation. Radiographs should always be made to detect associated fractures and identify the degree of osteoarthritis in chronic cases. Although closed reduction may be difficult to achieve, the results are good in most cases. After reduction of elbow luxation, the limb should be placed in a spica splint. Keeping the elbow extended maintains the anconeal process in the olecranon fossa, which increases joint stability.
39. **a** Pubic fractures are rarely, if ever, repaired. An ischial fracture is usually not repaired unless repair would contribute to stability of other pelvic fractures or if impingement on the sciatic nerve is a concern. Minimally displaced sacroiliac luxations are often treated conservatively, especially if there is no narrowing of the pelvic canal and no injuries to other limbs. Surgical correction of sacroiliac luxation should be considered when the pelvic canal is narrowed. Stabilization should be considered because it is unstable bilaterally. Acetabular fractures in the cranial two thirds of the joint should always be surgically stabilized. Acetabular fractures in the caudal one-third of the joint may be treated conservatively. Ilial fractures are best treated surgically, even with minimal displacement.
40. **b** A Velpeau sling is used on the front limb for some congenital shoulder luxations and scapular fractures. A Robinson sling allows movement of the joints. A 90-90 flexion sling is used primarily to prevent quadriceps tie-down. A spica splint is a fortified Robert Jones bandage, extending over the torso. It is used for temporary preoperative stabilization of humeral or femoral fractures.
41. **c** Meniscal damage is more common medially than laterally.
42. **d** Schroeder-Thomas splints should be avoided for proximal limb fractures because they can act as a fulcrum to further displace the fracture. Radial fractures in small-breed dogs are prone to nonunion and are best fixed with internal fixation. It is not possible to put a Schroeder-Thomas splint on the mandible.
43. **a** An intramedullary pin would not provide rotational stability. Cerclage wire cannot be applied to transverse fractures. Schroeder-Thomas splints are not recommended for femoral fractures because the proximal frame may act as a fulcrum to displace the fracture. External fixators are usually not desirable as the sole fixation for a humeral or femoral fracture. A type-I or type-Ib fixator could be placed, but this would not be as stable as a bone plate. In addition, there is increased morbidity with a fixator placed on the proximal portion of a limb because of the large muscle mass the pins must penetrate.
44. **a** The distal ulnar physis tends to be the most susceptible to premature closure. Although the deformity described in answer a would occur with closure of the proximal radial physis, it is much less common. Premature closure of the distal radial physis is uncommon. Asymmetric closure of the distal radius is more common than complete symmetric closure; the signs described in answer c would be seen with asymmetric closure of the lateral distal radial physis. Varus deformity may be seen with asymmetric premature closure of the medial distal radial physis. There may be caudal radial and ulnar bowing as well.

45. **c** Flexing the neck ventrally could result in respiratory paralysis and death if the dens is intact. Congenital atlantoaxial luxation almost exclusively affects toy-breed dogs of either gender. There is usually no history of trauma. Signs often develop during normal activity. Tetraparalysis rarely occurs because affected dogs die from respiratory paralysis first.
46. **e** The ventral longitudinal ligament is ventral to the vertebral bodies and would not impinge on the spinal canal even if it were hypertrophied.
47. **e** With the first episode of neck pain, conservative management should be tried. Surgery is indicated if there are repeated episodes of neck pain or unrelenting pain. It is not necessary to wait until neurologic deficits develop, as with thoracolumbar disk herniation.
48. **d** A lesion at C1-5 would also cause upper motor neuron signs in the front limbs. A lesion at C6-T2 would also cause lower motor neuron signs in the front limbs. Although a disk rupture would most likely occur at T10-L3, the lesion cannot be localized this accurately with this neurologic examination. A lesion at L4-S2 would cause lower motor neuron signs in the hind limbs.
49. **a** Other findings help to localize the lesion, but the pain sensation indicates that the spinal cord is functionally intact.
50. **e** Easy bladder expression would be expected with a lower motor neuron bladder. Dribbling of urine would be expected with a lower motor neuron bladder. (A dog with an upper motor neuron bladder may dribble urine if the bladder is overfilled.) A lesion at S1-3 would cause a lower motor neuron bladder.
51. **c** The Cushing pattern is continuous and inverting and does not expose suture material to the lumen. The Connell pattern exposes suture material to the lumen. The Halsted pattern is not a continuous pattern.
52. **b** Chlorhexidine's activity is maintained in the presence of blood.
53. **a** Povidon-iodine has sporicidal action in addition to its gram-positive and gram-negative antibacterial activity.
54. **d** Isopropyl alcohol kills bacteria by coagulation of proteins.
55. **e** Sodium hypochlorite (Clorox) is more commonly used to disinfect environmental surfaces.
56. **c** Alcohol eliminates the cumulative antibacterial action of hexachlorophene.
57. **b** Hypertrophic osteopathy is characterized by multiple-limb lameness and pain on palpation of distal limbs. It usually occurs in older animals secondary to a space-occupying mass in the thoracic or abdominal cavity.
58. **d** Radiographs of the elbow would be sufficient to display the likely lesions. Resolution of bone scintigraphy is not sufficient to differentiate these diseases. Fluid from elbow arthrocentesis might be normal or indicate only mild degenerative change.
59. **b** Removal of the anconeal process through a lateral arthrotomy results in quick resolution of clinical signs.
60. **a** Osteochondrosis has not been reported in the temporomandibular joint of dogs.
61. **e** Osteochondrosis is most commonly found on the medial aspect of the lateral condyle of the femur and on the medial trochlear ridge of the talus.
62. **d** Coxa valga leads to lateral patellar luxation, whereas coxa vara predisposes to medial patellar luxation.
63. **d** Grade-IV patellar luxation is characterized by a patella that remains luxated and cannot be manually reduced.
64. **e** Patellectomy generally results in severe stifle degenerative changes and should only be used for severe patellar fractures that cannot be repaired.
65. **a** Sound principles of joint arthrodesis include primary closure of the joint to maintain aseptic conditions postoperatively.
66. **c** Cranial cruciate ligament rupture are rare in dogs less than 1 year of age. Ligaments are generally stronger than the bone in young dogs, so injuries in young dogs are more commonly physeal fractures.
67. **b** Fractures of the pubis are not commonly repaired in dogs unless they result in a caudal abdominal hernia.
68. **b** Vitamin C is not useful for treatment of hip dysplasia, either in growing or adult animals.
69. **d** The thumb is not displaced when the hip is luxated craniodorsally and the limb is externally rotated.
70. **b** Avascular necrosis commonly occurs in young (8 to 12 months old) toy-breed dogs.
71. **b** Salter-II physeal fracture is one in which the distal fragment includes all of the epiphysis and a portion of the metaphysis.

72. **c** Bending over the twist results in loss of tension in the wire (loosens the wire).
73. **e** The remnants of the ligamentum teres are generally inadequate to hold sutures or provide support.
74. **a** The long digital extensor muscle traverses the lateral aspect of the tibia.
75. **e** The hip joint should be extended and the limb adducted.
76. **d** This dog shows lower motor neuron front limb signs and upper motor neuron rear limb signs.
77. **b** An intradural spinal neoplasm would be an unlikely cause for these signs because of the acute onset noted.
78. **e** Ultrasonography cannot be used to adequately evaluate spinal structures because of the bony structures surrounding them.
79. **c** Ventral slot decompression would allow removal of disk material from the spinal canal at C6-7.
80. **d** The intervertebral disk at T4-5 is unlikely to rupture because of the added stability provided by the intercapital ligaments in that region.
81. **a** A single intramedullary pin would not provide any rotational stability in a mid-shaft transverse fracture.
82. **d** Joint immobilization leads to joint contracture, muscle atrophy, and other aspects of "fracture disease."
83. **b** Polypropylene is a nonabsorbable, very inert suture material.
84. **e** Polyglyconate is the strongest absorbable material at implantation but degrades faster than polydiaxanone.
85. **d** Nylon is considered nonabsorbable but does slowly degrade, releasing antibacterial degradation products.
86. **c** Stainless steel is the strongest available suture material.
87. **a** Degeneration of polyglycolic acid is accelerated on exposure to urine.
88. **e** Nonsurgical treatment of cranial cruciate ruptures in large dogs generally results in severe, progressive degenerative joint disease.
89. **a** Circumcostal gastropexy provides the strongest adhesion of stomach to body wall and decreases recurrence.
90. **c** Increasing the number of drain lumina (e.g., from single-lumen tube drains to triple-lumen sump drain) increases the drainage of fluid.
91. **a** Dogs that are DEA 1 negative (40% of the population) can serve as universal donors.
92. **e** Immediate rigid fixation is not necessary for proper treatment of open fractures. If the wound is adequately cleaned, débrided, lavaged, and bandaged, definitive fracture repair may be postponed.
93. **d** The Type-III configuration of external fixation devices provides rigid stability for most applications.
94. **b** The rectus femoris originates on the ilium just cranial to the acetabulum. The semitindinosus is a not a member of the quadriceps group. The three vastus muscles originate on the proximal femur.
95. **b** Olecranon osteotomy provides excellent visualization of the distal articular surface of the humerus and allows for more secure fixation in a mature dog than triceps tenotomy.
96. **c** The cell count, differential count, and mucin clot strongly implicate septic arthritis as a cause.
97. **d** Hypertrophic osteodystrophy is characterized by hot, swollen metaphyses, multiple-limb lameness, and a "double physeal line" on radiographs.
98. **e** Isografts are grafts between identical twins or cloned individuals.
99. **b** Osteoconduction is the process by which the former bone graft acts as a scaffold for the construction of new bone.
100. **a** Hind limb amputation by coxofemoral disarticulation is cosmetically undesirable, because it leaves little muscle coverage for pelvic prominences after muscle atrophy and it results in exposure of the genitals in male dogs.
101. **e** Examples include cefmetazole and cefoxitin.
102. **e** Most animals in need of surgery are hypernatremic, with dehydration of the hypertonic type.
103. **b** Pyloric obstruction typically causes metabolic alkalosis with low potassium and chloride levels.
104. **b** Normal saline is most appropriate for rehydration of these cats.
105. **b** Most cats have low blood calcium levels after thyroid removal.
106. **a** The approach is made on the left, at the fourth intercostal space.

107. **a** Diaphragmatic hernia rarely needs to be surgically corrected on an emergency basis. Initial treatment of these patients should include fluid and electrolyte support and supplemental oxygen as needed. Many affected cats have underlying lung lesions, such as hemothorax or pulmonary contusions. Fluids should be infused very cautiously to these patients, because they are predisposed to pulmonary edema. It is ideal to wait at least 48 to 72 hours before performing surgery. Occasionally, life-threatening situations, such as those posed by strangulated bowel, encroachment of the lungs by abdominal viscera, stomach dilation, or failure of the cat to respond to initial therapy, dictate the need for earlier surgical intervention (herniorrhaphy). The prognosis in these cases is generally worse.
108. **b** The sinus space is filled with pieces of the patient's fat, and the space is obliterated over time.
109. **a** This artery could be severed during entry into the thorax.
110. **c** The pulmonary ligament is severed to allow resection of the left caudal lung lobe.
111. **e** This approach provides the best exposure to the mesenteric lymphatics.
112. **d** Chylothorax is commonly caused by thoracic duct obstruction.
113. **d** Pulmonary edema is a common postoperative complication.
114. **b** A portion of the diaphragm is sometimes formed into an advancement flap to cover these defects.
115. **e** Ultra-short-acting barbiturates, such as thiamylal sodium, require biotransformation by the liver for elimination. Methoxyflurane, halothane, and ether require a greater amount of hepatic biotransformation than isoflurane and therefore are not as ideal for use in a patient with liver disease.
116. **d** Section of the recurrent laryngeal nerve denervates the cricoarytenoideus muscle.
117. **b** The sternohyoideus muscle is located medially.
118. **b** Fluid accumulated in the stomach may pass up the esophagus and be aspirated, causing pneumonia.
119. **c** In most cases of megacolon, the cause is unknown.
120. **d** Oral squamous-cell carcinoma is treated by resection.
121. **c** The approach should be made on the right, at the second or third intercostal space.
122. **b** A buccal flap is used to close these defects.
123. **d** The mandibular artery is ligated as it enters at the caudal end of the mandible, medially.
124. **b** Hemimandibulectomy is most likely to prevent recurrence.
125. **a** Contrast medium in the trachea indicates a connection between the esophagus and trachea.
126. **c** When an animal spontaneously begins to regurgitate, an acquired esophageal disorder should be suspected. If the animal has no history of regurgitation before an anesthetic or a surgical episode but shows these signs after such an experience, reflux esophagitis must be a primary differential diagnosis. Reflux of gastric contents into the esophagus during anesthesia can result in prolonged contact of gastric contents (acid, bile, pancreatic juices) with the esophageal mucosa. This can cause extensive mucosal damage and, if severe enough, could result in a stricture once healing is complete. Contrast esophagography and endoscopy will confirm the diagnosis of stricture.
127. **b** The esophageal mucosa has relatively good suture-retaining qualities.
128. **c** The azygos vein courses over the esophagus at this location.
129. **d** This procedure has been used with varying success.
130. **b** Scarring in this area is likely related to infection with liver flukes, which are prevalent in Florida.
131. **b** Cryptococcosis is the most common nasal fungal infection in cats.
132. **c** The ipsilateral inguinal lymph node should be removed during this procedure.
133. **e** The external artery and vein must be ligated during removal of the fifth mammary gland.
134. **b** Although the incision is made under aseptic conditions, the respiratory tract is in direct contact with the external environment and hence is considered contaminated.
135. **b** The ethmoturbinates are contiguous with the cribriform plate.
136. **c** Air commonly dissects along subcutaneous tissue planes after rhinotomy.

137. **b** Lack of an air-tight seal following rhinotomy may allow air to escape into the subcutaneous tissues around the head and neck. This subcutaneous emphysema may extend through the thoracic inlet and collect within the mediastinal space. If air continues to accumulate, the mediastinal barrier will be lost and air will escape into the pleural space, resulting in pneumothorax.
138. **d** Ventral bulla osteotomy is required to resect such polyps.
139. **c** These procedures widen the narrowed airway.
140. **b** This portion of the trachea is approached through the left third intercostal space.
141. **d** Tracheostomy tubes tend to become quickly obstructed with mucus unless kept clean.
142. **b** Tension across the suture line should be minimized to prevent stricture.
143. **c** Postoperative stricture is least likely to occur after incision in this area.
144. **c** It is best to remove the affected rib, along with one rib on either side.
145. **b** These defects can be filled with an omental pedicle flap.
146. **c** Doubling-over of the implant edges improves holding power of the sutures.
147. **e** The sublingual and mandibular salivary glands must be resected to resolve mucoceles in cats.
148. **b** The sublingual salivary gland is most often involved in mucocele.
149. **d** These veins can be seen after the hair has been shaved and the skin prepared.
150. **a** Mucoceles may occur in the pharynx, under the tongue, and under the skin of the neck.
151. **c** A sublingual mucocele is termed a *ranula.*
152. **d** Omental patches are used to reinforce closures in enterotomy and anastomosis.
153. **d** The jejunum is used as a reinforcing serosal patch.
154. **d** Extensive resection of small intestine may result in malabsorption.
155. **d** Periodic closure of the ileocolic valve delays transit of ingesta and allows time for absorption of nutrients and water.
156. **a** The horizontal mattress suture is an everting pattern.
157. **a** Cushing and Lembert sutures are inverting patterns.
158. **b** Pancreatic gastrinomas secrete excessive gastrin, stimulating release of gastric acid and leading to duodenal ulceration.
159. **c** Hypercalcemia is a common finding in cats with intestinal lymphosarcoma.
160. **a** Cats may survive up to 6 months after tumor resection.
161. **d** These findings are characteristic of lymphosarcoma.
162. **b** A mid-duodenal obstruction results in a tremendous loss of the bicarbonate present in pancreatic juices and bile. This also decreases the amount of bicarbonate ion available for absorption from the intestinal tract. This loss of bicarbonate ion may result in metabolic acidosis if vomiting is severe.
163. **e** The sternohyoideus muscle can be used to reinforce cervical esophageal suture lines.
164. **e** Strictures related to reflux esophagitis typically occur at the thoracic inlet.
165. **d** Of those defects listed, persistent right aortic arch is most likely to cause regurgitation in cats.
166. **a** Most hiatal hernias in cats are of the axial sliding type.
167. **d** A 360-degree fundoplication is used to prevent gastric reflux in cats.
168. **e** Gastric foreign bodies are relatively common in cats.
169. **c** Impaired passage of ingesta through the pylorus results in vomiting.
170. **b** This procedure widens the pyloric outflow tract.
171. **c** The Gambee suture is a modified simple interrupted suture pattern.
172. **e** Good tissue color, presence of peristalsis, and arterial pulsations are indications of viable bowel.
173. **a** The intussusceptum is invaginated into the intussuscipiens.
174. **d** Intussusceptions most commonly occur in the ileocolic valve area.
175. **b** Adenocarcinomas most commonly affect the ileum of cats.
176. **e** The atonic section of colon is resected.
177. **d** Gram-negative enteric and anaerobic bacteria can cause complications after large-bowel surgery.

178. **d** The microbes targeted in the colon are gram-negative enterics and anaerobes. Of the drugs listed, the one that will cover the spectrum of activity needed is a second-generation cephalosporin, such as cefoxitin or cefmetazole.
179. **d** Hemostasis is critical after liver biopsy.
180. **c** Hypersalivation is associated with portosystemic shunts in cats more often than in dogs.
181. **e** Portal hypertension leads to production of ascitic fluid.
182. **b** The cranial mesenteric vein supplies most of the portal blood flow.
183. **a** None of the other answers is accurate.
184. **e** Lactulose, neomycin, and a low-protein diet all contribute to decreasing the hyperammonemia present in affected animals. Lactulose changes the pH to a more acidic environment, preventing conversion of ammonium ions to ammonia, which is freely diffusible across the enteric mucosa. Neomycin kills colonic urease-producing bacteria that are responsible for converting intraluminal urea to ammonia. A low-protein diet makes fewer amino acids available, which act as a substrate for production of ammonia and other nitrogenous toxins.
185. **c** Furosemide use may result in hypokalemia and alkalosis. Excessive loss of potassium increases renal output of ammonia. Alkalosis enhances transfer of ammonia into the central nervous system, which may worsen hepatoencephalopathy.
186. **d** When isolating the pancreas for removal, the blood supply common to both the duodenum and the pancreas is the pancreaticoduodenal artery and vein. Disruption of these vessels during pancreatotomy may result in loss of viability of the adjacent duodenum.
187. **c** Pancreatic trauma may result from rough handling of the pancreas by the surgeon. A potential sequela is pancreatitis.
188. **b** The cranial thyroid artery arises from the common carotid artery.
189. **a** If an extracapsular technique of bilateral thyroidectomy is used, parathyroid tissue may be removed as well. Loss of the parathyroid glands can result in hypoparathyroidism and decreased serum calcium levels.
190. **c** The intracapsular technique for thyroidectomy is used to preserve parathyroid tissue and prevent hypocalcemia. Although this more conservative approach may preserve parathyroid function, it may result in incomplete removal of thyroid tissue, which could lead to recurrence of signs related to hyperthyroidism.
191. **d** Signs of hypocalcemia typically develop 1 to 3 days after thyroidectomy.
192. **b** Overly tight application of the tourniquet may damage the radial nerve.
193. **e** The ischiatic nerve courses through this area and may become entrapped during fracture repair.
194. **c** This is the only way to prevent recurrence.
195. **c** Increased hydrostatic pressure in the ipsilateral kidney leads to dysfunction over the ensuing 4 to 5 weeks.
196. **b** The renal artery can be safely occluded for up to 25 minutes without damaging the kidney.
197. **e** The ischiocavernosus muscle must be resected during urethrostomy.
198. **c** "Blocked" cats typically show metabolic acidosis, with elevated potassium and blood urea nitrogen (BUN) levels.
199. **d** Bladder wall incisions are closed with inverting Lembert sutures.
200. **d** The bulbourethral glands indicate the most caudal portion of the pelvic urethra.
201. **a** Stricture of the incision can lead to recurrent obstruction.
202. **e** Antepubic urethrostomy bypasses the narrowed or damaged portion of the urethra.
203. **d** This is the most likely cause of vulvar bleeding 3 weeks after queening.
204. **d** *E. coli* is most commonly isolated from pyometra fluid samples.
205. **d** *E. coli* is most likely to be involved with pyometra. The drug with the most efficacy against this microbe should be chosen. Of the choices available, a second-generation cephalosporin would be most effective.
206. **c** This procedure is typically used in resecting otic tumors.
207. **d** The parietal vaginal tunic is incised in "open" castrations.
208. **c** Urine spraying behavior and territoriality are inconsistent and may be present even in castrated cats. Castration has no effect on the prevalence of urethral obstruction. Similarly, the retractor penis muscle is not affected by the absence or presence of male hormones. Therefore the only consistently predictable sign of retained testicles is the spines on the penis.

209. **a** Viable sperm may be ejaculated for up to 50 days after castration.
210. **d** This describes the round ligament of the uterus.
211. **d** Removing a portion of the genital tract is not likely to correct a uterine prolapse. Suturing the uretus to the colon is not likely to help because the colon is moveable. The technical difficulty of placing a pursestring suture in the vaginal vault, combined with the unpredictable results, makes this a poor choice of therapy for this condition. Hysteropexy gives good results and is relatively simple to perform.
212. **c** Episiotomy is done to widen the vaginal opening for delivery of fetuses and for some surgical procedures.
213. **e** Mammary tumors in cats are usually highly malignant. For this reason, increased disease-free intervals and longevity are best served by an aggressive surgical approach. This involves a complete chain mastectomy with regional lymph node removal, followed by removal of the opposite chain 3 to 4 weeks later.
214. **b** Tissue macrophages, fibroblasts, granulocytes, and capillary buds are all components of wound healing.
215. **c** Macrophages direct early wound repair.
216. **c** Wound contraction occurs after influx of myofibroblasts.
217. **c** This phenomenon aids wound contraction to close large wounds.
218. **c** Zinc methionine can be given orally at 15 mg/10 kg of body weight.
219. **e** Axial-pattern flaps contain a cutaneous artery and vein.
220. **b** The myocutaneous flap is a composite flap of muscle and skin.
221. **b** The median nerve and brachial artery course through the supracondylar foramen in cats.
222. **a** The prevalence of cryptorchidism in Persian cats is approximately 15 to 20 times greater than in other breeds.
223. **d** Mammary hyperplasia-fibroadenoma complex is a benign condition of young, intact queens. Mammary hyperplasia typically occurs 2 to 4 weeks after estrus. Mammary neoplasia occurs in older cats. Mastitis and abscesses cause pain and often systemic signs of illness.
224. **e** The horizontal mattress suture is an everting pattern and should not be used for closure of an organ because healing is slower than with appositional and inverting patterns. The simple interrupted pattern is an appositional pattern. Lembert, Cushing, and Connell patterns are inverting patterns.
225. **c** Hyperkalemia, not hypokalemia, results from urinary tract obstruction.
226. **a** Cultures for aerobic and anaerobic bacteria, mycobacteria, *Mycoplasma,* and fungi are negative. Growth of organisms may be noticed when a specific L-form culture medium is used.
227. **c** L-forms are bacteria that have lost part of their cell wall and may revert to a parental form. Antibiotics that interfere with cell wall synthesis are ineffective. Patients usually respond to tetracycline therapy within 48 hours.
228. **d** Horner's syndrome occurs in up to 80% of cats undergoing this procedure, but it often resolves within 2 weeks of surgery. Otitis interna occurs in up to 40% of cases. Other complications are reportedly much less common.
229. **b** The sympathetic nerves enter the middle ear canal at the caudal edge of the promontory of the petrous temporal bone in the middle ear, course through the promontory, and exit the middle ear at the apex of the petrous temporal bone. Avoiding damage to the surface of the promontory of the petrous temporal bone during polyp removal reduces the incidence of Horner's syndrome.
230. **e** Propranolol is a β-adrenoceptor–blocking agent that helps to decrease the heart rate in cats with tachycardia. The other drugs listed are either inappropriate for management of sinus tachycardia in general or have a relatively low safety index in cats.
231. **c** Hypocalcemia may occur 1 to 3 days after bilateral thyroidectomy if the parathyroid glands have been compromised during surgery. The signs listed are typical of hypocalcemia in cats. Seizures may also occur.
232. **a** No attempt is made to preserve the internal parathyroid glands because they are difficult to find within the parenchyma of the thyroid gland. The external parathyroid glands are typically located on the cranial pole of the thyroid gland; care should be taken to preserve them. Special care should be taken to identify the parathyroid gland because occasionally it may be found on the caudal pole of the thyroid gland.

233. **b** The celiac artery is spared during colectomy. The other vessels listed supply blood to portions of the colon that are removed during colectomy.
234. **c** Barium is contraindicated if perforation of the gastrointestinal tract is suspected, because it may cause peritonitis.
235. **b** Adducting the femur and extending the coxofemoral joint allow the pin to exit the trochanteric fossa away from the sciatic nerve. Flexing the hip joint and/or abducting the femur place the pin closer to the nerve when driving the pin in retrograde fashion.
236. **e** Hemicerclage wiring is not appropriate to stabilize a separation of the proximal femoral epiphysis because the wire cannot be placed in a nonarticular location in the proximal femoral epiphysis; the resulting stability is poor.
237. **d** *Pasteurella,* streptococci, and anaerobic bacteria are commonly found in the feline oral cavity.
238. **a** Chronic progressive polyarthritis is the most likely diagnosis in this case. Rheumatoid arthritis is very rare in cats and is an erosive polyarthritis. Systemic lupus erythematosus is also rare and exhibits minimal, if any, radiographic changes. Polyarthritis as a result of *Mycoplasma* infection also produces minimal radiographic changes. Polyarthritis associated with calicivirus infection occurs in young kittens.
239. **e** The pubis and ischium are non-weight-bearing and nonarticular portions of the pelvis. Nearly all fractures of these bones may be managed conservatively. The ilium, sacroiliac joint, and acetabulum are weight-bearing and/or articular portions of the pelvis. Although some of these fractures may be managed conservatively with good results, they are much more likely to require surgical treatment for optimal results.
240. **c** The De Vita pinning technique is not recommended in cats because the straight ilium of cats precludes adequate seating of the pin into the ilium.
241. **b** A spica splint is appropriate to maintain the elbow in an extended position and stabilize the joints proximal and distal to the injury. Flexion of the elbow may allow reluxation.
242. **c** Approximately 25% of cats develop urinary tract infections following perineal urethrostomy; however, some cats may not display signs of urinary tract infection.
243. **a** Tonsillar squamous-cell carcinoma is the most likely diagnosis in an older cat with a unilateral mass in the oropharynx. Lymphosarcoma is also possible, but it is less common in this location and is usually bilateral.
244. **d** This combination of signs in a cat of this age is most consistent with a portosystemic shunt. The key signs are those associated with hepatic encephalopathy. Ptyalism is also common in cats with portosystemic shunts.
245. **b** Cats with portosystemic shunts may exhibit any of these laboratory findings except elevated blood urea nitrogen concentration. The blood urea nitrogen level would likely be subnormal in affected cats.
246. **c** Traumatic rupture of the cranial cruciate ligament is the most common cause of degenerative osteoarthritis of the canine stifle joint.
247. **d** Grade-IV medial patellar luxation is the classification characterized by the most severe bone lesions and clinical signs.
248. **e** Wedge resection of the trochlear groove deepens the femoral sulcus and maintains articular cartilage contact between the patella and femur.
249. **a** The stifle joint is a complex, condylar, synovial joint.
250. **b** A medial meniscal tear occurs in 40% to 60% of the cases involving rupture of the cranial cruciate ligament.
251. **b** Rupture of the cranial cruciate ligament causes cranial drawer motion of the tibia relative to the femur.
252. **b** Treatment for medial luxation of the patella requires a medial relief incision and lateral tightening procedures.
253. **a** A derotation, nonabsorbable suture between the lateral fabella and tibial tuberosity is classified as an extracapsular repair.
254. **a** Surgical treatments for cranial cruciate ligament injury include extracapsular or intracapsular repairs.
255. **e** Lateral patellar luxation in large dogs can be associated with ipsilateral hip dysplasia.
256. **d** A median sternotomy provides the greatest exposure for organs in the thoracic cavity.
257. **a** A left fourth intercostal thoracotomy is used most frequently for repair of a patent ductus arteriosus or patent ductus venosus.

258. **c** A persistent right aortic arch produces postprandial regurgitation at weaning.
259. **d** The most common congenital cardiac anomaly in dogs is patent ductus arteriosus.
260. **a** The most common congenital cardiac anomaly in cats is ventricular septal defect.
261. **b** Tetralogy of Fallot is the most common congenital cardiac disease causing cyanosis in dogs.
262. **a** Treatment for patent ductus arteriosus includes ligation of the shunt.
263. **e** Treatment for chylothorax includes avoidance of long-chain fatty acids in the diet.
264. **a** Flail chest is unstable thoracic wall segment associated with paradoxic chest motions.
265. **c** An arteriovenous fistula or shunt is an abnormal communication between an artery and a vein.
266. **d** Splenic neoplasia is most often and most easily treated by splenectomy.
267. **d** Gastric dilatation-volvulus occurs most frequently in large dogs that have exercised after eating.
268. **c** Intervertebral disk degeneration (disease) commonly produces signs of neurologic dysfunction, including pain, paresis, and paralysis.
269. **b** The signs of lumbosacral stenosis, including caudal pain and paresis, are not affected by vitamin E or selenium injections.
270. **a** Thoracolumbar disk herniation causes upper motor neuron signs (hyperreflexia and spasticity) in the hind limbs.
271. **b** Progressive cervical vertebral instability requires spinal cord decompression and vertebral stabilization.
272. **d** Degenerative myelopathy of German shepherds is a progressive, nonpainful condition characterized by hind limb paresis.
273. **c** The caudal thoracic intervertebral disks are frequently associated with degeneration and disease in chondrodystrophic dogs.
274. **a** Eustachian tube dilation is not associated with the brachycephalic syndrome.
275. **d** Ventral flexion of the neck is not associated with laryngeal surgery.
276. **c** Dorsal rhinotomy is the most common surgical procedure of the nasal cavity.
277. **c** Tracheostomy provides a passage for movement of air into the trachea and lungs, circumventing an upper air obstruction.
278. **b** An oronasal fistula associated with severe periodontal disease most frequently produces a communication between the oral and nasal cavities.
279. **c** Osteochondritis dissecans has not been reported in the carpal joints.
280. **c** Treatment for osteochondritis dissecans includes cartilage flap removal and subchondral bone curettage to stimulate fibrocartilage formation.
281. **c** A fragmented medial coronoid process associated with lameness in a rapidly growing dog should be excised.
282. **a** Traumatic hip luxations usually occur in a craniodorsal direction because of the pull of the gluteal muscles.
283. **e** A De Vita pin can be used to stabilize a traumatic hip luxation.
284. **e** A type-V Salter-Harris physeal injury associated with crushing of germinal cells warrants the poorest prognosis.
285. **b** In repair of epiphyseal fractures, the primary goal is articular cartilage congruency producing joint stability.
286. **e** An intramedullary pin can only provide axial alignment and resistance to bending forces.
287. **a** A dynamic compression plate secured by screws provides the greatest degree of compression across a fracture line.
288. **a** Primary bone union most frequently occurs when a fracture is stabilized with a bone plate and screws.
289. **d** A ruptured urinary bladder produces metabolic acidosis, hyperkalemia, and azotemia and should be repaired before definitive orthopedic surgery.
290. **c** A portosystemic shunt produces central nervous system derangements because of excessive accumulation of toxic metabolites normally handled by a liver perfused by the portal vein and its tributaries.
291. **e** Ectopic ureters are treated by ligation and reimplantation into the urinary bladder.
292. **b** Episioplasty refers to excision of redundant skin around the vulva that has caused a perivulvar dermatitis, especially in overweight dogs.
293. **c** Of the answers listed, only an external fixator can provide axial alignment, rotational stability, and interfragmentary compression.

294. **e** Prophylactic antibiotics should be administered intravenously immediately before surgery, after induction of general anesthesia.

295. **b** Of the answers listed, intravenous antibiotics provide the highest drug concentration in serum, plasma, and tissues.

296. **e** An insulinoma is a solitary tumor of the pancreas that causes profound hypoglycemia.

297. **c** A Robert Jones bandage can reduce soft tissue swelling and provide temporary stability for a fractured tibia.

298. **d** Corticosteroids, such as dexamethasone, can effectively reduce inflammation and spinal cord swelling in traumatic or disk-associated injuries.

299. **c** Chronic obstipation and megacolon in cats can be effectively treated by removal of the affected segment of colon.

300. **a** Perianal fistulae are abscesses around the anus and tail base in German shepherds. They require surgical treatment.

301. **c** This approach provides the greatest possible exposure to explore the abdominal contents.

302. **d** If the viability of small intestines is in question, resection and anastomosis are the preferred surgical approach. Attempting to move an irregularly shaped foreign body within devitalized intestine risks significant intestinal damage.

303. **a** The antimesenteric surface should be shorter than the mesenteric surface. This maximizes the blood supply to the antimesenteric surface.

304. **d** The simple interrupted pattern placed in a crushing manner is simple and effective. The suture locks on the submucosa, which is the layer with the greatest holding strength.

305. **b** Upper motor neuron lesions cause loss of inhibitory function. Reflexes are exaggerated, and postural reactions are depressed to the rear limbs.

306. **c** Exposure to the level of the transverse spinous processes allows fenestration.

307. **a** The last rib originates at the thirteenth thoracic vertebra and is directed caudally. The transverse spinous process of the first lumbar vertebra is directly cranially. It is easy to palpate and visualize these structures.

308. **e** Fat disappears from the epidural space at sites of spinal cord compression. Decompression should proceed both cranially and caudally until epidural fat is observed.

309. **b** In cats, castration is performed through two scrotal incisions, one directly over each testicle.

310. **a** In dogs, castration is performed through one prescrotal incision. The testicles are pushed cranially into the prescrotal subcutaneous tissue, and the incision is made on the midline just cranial to the scrotum.

311. **d** The skin incision for ovariohysterectomy in cats is made midway between the umbilicus and pubis. The anatomic structure that is most difficult to exteriorize is the uterine body; therefore the incision must be made more caudally (as compared with the incision for ovariohysterectomy in dogs) to allow exposure of the uterus.

312. **a** The skin incision for ovariohysterectomy in dogs is started at the umbilicus and continued caudally. The anatomic structure that is most difficult to exteriorize is the right ovary; therefore the incision must be made more cranially (as compared with the incision for ovariohysterectomy in cats) to allow exposure of the ovaries.

313. **e** The bulbourethral glands represent the junction of the dilated pelvic urethra and the constricted penile urethra. The new urethral orifice must be constructed using dilated pelvic urethral tissue.

314. **c** The ureter, passing obliquely through the bladder wall, is compressed as the bladder fills with urine. This reduces backflow of urine into the ureter and renal pelvis with increasing bladder pressure.

315. **d** When incisions parallel skin tension lines, only a minimal gap is created because of less tension pulling the wound apart. This reduces the likelihood of dehiscence.

316. **c** Suture material in the bladder lumen can serve as a nidus for formation of cystic calculi.

317. **a** A drain minimizes the chances for infection and scarring.

318. **d** This represents a dehiscence of the abdominal wall and requires repair. It will not heal without surgical closure.

319. **a** The degree of callus formation is inversely related to the stability of a fracture.

320. **d** Callus formation in bone healing is classified on the basis of location. Callus can be periosteal, intercortical, or medullary. With intramedullary pin stabilization, all three types of callus may form. With plate and screw fixation, the primary callus formed is intercortical. There may be some medullary callus formed with plate and screw fixation.

321. **e** Bone fragments should be incorporated into the repair. They should only be discarded if the wound is contaminated and the risk of infection is great. Fragments of cortical bone, even devoid of blood supply, function as autogenous bone grafts.
322. **c** The serratus dorsalis could not be in the surgical field in this procedure. It is located dorsal to the surgical field.
323. **a** The preferred closure of the esophagus is two layers. The first layer captures the mucosa and submucosa. The second layer closes the muscularis and adventitia.
324. **d** Correcting and preventing recurrence of salivary mucocele generally do not involve excision of the cyst itself. The responsible salivary glands (mandibular and sublingual) are excised, and the cyst is drained.
325. **b** Connell sutures penetrate all layers and enter the lumen. Cushing sutures do not enter the lumen.
326. **a** Heller's myotomy is used to expand the esophageal-gastric junction. The other four procedures may be used to expand the lumen of the pyloric-intestinal junction.
327. **b** Suturing a longitudinal incision transversely expands the diameter of the intestine at that site.
328. **a** Omentum adheres to the intestinal incision rapidly, creating a fluid-tight seal.
329. **c** Elongated soft palate, laryngeal collapse, stenotic nares, and everting laryngeal saccules can all be managed surgically. There is no effective surgical management for tracheal hypoplasia.
330. **b** Osteochondritis dissecans of the right humeral head is the most likely cause, considering pain on extension of the shoulder and partial weight bearing.
331. **a** Contusions are classified as closed wounds.
332. **e** Puncture wounds are most likely to result in infection because of impeded egress of foreign material or exudates from the wound.
333. **e** Delayed closure of this wound would minimize scarring. Débridement and leaving the wound open until a healthy bed of granulation tissue develops would minimize infection.
334. **b** Allografts (also called homografts) are grafts between different animals of the same species.
335. **c** The stratum basale of the ungual crest contains germinal cells that give rise to the claw. These cells must be removed to prevent regrowth of the claw.
336. **b** A patent ductus arteriosus is best approached through the left fourth intercostal space.
337. **b** The thoracotomy approach for PRAA is the same as for patent ductus arteriosus (PDA) (left fourth).
338. **a** The problem associated with PRAA is that the ligamentum arteriosus creates a constriction of the thoracic esophagus. Your objective is to remove that constriction.
339. **e** Sialoliths are removed through an oral incision. The incisions are left open to drain saliva into the mouth.
340. **b** The caudal thoracic esophagus is best approached through a right eighth intercostal thoracotomy.
341. **d** Recent studies have failed to confirm the value of pyloroplasty in preventing recurrence of gastric dilatation-torsion.
342. **a** The transthoracic approach is generally preferred and is performed at the right seventh intercostal space. The transabdominal approach involves needle entry on the left between the xyphoid and the coastal arch.
343. **d** The most common sites for bone marrow aspiration are the iliac crest and the proximal femur.
344. **b** Partial splenic rupture is an indication for partial splenectomy. Partial splenectomy is contraindicated in splenic neoplasia, regardless of the location of the tumor.
345. **a** Hansen's type-I classification is chondroid metaplasia. It occurs in young chondrodystrophoid dogs and results in massive rupture.
346. **b** Many factors influence selection of the appropriate techniques for management of cervical intervertebral disk disease. Absence of clinical signs generally precludes surgical management, whereas the presence of motor or sensory deficits indicates the need for decompression.
347. **c** The calculi are exposed by longitudinal incision through the renal parenchyma.
348. **e** Cystotomy, combined with urethral backflushing, allows use of only one surgical procedure. The backflushing may be unsuccessful, at which point urethrotomy or urethrostomy may be indicated.
349. **a** Bone plates are most likely to neutralize all forces acting on a fracture.

350. **b** A single intramedullary pin by itself will not neutralize rotational forces.
351. **e** Diaphragmatic hernia, especially acute hernias with little chance of adhesion formation, are repaired through a ventral abdominal midline approach.
352. **c** The approach to incisional hernias should take advantage of the tissue already actively involved in the healing process. Débridement or excision of the existing wounds removes this advantage.
353. **a** The coccygeus, levator ani, external anal sphincter, and internal obturator muscles may all be used in repair of a perineal hernia. Of the muscles mentioned, only the rectococcygeus would not be involved.
354. **e** Perineal hernias occur most commonly in older male dogs. Several breeds, including collies and Boston terriers, are overrepresented.
355. **c** A left-to-right shunt causes dilation of the pulmonary artery, predisposing it to tearing or rupturing.
356. **d** Retrograde pinning implies that the pin is initially inserted at the fracture site, driven out the proximal end of the femur, and redirected distally. Positioning the limb in a normal weight-bearing position with slight adduction is necessary to minimize soft tissue injury and prevent impingement on the sciatic nerve.
357. **b** Eccentrically placed screws result in shear and loss of reduction.
358. **e** Buttress plates bridge defects in diaphyseal bone.
359. **a** Tension-band plates convert tensile forces into compressive forces.
360. **a** Compression plating to establish rigid fixation is the most appropriate choice. Débridement is not necessary as long as the bone ends are viable.
361. **b** In cases of nonhealing fractures complicated by osteomyelitis, implants providing rigid stability should not be removed unless they are keeping a sequestrum in place.
362. **a** Salter-I fractures are transverse fractures through the region of cartilage hypertrophy.
363. **b** Salter-II fractures are transverse fractures through the region of cartilage hypertrophy that extend into the metaphysis.
364. **e** Salter-V fractures are compression fractures of the epiphysis.
365. **c** Compression fractures of the ulnar epiphysis most likely result in radius curvis because of premature closure of the ulnar physis.
366. **d** The radial nerve crosses the humerus at the site of the fracture and must be reflected during surgical repair.
367. **d** The joint should be opened to visualize the reduction. The fracture should be stabilized with cancellous bone screws.
368. **a** Trochanteric osteotomy allows elevation of the gluteals and complete exposure of the dorsal aspect of the acetabulum.
369. **b** The cranial drawer sign is observed with cranial cruciate ligament damage.
370. **a** Tearing of the caudal body of the medial meniscus is the most common injury and the most difficult to detect on exploration of the stifle.
371. **e** Craniomandibular osteopathy is a noninflammatory, nonneoplastic proliferative bone disease occurring in young animals. It has a predilection for endochondral bone.
372. **c** Panosteitis causes shifting-leg lameness and long-bone pain in young growing dogs.
373. **b** The coronoid process is removed through a medial approach to the elbow joint.
374. **d** A comminuted fracture involves splintering or fragmentation, with multiple fracture lines converging on one point.
375. **b** Fractures on one side of the bone, with bending of the opposite side, are called *greenstick fractures.* They occur primarily in young growing dogs.
376. **a** Tension-band wires are applied in situations in which the bone fragments are distracted because of the pull of tendinous insertions of muscles.
377. **a** Osteochondrosis refers to an abnormality of endochondral ossification, with asymmetric maturation to bone. It may result in a horizontal cleft separating the articular cartilage from bone. Osteochondritis dissecans is a sequel to osteochondrosis, in which a vertical cleft arises and a cartilaginous flap pulls loose from underlying bone.
378. **c** Craniodorsal luxation is most common, with reports of 75% of greater incidence.
379. **c** The lumen diameter of the distal segment can be increased by cutting it at a more oblique angle.
380. **e** This foreign body should pass through the alimentary system of a large-breed dog with no problem. Good client education is important.

381. **b** Trimming the excess mucosa facilitates tissue apposition during the anastomosis.
382. **c** All four limbs show decreased proprioception and decreased reflexes.
383. **a** All four limbs show decreased proprioception and increased reflexes. The lesion is in the upper motor neuron to all four limbs.
384. **b** Upper motor neuron signs for all four limbs indicate a high cervical lesion.
385. **c** The wings of the atlas and the large ventral protuberance of the sixth cervical vertebra allow you to determine location. These landmarks can then be used to count cranially and caudally.
386. **d** Although some veterinarians use this technique, it is the most prone to complications.
387. **b** The right ovary is located more cranially than the left. Some surgeons prefer a right paramedian approach in canine ovariohysterectomy to reduce the difficulty in exteriorizing the right ovary.
388. **a** A dorsal incision in the uterine body is recommended. Incisions in the uterine horn may result in enough scarring to reduce future fertility.
389. **b** Stents can interfere with primary healing and increase risk of ascending infection.
390. **a** It is important to isolate and specifically clamp and ligate the bleeding vessel. The ureter is located in this area, and gross ligation could occlude the ureter.
391. **e** Cystocentesis reduces the size of the bladder and allows repositioning of the bladder back into a normal anatomic position.
392. **a** There is no technique described for preputial urethrostomy in dogs.
393. **c** Ammonium urate uroliths are associated with portal vascular anomalies.
394. **b** The Zepp procedure involves resection of the lateral cartilaginous wall of the vertical ear canal and formation of a ventral cartilaginous flap.
395. **e** Ventral bulla osteotomy provides the best means for drainage of the middle ear.
396. **b** The purpose of surgical management of PDA is to stop the left-to-right flow of blood. This is accomplished by ligation of the ductus.
397. **c** The purpose of surgical management of PRAA is transection of the ligamentum arteriosus, which forms a restrictive band of tissue occluding the esophagus.
398. **a** The central tendon of the diaphragm is stronger than the muscular portion and therefore tears less frequently.
399. **b** Stretching or breaking of the suspensory ligament is usually necessary for delivery of the ovaries into the surgical field.
400. **c** The incidence of perineal hernias is highest in older intact male dogs. Several breeds appear predisposed, including boxers.
401. **b** Polydioxanone is a monofilament synthetic absorbable sutures material.
402. **a** Polypropylene is a monofilament synthetic nonabsorbable suture material.
403. **d** Surgical catgut is a natural absorbable suture material.
404. **e** Stainless steel is inert in tissue.
405. **b** Plain catgut incites the most tissue reaction. Chromic catgut causes much less tissue reaction.
406. **c** The vertical mattress suture is everting.
407. **a** The Cushing pattern is an inverting pattern used on hollow organs.
408. **d** One of the basic principles of external fixation of fractures is immobilization of the joints proximal and distal to the fracture. Of the fractures listed, only the mid-diaphyseal fracture of the tibia could be treated with a Schroeder-Thomas splint.
409. **e** The Robert Jones bandage is the best technique to minimize soft tissue damage and provide temporary stability to a fracture distal to the stifle or elbow.
410. **b** The lumen diameter of the pylorus is increased by suturing a longitudinal incision transversely.
411. **b** The caudal border of the soft palate should be at the tip of the epiglottis.
412. **c** If a radiographically visible defect is present, surgical management is indicated. Curettage of the lesion is believed to stimulate filling of the defect.
413. **e** Panosteitis is a self-limiting disease of undetermined etiology. Analgesics are given as needed.
414. **e** The length of the surgical procedure, amount of tissue damage, amount of hemorrhage, and immunocompetence of the animal all influence the incidence of wound infection.
415. **a** A lacerated artery spurts blood under pressure.

416. **b** Arterial bleeders should be ligated.
417. **c** Bleeding in which blood oozes under low pressure at the time of incision is considered capillary/primary hemorrhage.
418. **e** Capillary bleeding can generally be stopped by applying light pressure with gauze sponges.
419. **c** Careful placement of subcutaneous sutures decreases dead space and can improve tissue apposition.
420. **d** An accidental wound, created in a nonsterile environment and of this duration, should be considered dirty.
421. **b** Current is concentrated at the active electrode and either cuts or coagulates tissue.
422. **d** Capillary action may draw bacteria from the underlying environment through the drapes.
423. **b** The falciform ligament is a fatty structure adherent to the linea alba just cranial to the umbilicus. Many surgeons recommend removal of this structure on closure of the abdominal wall.
424. **a** The ureter should be left with little or no blind stump. Ligation and transection should be done as close to the bladder as possible.
425. **c** Liquid nitrogen is the most commonly used cryogen in veterinary medicine because of its temperature, availability, and cost.
426. **b** Tissue that reaches -20° C or colder is most likely to under necrosis.
427. **d** The zone of edema is farthest from the tip of the laser instrument and eventually recovers.
428. **c** Holding the instrument perpendicular to the tissue prevents thermal injury in collateral tissues.
429. **d** The descending duodenum can be gently elevated and retracted to the left, providing improved exposure of the right kidney.
430. **c** The descending colon can be gently elevated and retracted to the right, providing improved exposure of the left kidney.
431. **b** Cellular death occurs by intracellular and extracellular formation of ice. Water content therefore is the factor that influences a tissue's reaction to cryosurgery.
432. **a** A conjunctival flap protects the inner layer of the cornea and provides a blood supply for more rapid healing.
433. **b** Second-intention healing is the process whereby the wound heals by granulation, contraction, and reepithelialization, without human intervention.
434. **c** Transplantation of the parotid duct is frequently effective in management of keratoconjunctivitis sicca.
435. **c** Current recommendations are for placement of three screws proximal and three distal to the fracture line.
436. **c** Third-intention healing involves delayed primary closure.
437. **e** The fibers of the rectus abdominis muscle parallel the linea alba and must be separated.
438. **b** A single lesion at C5-T2 would account for both sets of neurologic signs.
439. **d** A lesion at C1-5 would cause upper motor neuron signs to the front limbs. A lesion at L4-S3 would cause lower motor neuron signs to the rear limbs.
440. **e** The Connell suture pattern is inverting.
441. **d** The Ehmer sling prevents weight bearing and produces medial rotation of the femoral head into the acetabulum.
442. **c** The Velpeau bandage prevents weight bearing and holds the scapula firmly against the body wall.
443. **c** The Parker-Kerr pattern is an inverting continuous suture pattern used for closing transected tubular structures.
444. **d** Transplantation of the tibial crest may be indicated in patellar luxations but not in rupture of the cranial cruciate ligament.
445. **e** The Cushing suture pattern is placed parallel to the incision line. In the Lembert pattern the bites in the tissue are perpendicular to the incision line.
446. **c** The intercapital ligaments extend from the head of one rib to the head of the contralateral rib, passing ventral to the spinal cord and dorsal to the intervertebral disk. These ligaments prevent dorsal rupture of disk material.
447. **b** Amputation of the tail at Cy3-4 prevents fecal and urine soiling of the tail, minimizes the possibility of pain associated with motion of the tail, and preserves the origin of the muscles of the pelvic diaphragm.
448. **b** The femur is approached between the vastus lateralis and the biceps femoris.
449. **a** The incision should be made in an avascular area midway between the greater and lesser curvatures of the stomach and paralleling the long axis of the stomach.
450. **b** Stay sutures allow relatively atraumatic manipulation of tissue.

NOTES

SECTION

13

Theriogenology

K. Hinrichs

Recommended Reading

Feldman EC, Nelson RW: *Canine and feline endocrinology and reproduction,* ed 2, Philadelphia, 1996, WB Saunders.

Johnston SD, Olsen PN: *Canine & feline reproduction,* Philadelphia, 1997, WB Saunders.

Morrow DA: *Current therapy in theriogenology,* ed 2, Philadelphia, 1986, WB Saunders.

Practice answer sheet is on page 313.

Questions

1. *A bitch is presented because of a bloody vulvar discharge. The owners tell you that she was in heat 1 month ago, and they are puzzled about why she has the discharge now. The bitch is apparently healthy and has no fever. What are the most likely causes of these findings?*
   a. pyometra, split heat, and follicular cysts
   b. split heat, vaginal foreign body, and luteal cysts
   c. abortion, vaginitis, and split heat
   d. cystitis, abortion, and luteal cysts
   e. cystitis, pyometra, and short interestrus interval

2. *Estrogens (estradiol cypionate, ECP) can be used to prevent pregnancy in dogs. What are the major complications associated with estrogen treatment for this purpose?*
   a. short interestrus intervals and von Willebrand's disease
   b. pyometra and aplastic anemia
   c. nephrotoxicosis and hypoglycemia
   d. nymphomania, and raised tail head
   e. cleft palate in offspring

3. *What is a major difference in pregnancy in dogs and cats?*
   a. Cats show external signs of pregnancy in the first 2 to 3 weeks, but dogs do not.
   b. Ultrasonography can accurately diagnose pregnancy in cats at 11 days of gestation.
   c. Radiography cannot be used to diagnose pregnancy in cats.
   d. The gestation length from ovulation is 10 days shorter in cats than in dogs.
   e. Cats do not depend on luteal progesterone in early gestation to maintain pregnancy.

4. *Concerning reproductive physiology and endocrinology of unmated queens, which statement is most accurate?*
   a. Luteinizing hormone (LH) is released on day 2 of estrus.
   b. The queen shows periods of heat of approximately 1 week's duration, followed by interestrus periods lasting just over 1 week.
   c. Queens are nonseasonally polyestrous.
   d. The normal sequence of estrous cycle stages is proestrus, estrus, diestrus, interestrus, proestrus, etc.
   e. During proestrus, serum progesterone levels rise rapidly.

5. *Semen is typically collected from dogs by:*
   a. electroejaculation
   b. using a water-jacketed artificial vagina
   c. manually compressing the penis caudal to the bulbus glandis
   d. massaging the prostate gland digitally per rectum
   e. firmly grasping the tip of the penis caudal to the urethral orifice

6. *Which anatomic structure makes it difficult to cannulate the cervix of the bitch?*
   a. urethral orifice
   b. vestibular-vaginal fold
   c. vestibular fornix
   d. cervical rings
   e. dorsal median vaginal fold

7. *Serum progesterone levels begin to rise in the bitch:*
   a. on the first day of proestrus
   b. 2 days before ovulation
   c. on the day of ovulation
   d. 2 days after ovulation
   e. 7 days after ovulation

8. *A 3-year-old queen had two litters (March and September, 1996) with no complications. She was first taken to tom A on January 10, 1997. The pair was observed mating on several occasions over a period of 4 days. The queen was taken home on January 15 but was again in heat on March 1. The breeding procedure was repeated, and the pair was again observed mating on several occasions. However, the queen was again in heat on April 20, 1997. What is the most likely cause of reproductive failure?*
   a. incorrect breeding management
   b. ovulation failure
   c. cystic ovarian disease
   d. male infertility
   e. prolonged lactational anestrus

9. *Which criterion can be used to most accurately determine (ahead of time or in retrospect) the day of ovulation in a bitch?*
   a. first day of vulvar bleeding
   b. first day the bitch stands for the male
   c. first day of completely cornified cells in the vaginal smear
   d. first day of influx of parabasal cells in the vaginal smear
   e. first day the serum progesterone level reaches 10 ng/ml

10. *Which method is most effective for breeding management of dogs?*
   a. breed on the eleventh and thirteenth day after vulvar bleeding is first observed
   b. breed on the third and fifth days of standing heat
   c. breed on the first and second days of standing heat, to two different males
   d. breed every 2 or 3 days throughout standing heat
   e. repeated serum progesterone assays to detect the peak level

11. *How long, from the time of the first breeding, does gestation normally last in the bitch?*

    a. 62 to 64 days
    b. 70 to 75 days
    c. 58 to 62 days
    d. 62 to 68 days
    e. 58 to 72 days

12. *A bitch is presented because the owners have bred her on two heats and she seems to have lost her pregnancy, although they were not sure she was pregnant. Which test is most appropriate at this time, regardless of any additional aspects of the history, to determine the cause of infertility?*

    a. serum progesterone assay
    b. serum estrogen assay
    c. serum prolactin assay
    d. vaginal culture
    e. *Brucella* titer

13. *A bitch is presented 1 week after parturition. The bitch is depressed, febrile, and anorexic, and the pups are not thriving. What are the most likely causes of these findings?*

    a. metritis and subinvolution of placental sites
    b. metritis and mastitis
    c. galactostasis and subinvolution of placental sites
    d. mastitis and hypocalcemia
    e. galactostasis and hypocalcemia

14. *Which bacterium is most commonly associated with pyometra in the bitch?*

    a. *Actinomyces pyogenes*
    b. *Escherichia coli*
    c. *Streptococcus zooepidemicus*
    d. *Mycoplasma mycoides*
    e. *Brucella canis*

15. *Concerning "puppy vaginitis," which statement is most accurate?*

    a. It occurs in the bitch while she is lactating.
    b. It occurs in female puppies before their first heat and is usually self-limiting.
    c. It should be treated with broad-spectrum antibiotics.
    d. It causes depression, anorexia, and fever.
    e. It may be controlled by spaying.

16. *Concerning the estrous cycle of queens, which statement is most accurate?*

    a. Queens have one estrous cycle every season.
    b. Cervical stimulation causes estrogen release from the pituitary gland.
    c. The breeding season starts as periods of daylight begin to shorten.
    d. The amount of LH release depends on the day of the estrous cycle and the number of matings.
    e. After estrus, unmated queens have a 10-day diestrous period.

17. *Concerning dystocia in queens, which statement is most accurate?*

    a. Oxytocin treatment is always indicated.
    b. Posterior presentation is often a problem.
    c. Uterine inertia is the most common cause of dystocia.
    d. A Cray hook should be used for manipulation of kittens.
    e. Fetal malposition is a common cause of dystocia.

18. *Concerning use of mibolerone in the bitch, which statement is most accurate?*

    a. It is a progestogen.
    b. It can be given in the first 3 days of proestrus to prevent that heat.
    c. It may cause aplastic anemia in bitches.
    d. It must be given daily during the entire period that estrus is to be prevented.
    e. It must be given within 3 days of mismating.

19. *Pseudocyesis occurring 2 months after estrus in a bitch indicates:*

    a. a normal luteal phase
    b. an increased risk of pyometra
    c. luteal inadequacy
    d. split heats
    e. an abnormally short interestrus interval

Correct answers are on pages 280-281.

20. *You have scheduled a cesarean section for an English bulldog based on the time of breeding. You schedule the surgery at the latest date possible, to avoid removing the puppies prematurely. The owner is worried that the bitch will go into labor before the scheduled surgery. What is the most appropriate advice for this owner?*
    a. The bitch won't go into labor before the scheduled surgery date, so don't be concerned.
    b. Watch for signs of restlessness and nesting; then telephone to schedule the surgery.
    c. Monitor the rectal temperature; telephone to schedule the surgery if the temperature falls by 1° F or below 99° F.
    d. Watch for a watery vulvar discharge; then telephone to schedule the surgery.
    e. Watch for the onset of labor; then telephone to schedule the surgery.

21. *Which signs are most indicative of estrus in queens?*
    a. frequent urination and a bloody vulvar discharge
    b. increased affection, rolling, and calling
    c. switching of the tail and a clear, mucous vulvar discharge
    d. vulvar hyperemia and a raised tail head
    e. mounting other female cats and restlessness

22. *What type of placenta do cats have?*
    a. epitheliochorial
    b. trophochorial
    c. endotheliochorial
    d. hemochorial
    e. syndesmochorial

23. *How long do overt signs of heat (proestrus plus estrus) last in a bitch?*
    a. 4 days
    b. 7 days
    c. 10 days
    d. 14 days
    e. 18 days

24. *How long after parturition does lochia normally persist in the bitch?*
    a. 3 or 4 days
    b. 1 week
    c. 2 weeks
    d. 3 weeks
    e. 4 to 6 weeks

25. *A bitch is presented because of a mismating. The owners do not know the dog's stage of the estrous cycle. Microscopic examination of a vaginal smear shows that more than 90% of the cells are squamous. The serum progesterone level is 10 ng/ml (high). What is the most reasonable interpretation of these findings?*
    a. The bitch is in proestrus and likely has not conceived.
    b. The bitch is in estrus and has likely conceived.
    c. The bitch is in diestrus and likely has not conceived.
    d. The vaginal smear findings are not correlated with the serum progesterone level, and the bitch may have an ovarian cyst.
    e. The bitch may be in estrus but is unlikely to conceive, because the serum progesterone level is high.

Answers

1. **a** Pyometra can be manifested as a bloody vulvar discharge in the 3 months after estrus. Split heat indicates that the previous heat was anovulatory and the bitch is now in true heat. Follicular cysts can prolong vulvar bleeding.
2. **b** Estrogens increase progesterone receptors, and this increases progesterone's effects, which could lead to pyometra. Estrogens also induce bone marrow dysplasia.
3. **a** Cats show "pinking up" (hyperemia) of the nipples at 2 to 3 weeks of gestation.
4. **b** Cats are induced ovulators and do not ovulate or form a corpus luteum unless mated. An unmated queen has no diestrous period, but rather an "interestrus" between successive follicle waves.
5. **c** This penile compression mimics that of the bitch's vestibular muscles and stimulates erection and ejaculation.

6. **e** The dorsal medial vaginal fold reduces the diameter of the vagina cranial to the cervix and prevents direct cannulation of the cervical os.
7. **b** Preovulatory luteinization causes an increase in peripheral progesterone concentration 2 days before ovulation.
8. **d** The most likely explanation is that the tomcat is infertile. This queen is cycling normally. The cats are mating and ovulation is occurring, as seen by the delay in return to estrus.
9. **d** The predominant cell changes to parabasal reliably 6 days after ovulation. The other answers are variable in relation to ovulation.
10. **d** A bitch should be bred every 2 or 3 days throughout heat because the duration of heat (and therefore the time of ovulation) is variable.
11. **e** Conception can occur from a mating more than 7 days before ovulation to 5 days after ovulation.
12. **e** The *Brucella* titer should be determined for all bitches with a history of possible abortion.
13. **b** Metritis and mastitis typically develop in the first week postpartum and cause systemic illness.
14. **b** Pyometra may be associated with an ascending infection from the vagina, which is contaminated with intestinal *E. coli.*
15. **b** Vaginitis in puppies is resistant to antibiotic treatment but usually resolves spontaneously after the first heat.
16. **d** Multiple matings at peak follicular activity (e.g., day 2 of estrus) may be needed to stimulate LH release.
17. **c** In queens, fetal malpositioning or oversize is less common than uterine inertia.
18. **d** Mibolerone is an androgen contraceptive that must be given daily. Estrus occurs within weeks to a few months after withdrawal of the medication.
19. **a** Pseudocyesis (pseudopregnancy) is seen when serum progesterone levels fall, typically about 2 months after the end of estrus.
20. **c** The bitch should go into labor within 24 hours after the rectal temperature falls. The other signs mentioned are not as useful in estimating the time of whelping.
21. **b** These signs can be so extreme as to have a novice cat owner think that the cat is having convulsions.
22. **c** Dogs and cats have a zonary, endotheliochorial placenta, in which the maternal epithelium has eroded away to allow the surface of the fetal placenta (chorion) to contact the maternal capillary endothelium.
23. **e** In the bitch, proestrus typically lasts 9 or 10 days and estrus approximately 9 days.
24. **e** Lochia, the bloody or brown mucoid vulvar discharge with no foul odor, normally persists for up to 6 weeks postpartum in the bitch.
25. **b** The vaginal smear shows that the bitch is in estrus, because the cells are almost all squamous. Any mating during this time is likely to be fertile. Because progesterone levels begin to rise before ovulation and the bitch stays in cytologic estrus for 6 days after ovulation, the majority of estrus occurs while progesterone levels are high.

NOTES

NOTES

SECTION 1

Anesthesiology

Fill in a circled letter to indicate your answer choice.

1. ⓐ ⓑ ⓒ ⓓ ⓔ	11. ⓐ ⓑ ⓒ ⓓ ⓔ	21. ⓐ ⓑ ⓒ ⓓ ⓔ	
2. ⓐ ⓑ ⓒ ⓓ ⓔ	12. ⓐ ⓑ ⓒ ⓓ ⓔ	22. ⓐ ⓑ ⓒ ⓓ ⓔ	
3. ⓐ ⓑ ⓒ ⓓ ⓔ	13. ⓐ ⓑ ⓒ ⓓ ⓔ	23. ⓐ ⓑ ⓒ ⓓ ⓔ	
4. ⓐ ⓑ ⓒ ⓓ ⓔ	14. ⓐ ⓑ ⓒ ⓓ ⓔ	24. ⓐ ⓑ ⓒ ⓓ ⓔ	
5. ⓐ ⓑ ⓒ ⓓ ⓔ	15. ⓐ ⓑ ⓒ ⓓ ⓔ	25. ⓐ ⓑ ⓒ ⓓ ⓔ	
6. ⓐ ⓑ ⓒ ⓓ ⓔ	16. ⓐ ⓑ ⓒ ⓓ ⓔ		
7. ⓐ ⓑ ⓒ ⓓ ⓔ	17. ⓐ ⓑ ⓒ ⓓ ⓔ		
8. ⓐ ⓑ ⓒ ⓓ ⓔ	18. ⓐ ⓑ ⓒ ⓓ ⓔ		
9. ⓐ ⓑ ⓒ ⓓ ⓔ	19. ⓐ ⓑ ⓒ ⓓ ⓔ		
10. ⓐ ⓑ ⓒ ⓓ ⓔ	20. ⓐ ⓑ ⓒ ⓓ ⓔ		

SECTION 2

Cardiology

Fill in a circled letter to indicate your answer choice.

1. ⓐ ⓑ ⓒ ⓓ ⓔ	11. ⓐ ⓑ ⓒ ⓓ ⓔ	21. ⓐ ⓑ ⓒ ⓓ ⓔ	
2. ⓐ ⓑ ⓒ ⓓ ⓔ	12. ⓐ ⓑ ⓒ ⓓ ⓔ	22. ⓐ ⓑ ⓒ ⓓ ⓔ	
3. ⓐ ⓑ ⓒ ⓓ ⓔ	13. ⓐ ⓑ ⓒ ⓓ ⓔ	23. ⓐ ⓑ ⓒ ⓓ ⓔ	
4. ⓐ ⓑ ⓒ ⓓ ⓔ	14. ⓐ ⓑ ⓒ ⓓ ⓔ	24. ⓐ ⓑ ⓒ ⓓ ⓔ	
5. ⓐ ⓑ ⓒ ⓓ ⓔ	15. ⓐ ⓑ ⓒ ⓓ ⓔ	25. ⓐ ⓑ ⓒ ⓓ ⓔ	
6. ⓐ ⓑ ⓒ ⓓ ⓔ	16. ⓐ ⓑ ⓒ ⓓ ⓔ		
7. ⓐ ⓑ ⓒ ⓓ ⓔ	17. ⓐ ⓑ ⓒ ⓓ ⓔ		
8. ⓐ ⓑ ⓒ ⓓ ⓔ	18. ⓐ ⓑ ⓒ ⓓ ⓔ		
9. ⓐ ⓑ ⓒ ⓓ ⓔ	19. ⓐ ⓑ ⓒ ⓓ ⓔ		
10. ⓐ ⓑ ⓒ ⓓ ⓔ	20. ⓐ ⓑ ⓒ ⓓ ⓔ		

SECTION 3

Dentistry

Fill in a circled letter to indicate your answer choice.

1. ⓐ ⓑ ⓒ ⓓ ⓔ	11. ⓐ ⓑ ⓒ ⓓ ⓔ	21. ⓐ ⓑ ⓒ ⓓ ⓔ	
2. ⓐ ⓑ ⓒ ⓓ ⓔ	12. ⓐ ⓑ ⓒ ⓓ ⓔ	22. ⓐ ⓑ ⓒ ⓓ ⓔ	
3. ⓐ ⓑ ⓒ ⓓ ⓔ	13. ⓐ ⓑ ⓒ ⓓ ⓔ	23. ⓐ ⓑ ⓒ ⓓ ⓔ	
4. ⓐ ⓑ ⓒ ⓓ ⓔ	14. ⓐ ⓑ ⓒ ⓓ ⓔ	24. ⓐ ⓑ ⓒ ⓓ ⓔ	
5. ⓐ ⓑ ⓒ ⓓ ⓔ	15. ⓐ ⓑ ⓒ ⓓ ⓔ	25. ⓐ ⓑ ⓒ ⓓ ⓔ	
6. ⓐ ⓑ ⓒ ⓓ ⓔ	16. ⓐ ⓑ ⓒ ⓓ ⓔ		
7. ⓐ ⓑ ⓒ ⓓ ⓔ	17. ⓐ ⓑ ⓒ ⓓ ⓔ		
8. ⓐ ⓑ ⓒ ⓓ ⓔ	18. ⓐ ⓑ ⓒ ⓓ ⓔ		
9. ⓐ ⓑ ⓒ ⓓ ⓔ	19. ⓐ ⓑ ⓒ ⓓ ⓔ		
10. ⓐ ⓑ ⓒ ⓓ ⓔ	20. ⓐ ⓑ ⓒ ⓓ ⓔ		

SECTION 4

Dermatology

Fill in a circled letter to indicate your answer choice.

1. ⓐ ⓑ ⓒ ⓓ ⓔ	11. ⓐ ⓑ ⓒ ⓓ ⓔ	21. ⓐ ⓑ ⓒ ⓓ ⓔ	
2. ⓐ ⓑ ⓒ ⓓ ⓔ	12. ⓐ ⓑ ⓒ ⓓ ⓔ	22. ⓐ ⓑ ⓒ ⓓ ⓔ	
3. ⓐ ⓑ ⓒ ⓓ ⓔ	13. ⓐ ⓑ ⓒ ⓓ ⓔ	23. ⓐ ⓑ ⓒ ⓓ ⓔ	
4. ⓐ ⓑ ⓒ ⓓ ⓔ	14. ⓐ ⓑ ⓒ ⓓ ⓔ	24. ⓐ ⓑ ⓒ ⓓ ⓔ	
5. ⓐ ⓑ ⓒ ⓓ ⓔ	15. ⓐ ⓑ ⓒ ⓓ ⓔ	25. ⓐ ⓑ ⓒ ⓓ ⓔ	
6. ⓐ ⓑ ⓒ ⓓ ⓔ	16. ⓐ ⓑ ⓒ ⓓ ⓔ		
7. ⓐ ⓑ ⓒ ⓓ ⓔ	17. ⓐ ⓑ ⓒ ⓓ ⓔ		
8. ⓐ ⓑ ⓒ ⓓ ⓔ	18. ⓐ ⓑ ⓒ ⓓ ⓔ		
9. ⓐ ⓑ ⓒ ⓓ ⓔ	19. ⓐ ⓑ ⓒ ⓓ ⓔ		
10. ⓐ ⓑ ⓒ ⓓ ⓔ	20. ⓐ ⓑ ⓒ ⓓ ⓔ		

SECTION 6

Medical Diseases

Fill in a circled letter to indicate your answer choice.

1. ⓐ ⓑ ⓒ ⓓ ⓔ
2. ⓐ ⓑ ⓒ ⓓ ⓔ
3. ⓐ ⓑ ⓒ ⓓ ⓔ
4. ⓐ ⓑ ⓒ ⓓ ⓔ
5. ⓐ ⓑ ⓒ ⓓ ⓔ
6. ⓐ ⓑ ⓒ ⓓ ⓔ
7. ⓐ ⓑ ⓒ ⓓ ⓔ
8. ⓐ ⓑ ⓒ ⓓ ⓔ
9. ⓐ ⓑ ⓒ ⓓ ⓔ
10. ⓐ ⓑ ⓒ ⓓ ⓔ
11. ⓐ ⓑ ⓒ ⓓ ⓔ
12. ⓐ ⓑ ⓒ ⓓ ⓔ
13. ⓐ ⓑ ⓒ ⓓ ⓔ
14. ⓐ ⓑ ⓒ ⓓ ⓔ
15. ⓐ ⓑ ⓒ ⓓ ⓔ
16. ⓐ ⓑ ⓒ ⓓ ⓔ
17. ⓐ ⓑ ⓒ ⓓ ⓔ
18. ⓐ ⓑ ⓒ ⓓ ⓔ
19. ⓐ ⓑ ⓒ ⓓ ⓔ
20. ⓐ ⓑ ⓒ ⓓ ⓔ
21. ⓐ ⓑ ⓒ ⓓ ⓔ
22. ⓐ ⓑ ⓒ ⓓ ⓔ
23. ⓐ ⓑ ⓒ ⓓ ⓔ
24. ⓐ ⓑ ⓒ ⓓ ⓔ
25. ⓐ ⓑ ⓒ ⓓ ⓔ
26. ⓐ ⓑ ⓒ ⓓ ⓔ
27. ⓐ ⓑ ⓒ ⓓ ⓔ
28. ⓐ ⓑ ⓒ ⓓ ⓔ
29. ⓐ ⓑ ⓒ ⓓ ⓔ
30. ⓐ ⓑ ⓒ ⓓ ⓔ
31. ⓐ ⓑ ⓒ ⓓ ⓔ
32. ⓐ ⓑ ⓒ ⓓ ⓔ
33. ⓐ ⓑ ⓒ ⓓ ⓔ
34. ⓐ ⓑ ⓒ ⓓ ⓔ
35. ⓐ ⓑ ⓒ ⓓ ⓔ
36. ⓐ ⓑ ⓒ ⓓ ⓔ
37. ⓐ ⓑ ⓒ ⓓ ⓔ
38. ⓐ ⓑ ⓒ ⓓ ⓔ
39. ⓐ ⓑ ⓒ ⓓ ⓔ
40. ⓐ ⓑ ⓒ ⓓ ⓔ
41. ⓐ ⓑ ⓒ ⓓ ⓔ
42. ⓐ ⓑ ⓒ ⓓ ⓔ
43. ⓐ ⓑ ⓒ ⓓ ⓔ
44. ⓐ ⓑ ⓒ ⓓ ⓔ
45. ⓐ ⓑ ⓒ ⓓ ⓔ
46. ⓐ ⓑ ⓒ ⓓ ⓔ
47. ⓐ ⓑ ⓒ ⓓ ⓔ
48. ⓐ ⓑ ⓒ ⓓ ⓔ
49. ⓐ ⓑ ⓒ ⓓ ⓔ
50. ⓐ ⓑ ⓒ ⓓ ⓔ
51. ⓐ ⓑ ⓒ ⓓ ⓔ
52. ⓐ ⓑ ⓒ ⓓ ⓔ
53. ⓐ ⓑ ⓒ ⓓ ⓔ
54. ⓐ ⓑ ⓒ ⓓ ⓔ
55. ⓐ ⓑ ⓒ ⓓ ⓔ
56. ⓐ ⓑ ⓒ ⓓ ⓔ
57. ⓐ ⓑ ⓒ ⓓ ⓔ
58. ⓐ ⓑ ⓒ ⓓ ⓔ
59. ⓐ ⓑ ⓒ ⓓ ⓔ
60. ⓐ ⓑ ⓒ ⓓ ⓔ
61. ⓐ ⓑ ⓒ ⓓ ⓔ
62. ⓐ ⓑ ⓒ ⓓ ⓔ
63. ⓐ ⓑ ⓒ ⓓ ⓔ
64. ⓐ ⓑ ⓒ ⓓ ⓔ
65. ⓐ ⓑ ⓒ ⓓ ⓔ
66. ⓐ ⓑ ⓒ ⓓ ⓔ
67. ⓐ ⓑ ⓒ ⓓ ⓔ
68. ⓐ ⓑ ⓒ ⓓ ⓔ
69. ⓐ ⓑ ⓒ ⓓ ⓔ
70. ⓐ ⓑ ⓒ ⓓ ⓔ
71. ⓐ ⓑ ⓒ ⓓ ⓔ
72. ⓐ ⓑ ⓒ ⓓ ⓔ
73. ⓐ ⓑ ⓒ ⓓ ⓔ
74. ⓐ ⓑ ⓒ ⓓ ⓔ
75. ⓐ ⓑ ⓒ ⓓ ⓔ
76. ⓐ ⓑ ⓒ ⓓ ⓔ
77. ⓐ ⓑ ⓒ ⓓ ⓔ
78. ⓐ ⓑ ⓒ ⓓ ⓔ
79. ⓐ ⓑ ⓒ ⓓ ⓔ
80. ⓐ ⓑ ⓒ ⓓ ⓔ
81. ⓐ ⓑ ⓒ ⓓ ⓔ
82. ⓐ ⓑ ⓒ ⓓ ⓔ
83. ⓐ ⓑ ⓒ ⓓ ⓔ
84. ⓐ ⓑ ⓒ ⓓ ⓔ
85. ⓐ ⓑ ⓒ ⓓ ⓔ
86. ⓐ ⓑ ⓒ ⓓ ⓔ
87. ⓐ ⓑ ⓒ ⓓ ⓔ
88. ⓐ ⓑ ⓒ ⓓ ⓔ
89. ⓐ ⓑ ⓒ ⓓ ⓔ
90. ⓐ ⓑ ⓒ ⓓ ⓔ
91. ⓐ ⓑ ⓒ ⓓ ⓔ
92. ⓐ ⓑ ⓒ ⓓ ⓔ
93. ⓐ ⓑ ⓒ ⓓ ⓔ
94. ⓐ ⓑ ⓒ ⓓ ⓔ
95. ⓐ ⓑ ⓒ ⓓ ⓔ
96. ⓐ ⓑ ⓒ ⓓ ⓔ
97. ⓐ ⓑ ⓒ ⓓ ⓔ
98. ⓐ ⓑ ⓒ ⓓ ⓔ
99. ⓐ ⓑ ⓒ ⓓ ⓔ
100. ⓐ ⓑ ⓒ ⓓ ⓔ
101. ⓐ ⓑ ⓒ ⓓ ⓔ
102. ⓐ ⓑ ⓒ ⓓ ⓔ
103. ⓐ ⓑ ⓒ ⓓ ⓔ
104. ⓐ ⓑ ⓒ ⓓ ⓔ
105. ⓐ ⓑ ⓒ ⓓ ⓔ
106. ⓐ ⓑ ⓒ ⓓ ⓔ
107. ⓐ ⓑ ⓒ ⓓ ⓔ
108. ⓐ ⓑ ⓒ ⓓ ⓔ
109. ⓐ ⓑ ⓒ ⓓ ⓔ
110. ⓐ ⓑ ⓒ ⓓ ⓔ
111. ⓐ ⓑ ⓒ ⓓ ⓔ
112. ⓐ ⓑ ⓒ ⓓ ⓔ
113. ⓐ ⓑ ⓒ ⓓ ⓔ
114. ⓐ ⓑ ⓒ ⓓ ⓔ
115. ⓐ ⓑ ⓒ ⓓ ⓔ
116. ⓐ ⓑ ⓒ ⓓ ⓔ
117. ⓐ ⓑ ⓒ ⓓ ⓔ
118. ⓐ ⓑ ⓒ ⓓ ⓔ
119. ⓐ ⓑ ⓒ ⓓ ⓔ
120. ⓐ ⓑ ⓒ ⓓ ⓔ
121. ⓐ ⓑ ⓒ ⓓ ⓔ
122. ⓐ ⓑ ⓒ ⓓ ⓔ
123. ⓐ ⓑ ⓒ ⓓ ⓔ
124. ⓐ ⓑ ⓒ ⓓ ⓔ
125. ⓐ ⓑ ⓒ ⓓ ⓔ
126. ⓐ ⓑ ⓒ ⓓ ⓔ
127. ⓐ ⓑ ⓒ ⓓ ⓔ
128. ⓐ ⓑ ⓒ ⓓ ⓔ
129. ⓐ ⓑ ⓒ ⓓ ⓔ
130. ⓐ ⓑ ⓒ ⓓ ⓔ
131. ⓐ ⓑ ⓒ ⓓ ⓔ
132. ⓐ ⓑ ⓒ ⓓ ⓔ
133. ⓐ ⓑ ⓒ ⓓ ⓔ
134. ⓐ ⓑ ⓒ ⓓ ⓔ
135. ⓐ ⓑ ⓒ ⓓ ⓔ
136. ⓐ ⓑ ⓒ ⓓ ⓔ
137. ⓐ ⓑ ⓒ ⓓ ⓔ
138. ⓐ ⓑ ⓒ ⓓ ⓔ
139. ⓐ ⓑ ⓒ ⓓ ⓔ
140. ⓐ ⓑ ⓒ ⓓ ⓔ
141. ⓐ ⓑ ⓒ ⓓ ⓔ
142. ⓐ ⓑ ⓒ ⓓ ⓔ
143. ⓐ ⓑ ⓒ ⓓ ⓔ
144. ⓐ ⓑ ⓒ ⓓ ⓔ
145. ⓐ ⓑ ⓒ ⓓ ⓔ
146. ⓐ ⓑ ⓒ ⓓ ⓔ
147. ⓐ ⓑ ⓒ ⓓ ⓔ
148. ⓐ ⓑ ⓒ ⓓ ⓔ
149. ⓐ ⓑ ⓒ ⓓ ⓔ
150. ⓐ ⓑ ⓒ ⓓ ⓔ
151. ⓐ ⓑ ⓒ ⓓ ⓔ
152. ⓐ ⓑ ⓒ ⓓ ⓔ

Continued

Medical Diseases—*cont'd*

153. ⓐ ⓑ ⓒ ⓓ ⓔ	195. ⓐ ⓑ ⓒ ⓓ ⓔ	237. ⓐ ⓑ ⓒ ⓓ ⓔ	279. ⓐ ⓑ ⓒ ⓓ ⓔ
154. ⓐ ⓑ ⓒ ⓓ ⓔ	196. ⓐ ⓑ ⓒ ⓓ ⓔ	238. ⓐ ⓑ ⓒ ⓓ ⓔ	280. ⓐ ⓑ ⓒ ⓓ ⓔ
155. ⓐ ⓑ ⓒ ⓓ ⓔ	197. ⓐ ⓑ ⓒ ⓓ ⓔ	239. ⓐ ⓑ ⓒ ⓓ ⓔ	281. ⓐ ⓑ ⓒ ⓓ ⓔ
156. ⓐ ⓑ ⓒ ⓓ ⓔ	198. ⓐ ⓑ ⓒ ⓓ ⓔ	240. ⓐ ⓑ ⓒ ⓓ ⓔ	282. ⓐ ⓑ ⓒ ⓓ ⓔ
157. ⓐ ⓑ ⓒ ⓓ ⓔ	199. ⓐ ⓑ ⓒ ⓓ ⓔ	241. ⓐ ⓑ ⓒ ⓓ ⓔ	283. ⓐ ⓑ ⓒ ⓓ ⓔ
158. ⓐ ⓑ ⓒ ⓓ ⓔ	200. ⓐ ⓑ ⓒ ⓓ ⓔ	242. ⓐ ⓑ ⓒ ⓓ ⓔ	284. ⓐ ⓑ ⓒ ⓓ ⓔ
159. ⓐ ⓑ ⓒ ⓓ ⓔ	201. ⓐ ⓑ ⓒ ⓓ ⓔ	243. ⓐ ⓑ ⓒ ⓓ ⓔ	285. ⓐ ⓑ ⓒ ⓓ ⓔ
160. ⓐ ⓑ ⓒ ⓓ ⓔ	202. ⓐ ⓑ ⓒ ⓓ ⓔ	244. ⓐ ⓑ ⓒ ⓓ ⓔ	286. ⓐ ⓑ ⓒ ⓓ ⓔ
161. ⓐ ⓑ ⓒ ⓓ ⓔ	203. ⓐ ⓑ ⓒ ⓓ ⓔ	245. ⓐ ⓑ ⓒ ⓓ ⓔ	287. ⓐ ⓑ ⓒ ⓓ ⓔ
162. ⓐ ⓑ ⓒ ⓓ ⓔ	204. ⓐ ⓑ ⓒ ⓓ ⓔ	246. ⓐ ⓑ ⓒ ⓓ ⓔ	288. ⓐ ⓑ ⓒ ⓓ ⓔ
163. ⓐ ⓑ ⓒ ⓓ ⓔ	205. ⓐ ⓑ ⓒ ⓓ ⓔ	247. ⓐ ⓑ ⓒ ⓓ ⓔ	289. ⓐ ⓑ ⓒ ⓓ ⓔ
164. ⓐ ⓑ ⓒ ⓓ ⓔ	206. ⓐ ⓑ ⓒ ⓓ ⓔ	248. ⓐ ⓑ ⓒ ⓓ ⓔ	290. ⓐ ⓑ ⓒ ⓓ ⓔ
165. ⓐ ⓑ ⓒ ⓓ ⓔ	207. ⓐ ⓑ ⓒ ⓓ ⓔ	249. ⓐ ⓑ ⓒ ⓓ ⓔ	291. ⓐ ⓑ ⓒ ⓓ ⓔ
166. ⓐ ⓑ ⓒ ⓓ ⓔ	208. ⓐ ⓑ ⓒ ⓓ ⓔ	250. ⓐ ⓑ ⓒ ⓓ ⓔ	292. ⓐ ⓑ ⓒ ⓓ ⓔ
167. ⓐ ⓑ ⓒ ⓓ ⓔ	209. ⓐ ⓑ ⓒ ⓓ ⓔ	251. ⓐ ⓑ ⓒ ⓓ ⓔ	293. ⓐ ⓑ ⓒ ⓓ ⓔ
168. ⓐ ⓑ ⓒ ⓓ ⓔ	210. ⓐ ⓑ ⓒ ⓓ ⓔ	252. ⓐ ⓑ ⓒ ⓓ ⓔ	294. ⓐ ⓑ ⓒ ⓓ ⓔ
169. ⓐ ⓑ ⓒ ⓓ ⓔ	211. ⓐ ⓑ ⓒ ⓓ ⓔ	253. ⓐ ⓑ ⓒ ⓓ ⓔ	295. ⓐ ⓑ ⓒ ⓓ ⓔ
170. ⓐ ⓑ ⓒ ⓓ ⓔ	212. ⓐ ⓑ ⓒ ⓓ ⓔ	254. ⓐ ⓑ ⓒ ⓓ ⓔ	296. ⓐ ⓑ ⓒ ⓓ ⓔ
171. ⓐ ⓑ ⓒ ⓓ ⓔ	213. ⓐ ⓑ ⓒ ⓓ ⓔ	255. ⓐ ⓑ ⓒ ⓓ ⓔ	297. ⓐ ⓑ ⓒ ⓓ ⓔ
172. ⓐ ⓑ ⓒ ⓓ ⓔ	214. ⓐ ⓑ ⓒ ⓓ ⓔ	256. ⓐ ⓑ ⓒ ⓓ ⓔ	298. ⓐ ⓑ ⓒ ⓓ ⓔ
173. ⓐ ⓑ ⓒ ⓓ ⓔ	215. ⓐ ⓑ ⓒ ⓓ ⓔ	257. ⓐ ⓑ ⓒ ⓓ ⓔ	299. ⓐ ⓑ ⓒ ⓓ ⓔ
174. ⓐ ⓑ ⓒ ⓓ ⓔ	216. ⓐ ⓑ ⓒ ⓓ ⓔ	258. ⓐ ⓑ ⓒ ⓓ ⓔ	300. ⓐ ⓑ ⓒ ⓓ ⓔ
175. ⓐ ⓑ ⓒ ⓓ ⓔ	217. ⓐ ⓑ ⓒ ⓓ ⓔ	259. ⓐ ⓑ ⓒ ⓓ ⓔ	301. ⓐ ⓑ ⓒ ⓓ ⓔ
176. ⓐ ⓑ ⓒ ⓓ ⓔ	218. ⓐ ⓑ ⓒ ⓓ ⓔ	260. ⓐ ⓑ ⓒ ⓓ ⓔ	302. ⓐ ⓑ ⓒ ⓓ ⓔ
177. ⓐ ⓑ ⓒ ⓓ ⓔ	219. ⓐ ⓑ ⓒ ⓓ ⓔ	261. ⓐ ⓑ ⓒ ⓓ ⓔ	303. ⓐ ⓑ ⓒ ⓓ ⓔ
178. ⓐ ⓑ ⓒ ⓓ ⓔ	220. ⓐ ⓑ ⓒ ⓓ ⓔ	262. ⓐ ⓑ ⓒ ⓓ ⓔ	304. ⓐ ⓑ ⓒ ⓓ ⓔ
179. ⓐ ⓑ ⓒ ⓓ ⓔ	221. ⓐ ⓑ ⓒ ⓓ ⓔ	263. ⓐ ⓑ ⓒ ⓓ ⓔ	305. ⓐ ⓑ ⓒ ⓓ ⓔ
180. ⓐ ⓑ ⓒ ⓓ ⓔ	222. ⓐ ⓑ ⓒ ⓓ ⓔ	264. ⓐ ⓑ ⓒ ⓓ ⓔ	306. ⓐ ⓑ ⓒ ⓓ ⓔ
181. ⓐ ⓑ ⓒ ⓓ ⓔ	223. ⓐ ⓑ ⓒ ⓓ ⓔ	265. ⓐ ⓑ ⓒ ⓓ ⓔ	307. ⓐ ⓑ ⓒ ⓓ ⓔ
182. ⓐ ⓑ ⓒ ⓓ ⓔ	224. ⓐ ⓑ ⓒ ⓓ ⓔ	266. ⓐ ⓑ ⓒ ⓓ ⓔ	308. ⓐ ⓑ ⓒ ⓓ ⓔ
183. ⓐ ⓑ ⓒ ⓓ ⓔ	225. ⓐ ⓑ ⓒ ⓓ ⓔ	267. ⓐ ⓑ ⓒ ⓓ ⓔ	309. ⓐ ⓑ ⓒ ⓓ ⓔ
184. ⓐ ⓑ ⓒ ⓓ ⓔ	226. ⓐ ⓑ ⓒ ⓓ ⓔ	268. ⓐ ⓑ ⓒ ⓓ ⓔ	310. ⓐ ⓑ ⓒ ⓓ ⓔ
185. ⓐ ⓑ ⓒ ⓓ ⓔ	227. ⓐ ⓑ ⓒ ⓓ ⓔ	269. ⓐ ⓑ ⓒ ⓓ ⓔ	311. ⓐ ⓑ ⓒ ⓓ ⓔ
186. ⓐ ⓑ ⓒ ⓓ ⓔ	228. ⓐ ⓑ ⓒ ⓓ ⓔ	270. ⓐ ⓑ ⓒ ⓓ ⓔ	312. ⓐ ⓑ ⓒ ⓓ ⓔ
187. ⓐ ⓑ ⓒ ⓓ ⓔ	229. ⓐ ⓑ ⓒ ⓓ ⓔ	271. ⓐ ⓑ ⓒ ⓓ ⓔ	313. ⓐ ⓑ ⓒ ⓓ ⓔ
188. ⓐ ⓑ ⓒ ⓓ ⓔ	230. ⓐ ⓑ ⓒ ⓓ ⓔ	272. ⓐ ⓑ ⓒ ⓓ ⓔ	314. ⓐ ⓑ ⓒ ⓓ ⓔ
189. ⓐ ⓑ ⓒ ⓓ ⓔ	231. ⓐ ⓑ ⓒ ⓓ ⓔ	273. ⓐ ⓑ ⓒ ⓓ ⓔ	315. ⓐ ⓑ ⓒ ⓓ ⓔ
190. ⓐ ⓑ ⓒ ⓓ ⓔ	232. ⓐ ⓑ ⓒ ⓓ ⓔ	274. ⓐ ⓑ ⓒ ⓓ ⓔ	316. ⓐ ⓑ ⓒ ⓓ ⓔ
191. ⓐ ⓑ ⓒ ⓓ ⓔ	233. ⓐ ⓑ ⓒ ⓓ ⓔ	275. ⓐ ⓑ ⓒ ⓓ ⓔ	317. ⓐ ⓑ ⓒ ⓓ ⓔ
192. ⓐ ⓑ ⓒ ⓓ ⓔ	234. ⓐ ⓑ ⓒ ⓓ ⓔ	276. ⓐ ⓑ ⓒ ⓓ ⓔ	318. ⓐ ⓑ ⓒ ⓓ ⓔ
193. ⓐ ⓑ ⓒ ⓓ ⓔ	235. ⓐ ⓑ ⓒ ⓓ ⓔ	277. ⓐ ⓑ ⓒ ⓓ ⓔ	319. ⓐ ⓑ ⓒ ⓓ ⓔ
194. ⓐ ⓑ ⓒ ⓓ ⓔ	236. ⓐ ⓑ ⓒ ⓓ ⓔ	278. ⓐ ⓑ ⓒ ⓓ ⓔ	320. ⓐ ⓑ ⓒ ⓓ ⓔ

Medical Diseases—*cont'd*

321. ⓐ ⓑ ⓒ ⓓ ⓔ
322. ⓐ ⓑ ⓒ ⓓ ⓔ
323. ⓐ ⓑ ⓒ ⓓ ⓔ
324. ⓐ ⓑ ⓒ ⓓ ⓔ
325. ⓐ ⓑ ⓒ ⓓ ⓔ
326. ⓐ ⓑ ⓒ ⓓ ⓔ
327. ⓐ ⓑ ⓒ ⓓ ⓔ
328. ⓐ ⓑ ⓒ ⓓ ⓔ
329. ⓐ ⓑ ⓒ ⓓ ⓔ
330. ⓐ ⓑ ⓒ ⓓ ⓔ
331. ⓐ ⓑ ⓒ ⓓ ⓔ
332. ⓐ ⓑ ⓒ ⓓ ⓔ
333. ⓐ ⓑ ⓒ ⓓ ⓔ
334. ⓐ ⓑ ⓒ ⓓ ⓔ
335. ⓐ ⓑ ⓒ ⓓ ⓔ
336. ⓐ ⓑ ⓒ ⓓ ⓔ
337. ⓐ ⓑ ⓒ ⓓ ⓔ
338. ⓐ ⓑ ⓒ ⓓ ⓔ
339. ⓐ ⓑ ⓒ ⓓ ⓔ
340. ⓐ ⓑ ⓒ ⓓ ⓔ
341. ⓐ ⓑ ⓒ ⓓ ⓔ
342. ⓐ ⓑ ⓒ ⓓ ⓔ
343. ⓐ ⓑ ⓒ ⓓ ⓔ
344. ⓐ ⓑ ⓒ ⓓ ⓔ
345. ⓐ ⓑ ⓒ ⓓ ⓔ
346. ⓐ ⓑ ⓒ ⓓ ⓔ
347. ⓐ ⓑ ⓒ ⓓ ⓔ
348. ⓐ ⓑ ⓒ ⓓ ⓔ
349. ⓐ ⓑ ⓒ ⓓ ⓔ
350. ⓐ ⓑ ⓒ ⓓ ⓔ
351. ⓐ ⓑ ⓒ ⓓ ⓔ
352. ⓐ ⓑ ⓒ ⓓ ⓔ
353. ⓐ ⓑ ⓒ ⓓ ⓔ
354. ⓐ ⓑ ⓒ ⓓ ⓔ
355. ⓐ ⓑ ⓒ ⓓ ⓔ
356. ⓐ ⓑ ⓒ ⓓ ⓔ
357. ⓐ ⓑ ⓒ ⓓ ⓔ
358. ⓐ ⓑ ⓒ ⓓ ⓔ
359. ⓐ ⓑ ⓒ ⓓ ⓔ
360. ⓐ ⓑ ⓒ ⓓ ⓔ
361. ⓐ ⓑ ⓒ ⓓ ⓔ
362. ⓐ ⓑ ⓒ ⓓ ⓔ
363. ⓐ ⓑ ⓒ ⓓ ⓔ
364. ⓐ ⓑ ⓒ ⓓ ⓔ
365. ⓐ ⓑ ⓒ ⓓ ⓔ
366. ⓐ ⓑ ⓒ ⓓ ⓔ
367. ⓐ ⓑ ⓒ ⓓ ⓔ
368. ⓐ ⓑ ⓒ ⓓ ⓔ
369. ⓐ ⓑ ⓒ ⓓ ⓔ
370. ⓐ ⓑ ⓒ ⓓ ⓔ
371. ⓐ ⓑ ⓒ ⓓ ⓔ
372. ⓐ ⓑ ⓒ ⓓ ⓔ
373. ⓐ ⓑ ⓒ ⓓ ⓔ
374. ⓐ ⓑ ⓒ ⓓ ⓔ
375. ⓐ ⓑ ⓒ ⓓ ⓔ
376. ⓐ ⓑ ⓒ ⓓ ⓔ
377. ⓐ ⓑ ⓒ ⓓ ⓔ
378. ⓐ ⓑ ⓒ ⓓ ⓔ
379. ⓐ ⓑ ⓒ ⓓ ⓔ
380. ⓐ ⓑ ⓒ ⓓ ⓔ
381. ⓐ ⓑ ⓒ ⓓ ⓔ
382. ⓐ ⓑ ⓒ ⓓ ⓔ
383. ⓐ ⓑ ⓒ ⓓ ⓔ
384. ⓐ ⓑ ⓒ ⓓ ⓔ
385. ⓐ ⓑ ⓒ ⓓ ⓔ
386. ⓐ ⓑ ⓒ ⓓ ⓔ
387. ⓐ ⓑ ⓒ ⓓ ⓔ
388. ⓐ ⓑ ⓒ ⓓ ⓔ
389. ⓐ ⓑ ⓒ ⓓ ⓔ
390. ⓐ ⓑ ⓒ ⓓ ⓔ
391. ⓐ ⓑ ⓒ ⓓ ⓔ
392. ⓐ ⓑ ⓒ ⓓ ⓔ
393. ⓐ ⓑ ⓒ ⓓ ⓔ
394. ⓐ ⓑ ⓒ ⓓ ⓔ
395. ⓐ ⓑ ⓒ ⓓ ⓔ
396. ⓐ ⓑ ⓒ ⓓ ⓔ
397. ⓐ ⓑ ⓒ ⓓ ⓔ
398. ⓐ ⓑ ⓒ ⓓ ⓔ
399. ⓐ ⓑ ⓒ ⓓ ⓔ
400. ⓐ ⓑ ⓒ ⓓ ⓔ
401. ⓐ ⓑ ⓒ ⓓ ⓔ
402. ⓐ ⓑ ⓒ ⓓ ⓔ
403. ⓐ ⓑ ⓒ ⓓ ⓔ
404. ⓐ ⓑ ⓒ ⓓ ⓔ
405. ⓐ ⓑ ⓒ ⓓ ⓔ
406. ⓐ ⓑ ⓒ ⓓ ⓔ
407. ⓐ ⓑ ⓒ ⓓ ⓔ
408. ⓐ ⓑ ⓒ ⓓ ⓔ
409. ⓐ ⓑ ⓒ ⓓ ⓔ
410. ⓐ ⓑ ⓒ ⓓ ⓔ
411. ⓐ ⓑ ⓒ ⓓ ⓔ
412. ⓐ ⓑ ⓒ ⓓ ⓔ
413. ⓐ ⓑ ⓒ ⓓ ⓔ
414. ⓐ ⓑ ⓒ ⓓ ⓔ
415. ⓐ ⓑ ⓒ ⓓ ⓔ
416. ⓐ ⓑ ⓒ ⓓ ⓔ
417. ⓐ ⓑ ⓒ ⓓ ⓔ
418. ⓐ ⓑ ⓒ ⓓ ⓔ
419. ⓐ ⓑ ⓒ ⓓ ⓔ
420. ⓐ ⓑ ⓒ ⓓ ⓔ
421. ⓐ ⓑ ⓒ ⓓ ⓔ
422. ⓐ ⓑ ⓒ ⓓ ⓔ
423. ⓐ ⓑ ⓒ ⓓ ⓔ
424. ⓐ ⓑ ⓒ ⓓ ⓔ
425. ⓐ ⓑ ⓒ ⓓ ⓔ
426. ⓐ ⓑ ⓒ ⓓ ⓔ
427. ⓐ ⓑ ⓒ ⓓ ⓔ
428. ⓐ ⓑ ⓒ ⓓ ⓔ
429. ⓐ ⓑ ⓒ ⓓ ⓔ
430. ⓐ ⓑ ⓒ ⓓ ⓔ
431. ⓐ ⓑ ⓒ ⓓ ⓔ
432. ⓐ ⓑ ⓒ ⓓ ⓔ
433. ⓐ ⓑ ⓒ ⓓ ⓔ
434. ⓐ ⓑ ⓒ ⓓ ⓔ
435. ⓐ ⓑ ⓒ ⓓ ⓔ
436. ⓐ ⓑ ⓒ ⓓ ⓔ
437. ⓐ ⓑ ⓒ ⓓ ⓔ
438. ⓐ ⓑ ⓒ ⓓ ⓔ
439. ⓐ ⓑ ⓒ ⓓ ⓔ
440. ⓐ ⓑ ⓒ ⓓ ⓔ
441. ⓐ ⓑ ⓒ ⓓ ⓔ
442. ⓐ ⓑ ⓒ ⓓ ⓔ
443. ⓐ ⓑ ⓒ ⓓ ⓔ
444. ⓐ ⓑ ⓒ ⓓ ⓔ
445. ⓐ ⓑ ⓒ ⓓ ⓔ
446. ⓐ ⓑ ⓒ ⓓ ⓔ
447. ⓐ ⓑ ⓒ ⓓ ⓔ
448. ⓐ ⓑ ⓒ ⓓ ⓔ
449. ⓐ ⓑ ⓒ ⓓ ⓔ
450. ⓐ ⓑ ⓒ ⓓ ⓔ
451. ⓐ ⓑ ⓒ ⓓ ⓔ
452. ⓐ ⓑ ⓒ ⓓ ⓔ
453. ⓐ ⓑ ⓒ ⓓ ⓔ
454. ⓐ ⓑ ⓒ ⓓ ⓔ
455. ⓐ ⓑ ⓒ ⓓ ⓔ
456. ⓐ ⓑ ⓒ ⓓ ⓔ
457. ⓐ ⓑ ⓒ ⓓ ⓔ
458. ⓐ ⓑ ⓒ ⓓ ⓔ
459. ⓐ ⓑ ⓒ ⓓ ⓔ
460. ⓐ ⓑ ⓒ ⓓ ⓔ
461. ⓐ ⓑ ⓒ ⓓ ⓔ
462. ⓐ ⓑ ⓒ ⓓ ⓔ
463. ⓐ ⓑ ⓒ ⓓ ⓔ
464. ⓐ ⓑ ⓒ ⓓ ⓔ
465. ⓐ ⓑ ⓒ ⓓ ⓔ
466. ⓐ ⓑ ⓒ ⓓ ⓔ
467. ⓐ ⓑ ⓒ ⓓ ⓔ
468. ⓐ ⓑ ⓒ ⓓ ⓔ
469. ⓐ ⓑ ⓒ ⓓ ⓔ
470. ⓐ ⓑ ⓒ ⓓ ⓔ
471. ⓐ ⓑ ⓒ ⓓ ⓔ
472. ⓐ ⓑ ⓒ ⓓ ⓔ
473. ⓐ ⓑ ⓒ ⓓ ⓔ
474. ⓐ ⓑ ⓒ ⓓ ⓔ
475. ⓐ ⓑ ⓒ ⓓ ⓔ
476. ⓐ ⓑ ⓒ ⓓ ⓔ
477. ⓐ ⓑ ⓒ ⓓ ⓔ
478. ⓐ ⓑ ⓒ ⓓ ⓔ
479. ⓐ ⓑ ⓒ ⓓ ⓔ
480. ⓐ ⓑ ⓒ ⓓ ⓔ
481. ⓐ ⓑ ⓒ ⓓ ⓔ
482. ⓐ ⓑ ⓒ ⓓ ⓔ
483. ⓐ ⓑ ⓒ ⓓ ⓔ
484. ⓐ ⓑ ⓒ ⓓ ⓔ
485. ⓐ ⓑ ⓒ ⓓ ⓔ
486. ⓐ ⓑ ⓒ ⓓ ⓔ
487. ⓐ ⓑ ⓒ ⓓ ⓔ
488. ⓐ ⓑ ⓒ ⓓ ⓔ

Continued

Medical Diseases—*cont'd*

489. ⓐ ⓑ ⓒ ⓓ ⓔ
490. ⓐ ⓑ ⓒ ⓓ ⓔ
491. ⓐ ⓑ ⓒ ⓓ ⓔ
492. ⓐ ⓑ ⓒ ⓓ ⓔ
493. ⓐ ⓑ ⓒ ⓓ ⓔ
494. ⓐ ⓑ ⓒ ⓓ ⓔ
495. ⓐ ⓑ ⓒ ⓓ ⓔ
496. ⓐ ⓑ ⓒ ⓓ ⓔ
497. ⓐ ⓑ ⓒ ⓓ ⓔ
498. ⓐ ⓑ ⓒ ⓓ ⓔ
499. ⓐ ⓑ ⓒ ⓓ ⓔ
500. ⓐ ⓑ ⓒ ⓓ ⓔ
501. ⓐ ⓑ ⓒ ⓓ ⓔ
502. ⓐ ⓑ ⓒ ⓓ ⓔ
503. ⓐ ⓑ ⓒ ⓓ ⓔ
504. ⓐ ⓑ ⓒ ⓓ ⓔ
505. ⓐ ⓑ ⓒ ⓓ ⓔ
506. ⓐ ⓑ ⓒ ⓓ ⓔ
507. ⓐ ⓑ ⓒ ⓓ ⓔ
508. ⓐ ⓑ ⓒ ⓓ ⓔ
509. ⓐ ⓑ ⓒ ⓓ ⓔ
510. ⓐ ⓑ ⓒ ⓓ ⓔ
511. ⓐ ⓑ ⓒ ⓓ ⓔ
512. ⓐ ⓑ ⓒ ⓓ ⓔ
513. ⓐ ⓑ ⓒ ⓓ ⓔ
514. ⓐ ⓑ ⓒ ⓓ ⓔ
515. ⓐ ⓑ ⓒ ⓓ ⓔ
516. ⓐ ⓑ ⓒ ⓓ ⓔ
517. ⓐ ⓑ ⓒ ⓓ ⓔ
518. ⓐ ⓑ ⓒ ⓓ ⓔ
519. ⓐ ⓑ ⓒ ⓓ ⓔ
520. ⓐ ⓑ ⓒ ⓓ ⓔ
521. ⓐ ⓑ ⓒ ⓓ ⓔ
522. ⓐ ⓑ ⓒ ⓓ ⓔ
523. ⓐ ⓑ ⓒ ⓓ ⓔ
524. ⓐ ⓑ ⓒ ⓓ ⓔ
525. ⓐ ⓑ ⓒ ⓓ ⓔ
526. ⓐ ⓑ ⓒ ⓓ ⓔ
527. ⓐ ⓑ ⓒ ⓓ ⓔ
528. ⓐ ⓑ ⓒ ⓓ ⓔ
529. ⓐ ⓑ ⓒ ⓓ ⓔ
530. ⓐ ⓑ ⓒ ⓓ ⓔ
531. ⓐ ⓑ ⓒ ⓓ ⓔ
532. ⓐ ⓑ ⓒ ⓓ ⓔ
533. ⓐ ⓑ ⓒ ⓓ ⓔ
534. ⓐ ⓑ ⓒ ⓓ ⓔ
535. ⓐ ⓑ ⓒ ⓓ ⓔ
536. ⓐ ⓑ ⓒ ⓓ ⓔ
537. ⓐ ⓑ ⓒ ⓓ ⓔ
538. ⓐ ⓑ ⓒ ⓓ ⓔ
539. ⓐ ⓑ ⓒ ⓓ ⓔ
540. ⓐ ⓑ ⓒ ⓓ ⓔ
541. ⓐ ⓑ ⓒ ⓓ ⓔ
542. ⓐ ⓑ ⓒ ⓓ ⓔ
543. ⓐ ⓑ ⓒ ⓓ ⓔ
544. ⓐ ⓑ ⓒ ⓓ ⓔ
545. ⓐ ⓑ ⓒ ⓓ ⓔ
546. ⓐ ⓑ ⓒ ⓓ ⓔ
547. ⓐ ⓑ ⓒ ⓓ ⓔ
548. ⓐ ⓑ ⓒ ⓓ ⓔ
549. ⓐ ⓑ ⓒ ⓓ ⓔ
550. ⓐ ⓑ ⓒ ⓓ ⓔ
551. ⓐ ⓑ ⓒ ⓓ ⓔ
552. ⓐ ⓑ ⓒ ⓓ ⓔ
553. ⓐ ⓑ ⓒ ⓓ ⓔ
554. ⓐ ⓑ ⓒ ⓓ ⓔ
555. ⓐ ⓑ ⓒ ⓓ ⓔ
556. ⓐ ⓑ ⓒ ⓓ ⓔ
557. ⓐ ⓑ ⓒ ⓓ ⓔ
558. ⓐ ⓑ ⓒ ⓓ ⓔ
559. ⓐ ⓑ ⓒ ⓓ ⓔ
560. ⓐ ⓑ ⓒ ⓓ ⓔ
561. ⓐ ⓑ ⓒ ⓓ ⓔ
562. ⓐ ⓑ ⓒ ⓓ ⓔ
563. ⓐ ⓑ ⓒ ⓓ ⓔ
564. ⓐ ⓑ ⓒ ⓓ ⓔ
565. ⓐ ⓑ ⓒ ⓓ ⓔ
566. ⓐ ⓑ ⓒ ⓓ ⓔ
567. ⓐ ⓑ ⓒ ⓓ ⓔ
568. ⓐ ⓑ ⓒ ⓓ ⓔ
569. ⓐ ⓑ ⓒ ⓓ ⓔ
570. ⓐ ⓑ ⓒ ⓓ ⓔ
571. ⓐ ⓑ ⓒ ⓓ ⓔ
572. ⓐ ⓑ ⓒ ⓓ ⓔ
573. ⓐ ⓑ ⓒ ⓓ ⓔ
574. ⓐ ⓑ ⓒ ⓓ ⓔ
575. ⓐ ⓑ ⓒ ⓓ ⓔ
576. ⓐ ⓑ ⓒ ⓓ ⓔ
577. ⓐ ⓑ ⓒ ⓓ ⓔ
578. ⓐ ⓑ ⓒ ⓓ ⓔ
579. ⓐ ⓑ ⓒ ⓓ ⓔ
580. ⓐ ⓑ ⓒ ⓓ ⓔ
581. ⓐ ⓑ ⓒ ⓓ ⓔ
582. ⓐ ⓑ ⓒ ⓓ ⓔ
583. ⓐ ⓑ ⓒ ⓓ ⓔ
584. ⓐ ⓑ ⓒ ⓓ ⓔ
585. ⓐ ⓑ ⓒ ⓓ ⓔ
586. ⓐ ⓑ ⓒ ⓓ ⓔ
587. ⓐ ⓑ ⓒ ⓓ ⓔ
588. ⓐ ⓑ ⓒ ⓓ ⓔ
589. ⓐ ⓑ ⓒ ⓓ ⓔ
590. ⓐ ⓑ ⓒ ⓓ ⓔ
591. ⓐ ⓑ ⓒ ⓓ ⓔ
592. ⓐ ⓑ ⓒ ⓓ ⓔ
593. ⓐ ⓑ ⓒ ⓓ ⓔ
594. ⓐ ⓑ ⓒ ⓓ ⓔ
595. ⓐ ⓑ ⓒ ⓓ ⓔ
596. ⓐ ⓑ ⓒ ⓓ ⓔ
597. ⓐ ⓑ ⓒ ⓓ ⓔ
598. ⓐ ⓑ ⓒ ⓓ ⓔ
599. ⓐ ⓑ ⓒ ⓓ ⓔ
600. ⓐ ⓑ ⓒ ⓓ ⓔ
601. ⓐ ⓑ ⓒ ⓓ ⓔ
602. ⓐ ⓑ ⓒ ⓓ ⓔ
603. ⓐ ⓑ ⓒ ⓓ ⓔ
604. ⓐ ⓑ ⓒ ⓓ ⓔ
605. ⓐ ⓑ ⓒ ⓓ ⓔ
606. ⓐ ⓑ ⓒ ⓓ ⓔ
607. ⓐ ⓑ ⓒ ⓓ ⓔ
608. ⓐ ⓑ ⓒ ⓓ ⓔ
609. ⓐ ⓑ ⓒ ⓓ ⓔ
610. ⓐ ⓑ ⓒ ⓓ ⓔ
611. ⓐ ⓑ ⓒ ⓓ ⓔ
612. ⓐ ⓑ ⓒ ⓓ ⓔ
613. ⓐ ⓑ ⓒ ⓓ ⓔ
614. ⓐ ⓑ ⓒ ⓓ ⓔ
615. ⓐ ⓑ ⓒ ⓓ ⓔ
616. ⓐ ⓑ ⓒ ⓓ ⓔ
617. ⓐ ⓑ ⓒ ⓓ ⓔ
618. ⓐ ⓑ ⓒ ⓓ ⓔ
619. ⓐ ⓑ ⓒ ⓓ ⓔ
620. ⓐ ⓑ ⓒ ⓓ ⓔ
621. ⓐ ⓑ ⓒ ⓓ ⓔ
622. ⓐ ⓑ ⓒ ⓓ ⓔ
623. ⓐ ⓑ ⓒ ⓓ ⓔ
624. ⓐ ⓑ ⓒ ⓓ ⓔ
625. ⓐ ⓑ ⓒ ⓓ ⓔ
626. ⓐ ⓑ ⓒ ⓓ ⓔ
627. ⓐ ⓑ ⓒ ⓓ ⓔ
628. ⓐ ⓑ ⓒ ⓓ ⓔ
629. ⓐ ⓑ ⓒ ⓓ ⓔ
630. ⓐ ⓑ ⓒ ⓓ ⓔ
631. ⓐ ⓑ ⓒ ⓓ ⓔ
632. ⓐ ⓑ ⓒ ⓓ ⓔ
633. ⓐ ⓑ ⓒ ⓓ ⓔ
634. ⓐ ⓑ ⓒ ⓓ ⓔ
635. ⓐ ⓑ ⓒ ⓓ ⓔ
636. ⓐ ⓑ ⓒ ⓓ ⓔ
637. ⓐ ⓑ ⓒ ⓓ ⓔ
638. ⓐ ⓑ ⓒ ⓓ ⓔ
639. ⓐ ⓑ ⓒ ⓓ ⓔ
640. ⓐ ⓑ ⓒ ⓓ ⓔ
641. ⓐ ⓑ ⓒ ⓓ ⓔ
642. ⓐ ⓑ ⓒ ⓓ ⓔ
643. ⓐ ⓑ ⓒ ⓓ ⓔ
644. ⓐ ⓑ ⓒ ⓓ ⓔ
645. ⓐ ⓑ ⓒ ⓓ ⓔ
646. ⓐ ⓑ ⓒ ⓓ ⓔ
647. ⓐ ⓑ ⓒ ⓓ ⓔ
648. ⓐ ⓑ ⓒ ⓓ ⓔ
649. ⓐ ⓑ ⓒ ⓓ ⓔ
650. ⓐ ⓑ ⓒ ⓓ ⓔ
651. ⓐ ⓑ ⓒ ⓓ ⓔ
652. ⓐ ⓑ ⓒ ⓓ ⓔ
653. ⓐ ⓑ ⓒ ⓓ ⓔ
654. ⓐ ⓑ ⓒ ⓓ ⓔ
655. ⓐ ⓑ ⓒ ⓓ ⓔ
656. ⓐ ⓑ ⓒ ⓓ ⓔ

Medical Diseases—*cont'd*

657. ⓐ ⓑ ⓒ ⓓ ⓔ	699. ⓐ ⓑ ⓒ ⓓ ⓔ	741. ⓐ ⓑ ⓒ ⓓ ⓔ	783. ⓐ ⓑ ⓒ ⓓ ⓔ
658. ⓐ ⓑ ⓒ ⓓ ⓔ	700. ⓐ ⓑ ⓒ ⓓ ⓔ	742. ⓐ ⓑ ⓒ ⓓ ⓔ	784. ⓐ ⓑ ⓒ ⓓ ⓔ
659. ⓐ ⓑ ⓒ ⓓ ⓔ	701. ⓐ ⓑ ⓒ ⓓ ⓔ	743. ⓐ ⓑ ⓒ ⓓ ⓔ	785. ⓐ ⓑ ⓒ ⓓ ⓔ
660. ⓐ ⓑ ⓒ ⓓ ⓔ	702. ⓐ ⓑ ⓒ ⓓ ⓔ	744. ⓐ ⓑ ⓒ ⓓ ⓔ	786. ⓐ ⓑ ⓒ ⓓ ⓔ
661. ⓐ ⓑ ⓒ ⓓ ⓔ	703. ⓐ ⓑ ⓒ ⓓ ⓔ	745. ⓐ ⓑ ⓒ ⓓ ⓔ	787. ⓐ ⓑ ⓒ ⓓ ⓔ
662. ⓐ ⓑ ⓒ ⓓ ⓔ	704. ⓐ ⓑ ⓒ ⓓ ⓔ	746. ⓐ ⓑ ⓒ ⓓ ⓔ	788. ⓐ ⓑ ⓒ ⓓ ⓔ
663. ⓐ ⓑ ⓒ ⓓ ⓔ	705. ⓐ ⓑ ⓒ ⓓ ⓔ	747. ⓐ ⓑ ⓒ ⓓ ⓔ	789. ⓐ ⓑ ⓒ ⓓ ⓔ
664. ⓐ ⓑ ⓒ ⓓ ⓔ	706. ⓐ ⓑ ⓒ ⓓ ⓔ	748. ⓐ ⓑ ⓒ ⓓ ⓔ	790. ⓐ ⓑ ⓒ ⓓ ⓔ
665. ⓐ ⓑ ⓒ ⓓ ⓔ	707. ⓐ ⓑ ⓒ ⓓ ⓔ	749. ⓐ ⓑ ⓒ ⓓ ⓔ	791. ⓐ ⓑ ⓒ ⓓ ⓔ
666. ⓐ ⓑ ⓒ ⓓ ⓔ	708. ⓐ ⓑ ⓒ ⓓ ⓔ	750. ⓐ ⓑ ⓒ ⓓ ⓔ	792. ⓐ ⓑ ⓒ ⓓ ⓔ
667. ⓐ ⓑ ⓒ ⓓ ⓔ	709. ⓐ ⓑ ⓒ ⓓ ⓔ	751. ⓐ ⓑ ⓒ ⓓ ⓔ	793. ⓐ ⓑ ⓒ ⓓ ⓔ
668. ⓐ ⓑ ⓒ ⓓ ⓔ	710. ⓐ ⓑ ⓒ ⓓ ⓔ	752. ⓐ ⓑ ⓒ ⓓ ⓔ	794. ⓐ ⓑ ⓒ ⓓ ⓔ
669. ⓐ ⓑ ⓒ ⓓ ⓔ	711. ⓐ ⓑ ⓒ ⓓ ⓔ	753. ⓐ ⓑ ⓒ ⓓ ⓔ	795. ⓐ ⓑ ⓒ ⓓ ⓔ
670. ⓐ ⓑ ⓒ ⓓ ⓔ	712. ⓐ ⓑ ⓒ ⓓ ⓔ	754. ⓐ ⓑ ⓒ ⓓ ⓔ	796. ⓐ ⓑ ⓒ ⓓ ⓔ
671. ⓐ ⓑ ⓒ ⓓ ⓔ	713. ⓐ ⓑ ⓒ ⓓ ⓔ	755. ⓐ ⓑ ⓒ ⓓ ⓔ	797. ⓐ ⓑ ⓒ ⓓ ⓔ
672. ⓐ ⓑ ⓒ ⓓ ⓔ	714. ⓐ ⓑ ⓒ ⓓ ⓔ	756. ⓐ ⓑ ⓒ ⓓ ⓔ	798. ⓐ ⓑ ⓒ ⓓ ⓔ
673. ⓐ ⓑ ⓒ ⓓ ⓔ	715. ⓐ ⓑ ⓒ ⓓ ⓔ	757. ⓐ ⓑ ⓒ ⓓ ⓔ	799. ⓐ ⓑ ⓒ ⓓ ⓔ
674. ⓐ ⓑ ⓒ ⓓ ⓔ	716. ⓐ ⓑ ⓒ ⓓ ⓔ	758. ⓐ ⓑ ⓒ ⓓ ⓔ	800. ⓐ ⓑ ⓒ ⓓ ⓔ
675. ⓐ ⓑ ⓒ ⓓ ⓔ	717. ⓐ ⓑ ⓒ ⓓ ⓔ	759. ⓐ ⓑ ⓒ ⓓ ⓔ	801. ⓐ ⓑ ⓒ ⓓ ⓔ
676. ⓐ ⓑ ⓒ ⓓ ⓔ	718. ⓐ ⓑ ⓒ ⓓ ⓔ	760. ⓐ ⓑ ⓒ ⓓ ⓔ	802. ⓐ ⓑ ⓒ ⓓ ⓔ
677. ⓐ ⓑ ⓒ ⓓ ⓔ	719. ⓐ ⓑ ⓒ ⓓ ⓔ	761. ⓐ ⓑ ⓒ ⓓ ⓔ	803. ⓐ ⓑ ⓒ ⓓ ⓔ
678. ⓐ ⓑ ⓒ ⓓ ⓔ	720. ⓐ ⓑ ⓒ ⓓ ⓔ	762. ⓐ ⓑ ⓒ ⓓ ⓔ	804. ⓐ ⓑ ⓒ ⓓ ⓔ
679. ⓐ ⓑ ⓒ ⓓ ⓔ	721. ⓐ ⓑ ⓒ ⓓ ⓔ	763. ⓐ ⓑ ⓒ ⓓ ⓔ	805. ⓐ ⓑ ⓒ ⓓ ⓔ
680. ⓐ ⓑ ⓒ ⓓ ⓔ	722. ⓐ ⓑ ⓒ ⓓ ⓔ	764. ⓐ ⓑ ⓒ ⓓ ⓔ	806. ⓐ ⓑ ⓒ ⓓ ⓔ
681. ⓐ ⓑ ⓒ ⓓ ⓔ	723. ⓐ ⓑ ⓒ ⓓ ⓔ	765. ⓐ ⓑ ⓒ ⓓ ⓔ	807. ⓐ ⓑ ⓒ ⓓ ⓔ
682. ⓐ ⓑ ⓒ ⓓ ⓔ	724. ⓐ ⓑ ⓒ ⓓ ⓔ	766. ⓐ ⓑ ⓒ ⓓ ⓔ	808. ⓐ ⓑ ⓒ ⓓ ⓔ
683. ⓐ ⓑ ⓒ ⓓ ⓔ	725. ⓐ ⓑ ⓒ ⓓ ⓔ	767. ⓐ ⓑ ⓒ ⓓ ⓔ	809. ⓐ ⓑ ⓒ ⓓ ⓔ
684. ⓐ ⓑ ⓒ ⓓ ⓔ	726. ⓐ ⓑ ⓒ ⓓ ⓔ	768. ⓐ ⓑ ⓒ ⓓ ⓔ	810. ⓐ ⓑ ⓒ ⓓ ⓔ
685. ⓐ ⓑ ⓒ ⓓ ⓔ	727. ⓐ ⓑ ⓒ ⓓ ⓔ	769. ⓐ ⓑ ⓒ ⓓ ⓔ	811. ⓐ ⓑ ⓒ ⓓ ⓔ
686. ⓐ ⓑ ⓒ ⓓ ⓔ	728. ⓐ ⓑ ⓒ ⓓ ⓔ	770. ⓐ ⓑ ⓒ ⓓ ⓔ	812. ⓐ ⓑ ⓒ ⓓ ⓔ
687. ⓐ ⓑ ⓒ ⓓ ⓔ	729. ⓐ ⓑ ⓒ ⓓ ⓔ	771. ⓐ ⓑ ⓒ ⓓ ⓔ	813. ⓐ ⓑ ⓒ ⓓ ⓔ
688. ⓐ ⓑ ⓒ ⓓ ⓔ	730. ⓐ ⓑ ⓒ ⓓ ⓔ	772. ⓐ ⓑ ⓒ ⓓ ⓔ	814. ⓐ ⓑ ⓒ ⓓ ⓔ
689. ⓐ ⓑ ⓒ ⓓ ⓔ	731. ⓐ ⓑ ⓒ ⓓ ⓔ	773. ⓐ ⓑ ⓒ ⓓ ⓔ	815. ⓐ ⓑ ⓒ ⓓ ⓔ
690. ⓐ ⓑ ⓒ ⓓ ⓔ	732. ⓐ ⓑ ⓒ ⓓ ⓔ	774. ⓐ ⓑ ⓒ ⓓ ⓔ	816. ⓐ ⓑ ⓒ ⓓ ⓔ
691. ⓐ ⓑ ⓒ ⓓ ⓔ	733. ⓐ ⓑ ⓒ ⓓ ⓔ	775. ⓐ ⓑ ⓒ ⓓ ⓔ	817. ⓐ ⓑ ⓒ ⓓ ⓔ
692. ⓐ ⓑ ⓒ ⓓ ⓔ	734. ⓐ ⓑ ⓒ ⓓ ⓔ	776. ⓐ ⓑ ⓒ ⓓ ⓔ	818. ⓐ ⓑ ⓒ ⓓ ⓔ
693. ⓐ ⓑ ⓒ ⓓ ⓔ	735. ⓐ ⓑ ⓒ ⓓ ⓔ	777. ⓐ ⓑ ⓒ ⓓ ⓔ	819. ⓐ ⓑ ⓒ ⓓ ⓔ
694. ⓐ ⓑ ⓒ ⓓ ⓔ	736. ⓐ ⓑ ⓒ ⓓ ⓔ	778. ⓐ ⓑ ⓒ ⓓ ⓔ	820. ⓐ ⓑ ⓒ ⓓ ⓔ
695. ⓐ ⓑ ⓒ ⓓ ⓔ	737. ⓐ ⓑ ⓒ ⓓ ⓔ	779. ⓐ ⓑ ⓒ ⓓ ⓔ	821. ⓐ ⓑ ⓒ ⓓ ⓔ
696. ⓐ ⓑ ⓒ ⓓ ⓔ	738. ⓐ ⓑ ⓒ ⓓ ⓔ	780. ⓐ ⓑ ⓒ ⓓ ⓔ	822. ⓐ ⓑ ⓒ ⓓ ⓔ
697. ⓐ ⓑ ⓒ ⓓ ⓔ	739. ⓐ ⓑ ⓒ ⓓ ⓔ	781. ⓐ ⓑ ⓒ ⓓ ⓔ	823. ⓐ ⓑ ⓒ ⓓ ⓔ
698. ⓐ ⓑ ⓒ ⓓ ⓔ	740. ⓐ ⓑ ⓒ ⓓ ⓔ	782. ⓐ ⓑ ⓒ ⓓ ⓔ	824. ⓐ ⓑ ⓒ ⓓ ⓔ

Continued

Medical Diseases—*cont'd*

825. ⓐ ⓑ ⓒ ⓓ ⓔ	847. ⓐ ⓑ ⓒ ⓓ ⓔ	869. ⓐ ⓑ ⓒ ⓓ ⓔ	891. ⓐ ⓑ ⓒ ⓓ ⓔ
826. ⓐ ⓑ ⓒ ⓓ ⓔ	848. ⓐ ⓑ ⓒ ⓓ ⓔ	870. ⓐ ⓑ ⓒ ⓓ ⓔ	892. ⓐ ⓑ ⓒ ⓓ ⓔ
827. ⓐ ⓑ ⓒ ⓓ ⓔ	849. ⓐ ⓑ ⓒ ⓓ ⓔ	871. ⓐ ⓑ ⓒ ⓓ ⓔ	893. ⓐ ⓑ ⓒ ⓓ ⓔ
828. ⓐ ⓑ ⓒ ⓓ ⓔ	850. ⓐ ⓑ ⓒ ⓓ ⓔ	872. ⓐ ⓑ ⓒ ⓓ ⓔ	894. ⓐ ⓑ ⓒ ⓓ ⓔ
829. ⓐ ⓑ ⓒ ⓓ ⓔ	851. ⓐ ⓑ ⓒ ⓓ ⓔ	873. ⓐ ⓑ ⓒ ⓓ ⓔ	895. ⓐ ⓑ ⓒ ⓓ ⓔ
830. ⓐ ⓑ ⓒ ⓓ ⓔ	852. ⓐ ⓑ ⓒ ⓓ ⓔ	874. ⓐ ⓑ ⓒ ⓓ ⓔ	896. ⓐ ⓑ ⓒ ⓓ ⓔ
831. ⓐ ⓑ ⓒ ⓓ ⓔ	853. ⓐ ⓑ ⓒ ⓓ ⓔ	875. ⓐ ⓑ ⓒ ⓓ ⓔ	897. ⓐ ⓑ ⓒ ⓓ ⓔ
832. ⓐ ⓑ ⓒ ⓓ ⓔ	854. ⓐ ⓑ ⓒ ⓓ ⓔ	876. ⓐ ⓑ ⓒ ⓓ ⓔ	898. ⓐ ⓑ ⓒ ⓓ ⓔ
833. ⓐ ⓑ ⓒ ⓓ ⓔ	855. ⓐ ⓑ ⓒ ⓓ ⓔ	877. ⓐ ⓑ ⓒ ⓓ ⓔ	899. ⓐ ⓑ ⓒ ⓓ ⓔ
834. ⓐ ⓑ ⓒ ⓓ ⓔ	856. ⓐ ⓑ ⓒ ⓓ ⓔ	878. ⓐ ⓑ ⓒ ⓓ ⓔ	900. ⓐ ⓑ ⓒ ⓓ ⓔ
835. ⓐ ⓑ ⓒ ⓓ ⓔ	857. ⓐ ⓑ ⓒ ⓓ ⓔ	879. ⓐ ⓑ ⓒ ⓓ ⓔ	
836. ⓐ ⓑ ⓒ ⓓ ⓔ	858. ⓐ ⓑ ⓒ ⓓ ⓔ	880. ⓐ ⓑ ⓒ ⓓ ⓔ	
837. ⓐ ⓑ ⓒ ⓓ ⓔ	859. ⓐ ⓑ ⓒ ⓓ ⓔ	881. ⓐ ⓑ ⓒ ⓓ ⓔ	
838. ⓐ ⓑ ⓒ ⓓ ⓔ	860. ⓐ ⓑ ⓒ ⓓ ⓔ	882. ⓐ ⓑ ⓒ ⓓ ⓔ	
839. ⓐ ⓑ ⓒ ⓓ ⓔ	861. ⓐ ⓑ ⓒ ⓓ ⓔ	883. ⓐ ⓑ ⓒ ⓓ ⓔ	
840. ⓐ ⓑ ⓒ ⓓ ⓔ	862. ⓐ ⓑ ⓒ ⓓ ⓔ	884. ⓐ ⓑ ⓒ ⓓ ⓔ	
841. ⓐ ⓑ ⓒ ⓓ ⓔ	863. ⓐ ⓑ ⓒ ⓓ ⓔ	885. ⓐ ⓑ ⓒ ⓓ ⓔ	
842. ⓐ ⓑ ⓒ ⓓ ⓔ	864. ⓐ ⓑ ⓒ ⓓ ⓔ	886. ⓐ ⓑ ⓒ ⓓ ⓔ	
843. ⓐ ⓑ ⓒ ⓓ ⓔ	865. ⓐ ⓑ ⓒ ⓓ ⓔ	887. ⓐ ⓑ ⓒ ⓓ ⓔ	
844. ⓐ ⓑ ⓒ ⓓ ⓔ	866. ⓐ ⓑ ⓒ ⓓ ⓔ	888. ⓐ ⓑ ⓒ ⓓ ⓔ	
845. ⓐ ⓑ ⓒ ⓓ ⓔ	867. ⓐ ⓑ ⓒ ⓓ ⓔ	889. ⓐ ⓑ ⓒ ⓓ ⓔ	
846. ⓐ ⓑ ⓒ ⓓ ⓔ	868. ⓐ ⓑ ⓒ ⓓ ⓔ	890. ⓐ ⓑ ⓒ ⓓ ⓔ	

SECTION 7

Nephrology and Urology

Fill in a circled letter to indicate your answer choice.

1. ⓐ ⓑ ⓒ ⓓ ⓔ	11. ⓐ ⓑ ⓒ ⓓ ⓔ	21. ⓐ ⓑ ⓒ ⓓ ⓔ	
2. ⓐ ⓑ ⓒ ⓓ ⓔ	12. ⓐ ⓑ ⓒ ⓓ ⓔ	22. ⓐ ⓑ ⓒ ⓓ ⓔ	
3. ⓐ ⓑ ⓒ ⓓ ⓔ	13. ⓐ ⓑ ⓒ ⓓ ⓔ	23. ⓐ ⓑ ⓒ ⓓ ⓔ	
4. ⓐ ⓑ ⓒ ⓓ ⓔ	14. ⓐ ⓑ ⓒ ⓓ ⓔ	24. ⓐ ⓑ ⓒ ⓓ ⓔ	
5. ⓐ ⓑ ⓒ ⓓ ⓔ	15. ⓐ ⓑ ⓒ ⓓ ⓔ	25. ⓐ ⓑ ⓒ ⓓ ⓔ	
6. ⓐ ⓑ ⓒ ⓓ ⓔ	16. ⓐ ⓑ ⓒ ⓓ ⓔ		
7. ⓐ ⓑ ⓒ ⓓ ⓔ	17. ⓐ ⓑ ⓒ ⓓ ⓔ		
8. ⓐ ⓑ ⓒ ⓓ ⓔ	18. ⓐ ⓑ ⓒ ⓓ ⓔ		
9. ⓐ ⓑ ⓒ ⓓ ⓔ	19. ⓐ ⓑ ⓒ ⓓ ⓔ		
10. ⓐ ⓑ ⓒ ⓓ ⓔ	20. ⓐ ⓑ ⓒ ⓓ ⓔ		

Practice Answer Sheet

SECTION 8

Neurology

Fill in a circled letter to indicate your answer choice.

1. ⓐ ⓑ ⓒ ⓓ ⓔ	11. ⓐ ⓑ ⓒ ⓓ ⓔ	21. ⓐ ⓑ ⓒ ⓓ ⓔ	
2. ⓐ ⓑ ⓒ ⓓ ⓔ	12. ⓐ ⓑ ⓒ ⓓ ⓔ	22. ⓐ ⓑ ⓒ ⓓ ⓔ	
3. ⓐ ⓑ ⓒ ⓓ ⓔ	13. ⓐ ⓑ ⓒ ⓓ ⓔ	23. ⓐ ⓑ ⓒ ⓓ ⓔ	
4. ⓐ ⓑ ⓒ ⓓ ⓔ	14. ⓐ ⓑ ⓒ ⓓ ⓔ	24. ⓐ ⓑ ⓒ ⓓ ⓔ	
5. ⓐ ⓑ ⓒ ⓓ ⓔ	15. ⓐ ⓑ ⓒ ⓓ ⓔ	25. ⓐ ⓑ ⓒ ⓓ ⓔ	
6. ⓐ ⓑ ⓒ ⓓ ⓔ	16. ⓐ ⓑ ⓒ ⓓ ⓔ		
7. ⓐ ⓑ ⓒ ⓓ ⓔ	17. ⓐ ⓑ ⓒ ⓓ ⓔ		
8. ⓐ ⓑ ⓒ ⓓ ⓔ	18. ⓐ ⓑ ⓒ ⓓ ⓔ		
9. ⓐ ⓑ ⓒ ⓓ ⓔ	19. ⓐ ⓑ ⓒ ⓓ ⓔ		
10. ⓐ ⓑ ⓒ ⓓ ⓔ	20. ⓐ ⓑ ⓒ ⓓ ⓔ		

SECTION 9

Oncology

Fill in a circled letter to indicate your answer choice.

1. ⓐ ⓑ ⓒ ⓓ ⓔ	11. ⓐ ⓑ ⓒ ⓓ ⓔ	21. ⓐ ⓑ ⓒ ⓓ ⓔ	
2. ⓐ ⓑ ⓒ ⓓ ⓔ	12. ⓐ ⓑ ⓒ ⓓ ⓔ	22. ⓐ ⓑ ⓒ ⓓ ⓔ	
3. ⓐ ⓑ ⓒ ⓓ ⓔ	13. ⓐ ⓑ ⓒ ⓓ ⓔ	23. ⓐ ⓑ ⓒ ⓓ ⓔ	
4. ⓐ ⓑ ⓒ ⓓ ⓔ	14. ⓐ ⓑ ⓒ ⓓ ⓔ	24. ⓐ ⓑ ⓒ ⓓ ⓔ	
5. ⓐ ⓑ ⓒ ⓓ ⓔ	15. ⓐ ⓑ ⓒ ⓓ ⓔ	25. ⓐ ⓑ ⓒ ⓓ ⓔ	
6. ⓐ ⓑ ⓒ ⓓ ⓔ	16. ⓐ ⓑ ⓒ ⓓ ⓔ		
7. ⓐ ⓑ ⓒ ⓓ ⓔ	17. ⓐ ⓑ ⓒ ⓓ ⓔ		
8. ⓐ ⓑ ⓒ ⓓ ⓔ	18. ⓐ ⓑ ⓒ ⓓ ⓔ		
9. ⓐ ⓑ ⓒ ⓓ ⓔ	19. ⓐ ⓑ ⓒ ⓓ ⓔ		
10. ⓐ ⓑ ⓒ ⓓ ⓔ	20. ⓐ ⓑ ⓒ ⓓ ⓔ		

Practice Answer Sheet

SECTION 10

Ophthalmology

Fill in a circled letter to indicate your answer choice.

1. ⓐ ⓑ ⓒ ⓓ ⓔ	11. ⓐ ⓑ ⓒ ⓓ ⓔ	21. ⓐ ⓑ ⓒ ⓓ ⓔ	
2. ⓐ ⓑ ⓒ ⓓ ⓔ	12. ⓐ ⓑ ⓒ ⓓ ⓔ	22. ⓐ ⓑ ⓒ ⓓ ⓔ	
3. ⓐ ⓑ ⓒ ⓓ ⓔ	13. ⓐ ⓑ ⓒ ⓓ ⓔ	23. ⓐ ⓑ ⓒ ⓓ ⓔ	
4. ⓐ ⓑ ⓒ ⓓ ⓔ	14. ⓐ ⓑ ⓒ ⓓ ⓔ	24. ⓐ ⓑ ⓒ ⓓ ⓔ	
5. ⓐ ⓑ ⓒ ⓓ ⓔ	15. ⓐ ⓑ ⓒ ⓓ ⓔ	25. ⓐ ⓑ ⓒ ⓓ ⓔ	
6. ⓐ ⓑ ⓒ ⓓ ⓔ	16. ⓐ ⓑ ⓒ ⓓ ⓔ		
7. ⓐ ⓑ ⓒ ⓓ ⓔ	17. ⓐ ⓑ ⓒ ⓓ ⓔ		
8. ⓐ ⓑ ⓒ ⓓ ⓔ	18. ⓐ ⓑ ⓒ ⓓ ⓔ		
9. ⓐ ⓑ ⓒ ⓓ ⓔ	19. ⓐ ⓑ ⓒ ⓓ ⓔ		
10. ⓐ ⓑ ⓒ ⓓ ⓔ	20. ⓐ ⓑ ⓒ ⓓ ⓔ		

SECTION 11

Preventive Medicine

Fill in a circled letter to indicate your answer choice.

1. ⓐ ⓑ ⓒ ⓓ ⓔ	11. ⓐ ⓑ ⓒ ⓓ ⓔ	21. ⓐ ⓑ ⓒ ⓓ ⓔ	
2. ⓐ ⓑ ⓒ ⓓ ⓔ	12. ⓐ ⓑ ⓒ ⓓ ⓔ	22. ⓐ ⓑ ⓒ ⓓ ⓔ	
3. ⓐ ⓑ ⓒ ⓓ ⓔ	13. ⓐ ⓑ ⓒ ⓓ ⓔ	23. ⓐ ⓑ ⓒ ⓓ ⓔ	
4. ⓐ ⓑ ⓒ ⓓ ⓔ	14. ⓐ ⓑ ⓒ ⓓ ⓔ	24. ⓐ ⓑ ⓒ ⓓ ⓔ	
5. ⓐ ⓑ ⓒ ⓓ ⓔ	15. ⓐ ⓑ ⓒ ⓓ ⓔ	25. ⓐ ⓑ ⓒ ⓓ ⓔ	
6. ⓐ ⓑ ⓒ ⓓ ⓔ	16. ⓐ ⓑ ⓒ ⓓ ⓔ		
7. ⓐ ⓑ ⓒ ⓓ ⓔ	17. ⓐ ⓑ ⓒ ⓓ ⓔ		
8. ⓐ ⓑ ⓒ ⓓ ⓔ	18. ⓐ ⓑ ⓒ ⓓ ⓔ		
9. ⓐ ⓑ ⓒ ⓓ ⓔ	19. ⓐ ⓑ ⓒ ⓓ ⓔ		
10. ⓐ ⓑ ⓒ ⓓ ⓔ	20. ⓐ ⓑ ⓒ ⓓ ⓔ		

Practice Answer Sheet

SECTION 12

Surgical Diseases

Fill in a circled letter to indicate your answer choice.

1. ⓐ ⓑ ⓒ ⓓ ⓔ	39. ⓐ ⓑ ⓒ ⓓ ⓔ	77. ⓐ ⓑ ⓒ ⓓ ⓔ	115. ⓐ ⓑ ⓒ ⓓ ⓔ
2. ⓐ ⓑ ⓒ ⓓ ⓔ	40. ⓐ ⓑ ⓒ ⓓ ⓔ	78. ⓐ ⓑ ⓒ ⓓ ⓔ	116. ⓐ ⓑ ⓒ ⓓ ⓔ
3. ⓐ ⓑ ⓒ ⓓ ⓔ	41. ⓐ ⓑ ⓒ ⓓ ⓔ	79. ⓐ ⓑ ⓒ ⓓ ⓔ	117. ⓐ ⓑ ⓒ ⓓ ⓔ
4. ⓐ ⓑ ⓒ ⓓ ⓔ	42. ⓐ ⓑ ⓒ ⓓ ⓔ	80. ⓐ ⓑ ⓒ ⓓ ⓔ	118. ⓐ ⓑ ⓒ ⓓ ⓔ
5. ⓐ ⓑ ⓒ ⓓ ⓔ	43. ⓐ ⓑ ⓒ ⓓ ⓔ	81. ⓐ ⓑ ⓒ ⓓ ⓔ	119. ⓐ ⓑ ⓒ ⓓ ⓔ
6. ⓐ ⓑ ⓒ ⓓ ⓔ	44. ⓐ ⓑ ⓒ ⓓ ⓔ	82. ⓐ ⓑ ⓒ ⓓ ⓔ	120. ⓐ ⓑ ⓒ ⓓ ⓔ
7. ⓐ ⓑ ⓒ ⓓ ⓔ	45. ⓐ ⓑ ⓒ ⓓ ⓔ	83. ⓐ ⓑ ⓒ ⓓ ⓔ	121. ⓐ ⓑ ⓒ ⓓ ⓔ
8. ⓐ ⓑ ⓒ ⓓ ⓔ	46. ⓐ ⓑ ⓒ ⓓ ⓔ	84. ⓐ ⓑ ⓒ ⓓ ⓔ	122. ⓐ ⓑ ⓒ ⓓ ⓔ
9. ⓐ ⓑ ⓒ ⓓ ⓔ	47. ⓐ ⓑ ⓒ ⓓ ⓔ	85. ⓐ ⓑ ⓒ ⓓ ⓔ	123. ⓐ ⓑ ⓒ ⓓ ⓔ
10. ⓐ ⓑ ⓒ ⓓ ⓔ	48. ⓐ ⓑ ⓒ ⓓ ⓔ	86. ⓐ ⓑ ⓒ ⓓ ⓔ	124. ⓐ ⓑ ⓒ ⓓ ⓔ
11. ⓐ ⓑ ⓒ ⓓ ⓔ	49. ⓐ ⓑ ⓒ ⓓ ⓔ	87. ⓐ ⓑ ⓒ ⓓ ⓔ	125. ⓐ ⓑ ⓒ ⓓ ⓔ
12. ⓐ ⓑ ⓒ ⓓ ⓔ	50. ⓐ ⓑ ⓒ ⓓ ⓔ	88. ⓐ ⓑ ⓒ ⓓ ⓔ	126. ⓐ ⓑ ⓒ ⓓ ⓔ
13. ⓐ ⓑ ⓒ ⓓ ⓔ	51. ⓐ ⓑ ⓒ ⓓ ⓔ	89. ⓐ ⓑ ⓒ ⓓ ⓔ	127. ⓐ ⓑ ⓒ ⓓ ⓔ
14. ⓐ ⓑ ⓒ ⓓ ⓔ	52. ⓐ ⓑ ⓒ ⓓ ⓔ	90. ⓐ ⓑ ⓒ ⓓ ⓔ	128. ⓐ ⓑ ⓒ ⓓ ⓔ
15. ⓐ ⓑ ⓒ ⓓ ⓔ	53. ⓐ ⓑ ⓒ ⓓ ⓔ	91. ⓐ ⓑ ⓒ ⓓ ⓔ	129. ⓐ ⓑ ⓒ ⓓ ⓔ
16. ⓐ ⓑ ⓒ ⓓ ⓔ	54. ⓐ ⓑ ⓒ ⓓ ⓔ	92. ⓐ ⓑ ⓒ ⓓ ⓔ	130. ⓐ ⓑ ⓒ ⓓ ⓔ
17. ⓐ ⓑ ⓒ ⓓ ⓔ	55. ⓐ ⓑ ⓒ ⓓ ⓔ	93. ⓐ ⓑ ⓒ ⓓ ⓔ	131. ⓐ ⓑ ⓒ ⓓ ⓔ
18. ⓐ ⓑ ⓒ ⓓ ⓔ	56. ⓐ ⓑ ⓒ ⓓ ⓔ	94. ⓐ ⓑ ⓒ ⓓ ⓔ	132. ⓐ ⓑ ⓒ ⓓ ⓔ
19. ⓐ ⓑ ⓒ ⓓ ⓔ	57. ⓐ ⓑ ⓒ ⓓ ⓔ	95. ⓐ ⓑ ⓒ ⓓ ⓔ	133. ⓐ ⓑ ⓒ ⓓ ⓔ
20. ⓐ ⓑ ⓒ ⓓ ⓔ	58. ⓐ ⓑ ⓒ ⓓ ⓔ	96. ⓐ ⓑ ⓒ ⓓ ⓔ	134. ⓐ ⓑ ⓒ ⓓ ⓔ
21. ⓐ ⓑ ⓒ ⓓ ⓔ	59. ⓐ ⓑ ⓒ ⓓ ⓔ	97. ⓐ ⓑ ⓒ ⓓ ⓔ	135. ⓐ ⓑ ⓒ ⓓ ⓔ
22. ⓐ ⓑ ⓒ ⓓ ⓔ	60. ⓐ ⓑ ⓒ ⓓ ⓔ	98. ⓐ ⓑ ⓒ ⓓ ⓔ	136. ⓐ ⓑ ⓒ ⓓ ⓔ
23. ⓐ ⓑ ⓒ ⓓ ⓔ	61. ⓐ ⓑ ⓒ ⓓ ⓔ	99. ⓐ ⓑ ⓒ ⓓ ⓔ	137. ⓐ ⓑ ⓒ ⓓ ⓔ
24. ⓐ ⓑ ⓒ ⓓ ⓔ	62. ⓐ ⓑ ⓒ ⓓ ⓔ	100. ⓐ ⓑ ⓒ ⓓ ⓔ	138. ⓐ ⓑ ⓒ ⓓ ⓔ
25. ⓐ ⓑ ⓒ ⓓ ⓔ	63. ⓐ ⓑ ⓒ ⓓ ⓔ	101. ⓐ ⓑ ⓒ ⓓ ⓔ	139. ⓐ ⓑ ⓒ ⓓ ⓔ
26. ⓐ ⓑ ⓒ ⓓ ⓔ	64. ⓐ ⓑ ⓒ ⓓ ⓔ	102. ⓐ ⓑ ⓒ ⓓ ⓔ	140. ⓐ ⓑ ⓒ ⓓ ⓔ
27. ⓐ ⓑ ⓒ ⓓ ⓔ	65. ⓐ ⓑ ⓒ ⓓ ⓔ	103. ⓐ ⓑ ⓒ ⓓ ⓔ	141. ⓐ ⓑ ⓒ ⓓ ⓔ
28. ⓐ ⓑ ⓒ ⓓ ⓔ	66. ⓐ ⓑ ⓒ ⓓ ⓔ	104. ⓐ ⓑ ⓒ ⓓ ⓔ	142. ⓐ ⓑ ⓒ ⓓ ⓔ
29. ⓐ ⓑ ⓒ ⓓ ⓔ	67. ⓐ ⓑ ⓒ ⓓ ⓔ	105. ⓐ ⓑ ⓒ ⓓ ⓔ	143. ⓐ ⓑ ⓒ ⓓ ⓔ
30. ⓐ ⓑ ⓒ ⓓ ⓔ	68. ⓐ ⓑ ⓒ ⓓ ⓔ	106. ⓐ ⓑ ⓒ ⓓ ⓔ	144. ⓐ ⓑ ⓒ ⓓ ⓔ
31. ⓐ ⓑ ⓒ ⓓ ⓔ	69. ⓐ ⓑ ⓒ ⓓ ⓔ	107. ⓐ ⓑ ⓒ ⓓ ⓔ	145. ⓐ ⓑ ⓒ ⓓ ⓔ
32. ⓐ ⓑ ⓒ ⓓ ⓔ	70. ⓐ ⓑ ⓒ ⓓ ⓔ	108. ⓐ ⓑ ⓒ ⓓ ⓔ	146. ⓐ ⓑ ⓒ ⓓ ⓔ
33. ⓐ ⓑ ⓒ ⓓ ⓔ	71. ⓐ ⓑ ⓒ ⓓ ⓔ	109. ⓐ ⓑ ⓒ ⓓ ⓔ	147. ⓐ ⓑ ⓒ ⓓ ⓔ
34. ⓐ ⓑ ⓒ ⓓ ⓔ	72. ⓐ ⓑ ⓒ ⓓ ⓔ	110. ⓐ ⓑ ⓒ ⓓ ⓔ	148. ⓐ ⓑ ⓒ ⓓ ⓔ
35. ⓐ ⓑ ⓒ ⓓ ⓔ	73. ⓐ ⓑ ⓒ ⓓ ⓔ	111. ⓐ ⓑ ⓒ ⓓ ⓔ	149. ⓐ ⓑ ⓒ ⓓ ⓔ
36. ⓐ ⓑ ⓒ ⓓ ⓔ	74. ⓐ ⓑ ⓒ ⓓ ⓔ	112. ⓐ ⓑ ⓒ ⓓ ⓔ	150. ⓐ ⓑ ⓒ ⓓ ⓔ
37. ⓐ ⓑ ⓒ ⓓ ⓔ	75. ⓐ ⓑ ⓒ ⓓ ⓔ	113. ⓐ ⓑ ⓒ ⓓ ⓔ	151. ⓐ ⓑ ⓒ ⓓ ⓔ
38. ⓐ ⓑ ⓒ ⓓ ⓔ	76. ⓐ ⓑ ⓒ ⓓ ⓔ	114. ⓐ ⓑ ⓒ ⓓ ⓔ	152. ⓐ ⓑ ⓒ ⓓ ⓔ

Continued

Surgical Diseases—*cont'd*

153. ⓐ ⓑ ⓒ ⓓ ⓔ	195. ⓐ ⓑ ⓒ ⓓ ⓔ	237. ⓐ ⓑ ⓒ ⓓ ⓔ	279. ⓐ ⓑ ⓒ ⓓ ⓔ
154. ⓐ ⓑ ⓒ ⓓ ⓔ	196. ⓐ ⓑ ⓒ ⓓ ⓔ	238. ⓐ ⓑ ⓒ ⓓ ⓔ	280. ⓐ ⓑ ⓒ ⓓ ⓔ
155. ⓐ ⓑ ⓒ ⓓ ⓔ	197. ⓐ ⓑ ⓒ ⓓ ⓔ	239. ⓐ ⓑ ⓒ ⓓ ⓔ	281. ⓐ ⓑ ⓒ ⓓ ⓔ
156. ⓐ ⓑ ⓒ ⓓ ⓔ	198. ⓐ ⓑ ⓒ ⓓ ⓔ	240. ⓐ ⓑ ⓒ ⓓ ⓔ	282. ⓐ ⓑ ⓒ ⓓ ⓔ
157. ⓐ ⓑ ⓒ ⓓ ⓔ	199. ⓐ ⓑ ⓒ ⓓ ⓔ	241. ⓐ ⓑ ⓒ ⓓ ⓔ	283. ⓐ ⓑ ⓒ ⓓ ⓔ
158. ⓐ ⓑ ⓒ ⓓ ⓔ	200. ⓐ ⓑ ⓒ ⓓ ⓔ	242. ⓐ ⓑ ⓒ ⓓ ⓔ	284. ⓐ ⓑ ⓒ ⓓ ⓔ
159. ⓐ ⓑ ⓒ ⓓ ⓔ	201. ⓐ ⓑ ⓒ ⓓ ⓔ	243. ⓐ ⓑ ⓒ ⓓ ⓔ	285. ⓐ ⓑ ⓒ ⓓ ⓔ
160. ⓐ ⓑ ⓒ ⓓ ⓔ	202. ⓐ ⓑ ⓒ ⓓ ⓔ	244. ⓐ ⓑ ⓒ ⓓ ⓔ	286. ⓐ ⓑ ⓒ ⓓ ⓔ
161. ⓐ ⓑ ⓒ ⓓ ⓔ	203. ⓐ ⓑ ⓒ ⓓ ⓔ	245. ⓐ ⓑ ⓒ ⓓ ⓔ	287. ⓐ ⓑ ⓒ ⓓ ⓔ
162. ⓐ ⓑ ⓒ ⓓ ⓔ	204. ⓐ ⓑ ⓒ ⓓ ⓔ	246. ⓐ ⓑ ⓒ ⓓ ⓔ	288. ⓐ ⓑ ⓒ ⓓ ⓔ
163. ⓐ ⓑ ⓒ ⓓ ⓔ	205. ⓐ ⓑ ⓒ ⓓ ⓔ	247. ⓐ ⓑ ⓒ ⓓ ⓔ	289. ⓐ ⓑ ⓒ ⓓ ⓔ
164. ⓐ ⓑ ⓒ ⓓ ⓔ	206. ⓐ ⓑ ⓒ ⓓ ⓔ	248. ⓐ ⓑ ⓒ ⓓ ⓔ	290. ⓐ ⓑ ⓒ ⓓ ⓔ
165. ⓐ ⓑ ⓒ ⓓ ⓔ	207. ⓐ ⓑ ⓒ ⓓ ⓔ	249. ⓐ ⓑ ⓒ ⓓ ⓔ	291. ⓐ ⓑ ⓒ ⓓ ⓔ
166. ⓐ ⓑ ⓒ ⓓ ⓔ	208. ⓐ ⓑ ⓒ ⓓ ⓔ	250. ⓐ ⓑ ⓒ ⓓ ⓔ	292. ⓐ ⓑ ⓒ ⓓ ⓔ
167. ⓐ ⓑ ⓒ ⓓ ⓔ	209. ⓐ ⓑ ⓒ ⓓ ⓔ	251. ⓐ ⓑ ⓒ ⓓ ⓔ	293. ⓐ ⓑ ⓒ ⓓ ⓔ
168. ⓐ ⓑ ⓒ ⓓ ⓔ	210. ⓐ ⓑ ⓒ ⓓ ⓔ	252. ⓐ ⓑ ⓒ ⓓ ⓔ	294. ⓐ ⓑ ⓒ ⓓ ⓔ
169. ⓐ ⓑ ⓒ ⓓ ⓔ	211. ⓐ ⓑ ⓒ ⓓ ⓔ	253. ⓐ ⓑ ⓒ ⓓ ⓔ	295. ⓐ ⓑ ⓒ ⓓ ⓔ
170. ⓐ ⓑ ⓒ ⓓ ⓔ	212. ⓐ ⓑ ⓒ ⓓ ⓔ	254. ⓐ ⓑ ⓒ ⓓ ⓔ	296. ⓐ ⓑ ⓒ ⓓ ⓔ
171. ⓐ ⓑ ⓒ ⓓ ⓔ	213. ⓐ ⓑ ⓒ ⓓ ⓔ	255. ⓐ ⓑ ⓒ ⓓ ⓔ	297. ⓐ ⓑ ⓒ ⓓ ⓔ
172. ⓐ ⓑ ⓒ ⓓ ⓔ	214. ⓐ ⓑ ⓒ ⓓ ⓔ	256. ⓐ ⓑ ⓒ ⓓ ⓔ	298. ⓐ ⓑ ⓒ ⓓ ⓔ
173. ⓐ ⓑ ⓒ ⓓ ⓔ	215. ⓐ ⓑ ⓒ ⓓ ⓔ	257. ⓐ ⓑ ⓒ ⓓ ⓔ	299. ⓐ ⓑ ⓒ ⓓ ⓔ
174. ⓐ ⓑ ⓒ ⓓ ⓔ	216. ⓐ ⓑ ⓒ ⓓ ⓔ	258. ⓐ ⓑ ⓒ ⓓ ⓔ	300. ⓐ ⓑ ⓒ ⓓ ⓔ
175. ⓐ ⓑ ⓒ ⓓ ⓔ	217. ⓐ ⓑ ⓒ ⓓ ⓔ	259. ⓐ ⓑ ⓒ ⓓ ⓔ	301. ⓐ ⓑ ⓒ ⓓ ⓔ
176. ⓐ ⓑ ⓒ ⓓ ⓔ	218. ⓐ ⓑ ⓒ ⓓ ⓔ	260. ⓐ ⓑ ⓒ ⓓ ⓔ	302. ⓐ ⓑ ⓒ ⓓ ⓔ
177. ⓐ ⓑ ⓒ ⓓ ⓔ	219. ⓐ ⓑ ⓒ ⓓ ⓔ	261. ⓐ ⓑ ⓒ ⓓ ⓔ	303. ⓐ ⓑ ⓒ ⓓ ⓔ
178. ⓐ ⓑ ⓒ ⓓ ⓔ	220. ⓐ ⓑ ⓒ ⓓ ⓔ	262. ⓐ ⓑ ⓒ ⓓ ⓔ	304. ⓐ ⓑ ⓒ ⓓ ⓔ
179. ⓐ ⓑ ⓒ ⓓ ⓔ	221. ⓐ ⓑ ⓒ ⓓ ⓔ	263. ⓐ ⓑ ⓒ ⓓ ⓔ	305. ⓐ ⓑ ⓒ ⓓ ⓔ
180. ⓐ ⓑ ⓒ ⓓ ⓔ	222. ⓐ ⓑ ⓒ ⓓ ⓔ	264. ⓐ ⓑ ⓒ ⓓ ⓔ	306. ⓐ ⓑ ⓒ ⓓ ⓔ
181. ⓐ ⓑ ⓒ ⓓ ⓔ	223. ⓐ ⓑ ⓒ ⓓ ⓔ	265. ⓐ ⓑ ⓒ ⓓ ⓔ	307. ⓐ ⓑ ⓒ ⓓ ⓔ
182. ⓐ ⓑ ⓒ ⓓ ⓔ	224. ⓐ ⓑ ⓒ ⓓ ⓔ	266. ⓐ ⓑ ⓒ ⓓ ⓔ	308. ⓐ ⓑ ⓒ ⓓ ⓔ
183. ⓐ ⓑ ⓒ ⓓ ⓔ	225. ⓐ ⓑ ⓒ ⓓ ⓔ	267. ⓐ ⓑ ⓒ ⓓ ⓔ	309. ⓐ ⓑ ⓒ ⓓ ⓔ
184. ⓐ ⓑ ⓒ ⓓ ⓔ	226. ⓐ ⓑ ⓒ ⓓ ⓔ	268. ⓐ ⓑ ⓒ ⓓ ⓔ	310. ⓐ ⓑ ⓒ ⓓ ⓔ
185. ⓐ ⓑ ⓒ ⓓ ⓔ	227. ⓐ ⓑ ⓒ ⓓ ⓔ	269. ⓐ ⓑ ⓒ ⓓ ⓔ	311. ⓐ ⓑ ⓒ ⓓ ⓔ
186. ⓐ ⓑ ⓒ ⓓ ⓔ	228. ⓐ ⓑ ⓒ ⓓ ⓔ	270. ⓐ ⓑ ⓒ ⓓ ⓔ	312. ⓐ ⓑ ⓒ ⓓ ⓔ
187. ⓐ ⓑ ⓒ ⓓ ⓔ	229. ⓐ ⓑ ⓒ ⓓ ⓔ	271. ⓐ ⓑ ⓒ ⓓ ⓔ	313. ⓐ ⓑ ⓒ ⓓ ⓔ
188. ⓐ ⓑ ⓒ ⓓ ⓔ	230. ⓐ ⓑ ⓒ ⓓ ⓔ	272. ⓐ ⓑ ⓒ ⓓ ⓔ	314. ⓐ ⓑ ⓒ ⓓ ⓔ
189. ⓐ ⓑ ⓒ ⓓ ⓔ	231. ⓐ ⓑ ⓒ ⓓ ⓔ	273. ⓐ ⓑ ⓒ ⓓ ⓔ	315. ⓐ ⓑ ⓒ ⓓ ⓔ
190. ⓐ ⓑ ⓒ ⓓ ⓔ	232. ⓐ ⓑ ⓒ ⓓ ⓔ	274. ⓐ ⓑ ⓒ ⓓ ⓔ	316. ⓐ ⓑ ⓒ ⓓ ⓔ
191. ⓐ ⓑ ⓒ ⓓ ⓔ	233. ⓐ ⓑ ⓒ ⓓ ⓔ	275. ⓐ ⓑ ⓒ ⓓ ⓔ	317. ⓐ ⓑ ⓒ ⓓ ⓔ
192. ⓐ ⓑ ⓒ ⓓ ⓔ	234. ⓐ ⓑ ⓒ ⓓ ⓔ	276. ⓐ ⓑ ⓒ ⓓ ⓔ	318. ⓐ ⓑ ⓒ ⓓ ⓔ
193. ⓐ ⓑ ⓒ ⓓ ⓔ	235. ⓐ ⓑ ⓒ ⓓ ⓔ	277. ⓐ ⓑ ⓒ ⓓ ⓔ	319. ⓐ ⓑ ⓒ ⓓ ⓔ
194. ⓐ ⓑ ⓒ ⓓ ⓔ	236. ⓐ ⓑ ⓒ ⓓ ⓔ	278. ⓐ ⓑ ⓒ ⓓ ⓔ	320. ⓐ ⓑ ⓒ ⓓ ⓔ

Surgical Diseases—*cont'd*

321. ⓐ ⓑ ⓒ ⓓ ⓔ	355. ⓐ ⓑ ⓒ ⓓ ⓔ	389. ⓐ ⓑ ⓒ ⓓ ⓔ	423. ⓐ ⓑ ⓒ ⓓ ⓔ
322. ⓐ ⓑ ⓒ ⓓ ⓔ	356. ⓐ ⓑ ⓒ ⓓ ⓔ	390. ⓐ ⓑ ⓒ ⓓ ⓔ	424. ⓐ ⓑ ⓒ ⓓ ⓔ
323. ⓐ ⓑ ⓒ ⓓ ⓔ	357. ⓐ ⓑ ⓒ ⓓ ⓔ	391. ⓐ ⓑ ⓒ ⓓ ⓔ	425. ⓐ ⓑ ⓒ ⓓ ⓔ
324. ⓐ ⓑ ⓒ ⓓ ⓔ	358. ⓐ ⓑ ⓒ ⓓ ⓔ	392. ⓐ ⓑ ⓒ ⓓ ⓔ	426. ⓐ ⓑ ⓒ ⓓ ⓔ
325. ⓐ ⓑ ⓒ ⓓ ⓔ	359. ⓐ ⓑ ⓒ ⓓ ⓔ	393. ⓐ ⓑ ⓒ ⓓ ⓔ	427. ⓐ ⓑ ⓒ ⓓ ⓔ
326. ⓐ ⓑ ⓒ ⓓ ⓔ	360. ⓐ ⓑ ⓒ ⓓ ⓔ	394. ⓐ ⓑ ⓒ ⓓ ⓔ	428. ⓐ ⓑ ⓒ ⓓ ⓔ
327. ⓐ ⓑ ⓒ ⓓ ⓔ	361. ⓐ ⓑ ⓒ ⓓ ⓔ	395. ⓐ ⓑ ⓒ ⓓ ⓔ	429. ⓐ ⓑ ⓒ ⓓ ⓔ
328. ⓐ ⓑ ⓒ ⓓ ⓔ	362. ⓐ ⓑ ⓒ ⓓ ⓔ	396. ⓐ ⓑ ⓒ ⓓ ⓔ	430. ⓐ ⓑ ⓒ ⓓ ⓔ
329. ⓐ ⓑ ⓒ ⓓ ⓔ	363. ⓐ ⓑ ⓒ ⓓ ⓔ	397. ⓐ ⓑ ⓒ ⓓ ⓔ	431. ⓐ ⓑ ⓒ ⓓ ⓔ
330. ⓐ ⓑ ⓒ ⓓ ⓔ	364. ⓐ ⓑ ⓒ ⓓ ⓔ	398. ⓐ ⓑ ⓒ ⓓ ⓔ	432. ⓐ ⓑ ⓒ ⓓ ⓔ
331. ⓐ ⓑ ⓒ ⓓ ⓔ	365. ⓐ ⓑ ⓒ ⓓ ⓔ	399. ⓐ ⓑ ⓒ ⓓ ⓔ	433. ⓐ ⓑ ⓒ ⓓ ⓔ
332. ⓐ ⓑ ⓒ ⓓ ⓔ	366. ⓐ ⓑ ⓒ ⓓ ⓔ	400. ⓐ ⓑ ⓒ ⓓ ⓔ	434. ⓐ ⓑ ⓒ ⓓ ⓔ
333. ⓐ ⓑ ⓒ ⓓ ⓔ	367. ⓐ ⓑ ⓒ ⓓ ⓔ	401. ⓐ ⓑ ⓒ ⓓ ⓔ	435. ⓐ ⓑ ⓒ ⓓ ⓔ
334. ⓐ ⓑ ⓒ ⓓ ⓔ	368. ⓐ ⓑ ⓒ ⓓ ⓔ	402. ⓐ ⓑ ⓒ ⓓ ⓔ	436. ⓐ ⓑ ⓒ ⓓ ⓔ
335. ⓐ ⓑ ⓒ ⓓ ⓔ	369. ⓐ ⓑ ⓒ ⓓ ⓔ	403. ⓐ ⓑ ⓒ ⓓ ⓔ	437. ⓐ ⓑ ⓒ ⓓ ⓔ
336. ⓐ ⓑ ⓒ ⓓ ⓔ	370. ⓐ ⓑ ⓒ ⓓ ⓔ	404. ⓐ ⓑ ⓒ ⓓ ⓔ	438. ⓐ ⓑ ⓒ ⓓ ⓔ
337. ⓐ ⓑ ⓒ ⓓ ⓔ	371. ⓐ ⓑ ⓒ ⓓ ⓔ	405. ⓐ ⓑ ⓒ ⓓ ⓔ	439. ⓐ ⓑ ⓒ ⓓ ⓔ
338. ⓐ ⓑ ⓒ ⓓ ⓔ	372. ⓐ ⓑ ⓒ ⓓ ⓔ	406. ⓐ ⓑ ⓒ ⓓ ⓔ	440. ⓐ ⓑ ⓒ ⓓ ⓔ
339. ⓐ ⓑ ⓒ ⓓ ⓔ	373. ⓐ ⓑ ⓒ ⓓ ⓔ	407. ⓐ ⓑ ⓒ ⓓ ⓔ	441. ⓐ ⓑ ⓒ ⓓ ⓔ
340. ⓐ ⓑ ⓒ ⓓ ⓔ	374. ⓐ ⓑ ⓒ ⓓ ⓔ	408. ⓐ ⓑ ⓒ ⓓ ⓔ	442. ⓐ ⓑ ⓒ ⓓ ⓔ
341. ⓐ ⓑ ⓒ ⓓ ⓔ	375. ⓐ ⓑ ⓒ ⓓ ⓔ	409. ⓐ ⓑ ⓒ ⓓ ⓔ	443. ⓐ ⓑ ⓒ ⓓ ⓔ
342. ⓐ ⓑ ⓒ ⓓ ⓔ	376. ⓐ ⓑ ⓒ ⓓ ⓔ	410. ⓐ ⓑ ⓒ ⓓ ⓔ	444. ⓐ ⓑ ⓒ ⓓ ⓔ
343. ⓐ ⓑ ⓒ ⓓ ⓔ	377. ⓐ ⓑ ⓒ ⓓ ⓔ	411. ⓐ ⓑ ⓒ ⓓ ⓔ	445. ⓐ ⓑ ⓒ ⓓ ⓔ
344. ⓐ ⓑ ⓒ ⓓ ⓔ	378. ⓐ ⓑ ⓒ ⓓ ⓔ	412. ⓐ ⓑ ⓒ ⓓ ⓔ	446. ⓐ ⓑ ⓒ ⓓ ⓔ
345. ⓐ ⓑ ⓒ ⓓ ⓔ	379. ⓐ ⓑ ⓒ ⓓ ⓔ	413. ⓐ ⓑ ⓒ ⓓ ⓔ	447. ⓐ ⓑ ⓒ ⓓ ⓔ
346. ⓐ ⓑ ⓒ ⓓ ⓔ	380. ⓐ ⓑ ⓒ ⓓ ⓔ	414. ⓐ ⓑ ⓒ ⓓ ⓔ	448. ⓐ ⓑ ⓒ ⓓ ⓔ
347. ⓐ ⓑ ⓒ ⓓ ⓔ	381. ⓐ ⓑ ⓒ ⓓ ⓔ	415. ⓐ ⓑ ⓒ ⓓ ⓔ	449. ⓐ ⓑ ⓒ ⓓ ⓔ
348. ⓐ ⓑ ⓒ ⓓ ⓔ	382. ⓐ ⓑ ⓒ ⓓ ⓔ	416. ⓐ ⓑ ⓒ ⓓ ⓔ	450. ⓐ ⓑ ⓒ ⓓ ⓔ
349. ⓐ ⓑ ⓒ ⓓ ⓔ	383. ⓐ ⓑ ⓒ ⓓ ⓔ	417. ⓐ ⓑ ⓒ ⓓ ⓔ	
350. ⓐ ⓑ ⓒ ⓓ ⓔ	384. ⓐ ⓑ ⓒ ⓓ ⓔ	418. ⓐ ⓑ ⓒ ⓓ ⓔ	
351. ⓐ ⓑ ⓒ ⓓ ⓔ	385. ⓐ ⓑ ⓒ ⓓ ⓔ	419. ⓐ ⓑ ⓒ ⓓ ⓔ	
352. ⓐ ⓑ ⓒ ⓓ ⓔ	386. ⓐ ⓑ ⓒ ⓓ ⓔ	420. ⓐ ⓑ ⓒ ⓓ ⓔ	
353. ⓐ ⓑ ⓒ ⓓ ⓔ	387. ⓐ ⓑ ⓒ ⓓ ⓔ	421. ⓐ ⓑ ⓒ ⓓ ⓔ	
354. ⓐ ⓑ ⓒ ⓓ ⓔ	388. ⓐ ⓑ ⓒ ⓓ ⓔ	422. ⓐ ⓑ ⓒ ⓓ ⓔ	

SECTION 13

Theriogenology

Fill in a circled letter to indicate your answer choice.

1. ⓐ ⓑ ⓒ ⓓ ⓔ	11. ⓐ ⓑ ⓒ ⓓ ⓔ	21. ⓐ ⓑ ⓒ ⓓ ⓔ	
2. ⓐ ⓑ ⓒ ⓓ ⓔ	12. ⓐ ⓑ ⓒ ⓓ ⓔ	22. ⓐ ⓑ ⓒ ⓓ ⓔ	
3. ⓐ ⓑ ⓒ ⓓ ⓔ	13. ⓐ ⓑ ⓒ ⓓ ⓔ	23. ⓐ ⓑ ⓒ ⓓ ⓔ	
4. ⓐ ⓑ ⓒ ⓓ ⓔ	14. ⓐ ⓑ ⓒ ⓓ ⓔ	24. ⓐ ⓑ ⓒ ⓓ ⓔ	
5. ⓐ ⓑ ⓒ ⓓ ⓔ	15. ⓐ ⓑ ⓒ ⓓ ⓔ	25. ⓐ ⓑ ⓒ ⓓ ⓔ	
6. ⓐ ⓑ ⓒ ⓓ ⓔ	16. ⓐ ⓑ ⓒ ⓓ ⓔ		
7. ⓐ ⓑ ⓒ ⓓ ⓔ	17. ⓐ ⓑ ⓒ ⓓ ⓔ		
8. ⓐ ⓑ ⓒ ⓓ ⓔ	18. ⓐ ⓑ ⓒ ⓓ ⓔ		
9. ⓐ ⓑ ⓒ ⓓ ⓔ	19. ⓐ ⓑ ⓒ ⓓ ⓔ		
10. ⓐ ⓑ ⓒ ⓓ ⓔ	20. ⓐ ⓑ ⓒ ⓓ ⓔ		

NOTES